AF678156

Molecular Biology of Atherosclerosis

Molecular Biology of Atherosclerosis

Proceedings of the Twentieth Steenbock Symposium
held June 3 through June 5, 1990
at the University of Wisconsin–Madison
Madison, Wisconsin, U.S.A.

Edited by
Alan D. Attie, Ph.D.
Associate Professor
Departments of Biochemistry and Comparative Biosciences
University of Wisconsin–Madison
Madison, Wisconsin, U.S.A.

Elsevier
New York • Amsterdam • London

No responsibility is assumed by the publisher for any injury and/or damage to persons or property as a matter of products liability, negligence, or otherwise, or from any use or operation of any methods, products, instructions, or ideas contained in the material herein. No suggested test or procedure should be carried out unless, in the reader's judgment, its risk is justified. Because of rapid advances in the medical sciences, we recommend that the independent verification of diagnosis and drug dosages should be made. Discussions, views, and recommendations as to medical procedures, choice of drugs, and drug dosages are the responsibility of the authors.

Elsevier Science Publishing Co., Inc.
655 Avenue of the Americas, New York, New York 10010

Sole distributors outside the United States and Canada:
Elsevier Science Publishers B.V.
P.O. Box 211, 1000 AE Amsterdam, The Netherlands

© 1990 by Elsevier Science Publishing Co., Inc.

This book has been registered with the Copyright Clearance Center, Inc.
For further information, please contact the Copyright Clearance Center, Inc., Salem, Massachusetts.

This book is printed on acid-free paper.

ISBN 0-444-01587-6

Current printing (last digit):
10 9 8 7 6 5 4 3 2 1

Manufactured in the United States of America

Contents

ANIMAL MODELS

APOLIPOPROTEIN STRUCTURE

Preface

Originally confined to events occurring at the arterial wall, atherosclerosis investigation also attends to events occurring in virtually all types of organ systems and blood cells. As a result of the revolution that made powerful molecular biology techniques available to all biologists and is beginning to transform diagnostic and clinical medicine, researchers approach atherosclerosis mindful of processes occurring on a molecular level. This trend, of course, is not unique to atherosclerosis research; it is prevalent in all of biomedical research.

The Steenbock Symposium on Molecular Biology of Atherosclerosis brought together a sampling of outstanding researchers representing levels of analysis spanning nucleic acids, lipids, proteins, whole cells, and whole animals.

Several papers describe practical and theoretical aspects of gene expression. John Taylor describes regulatory elements distant from the apo-E coding region necessary for liver expression in transgenic mice. Lorne Taichman describes the use of keratinocytes to express apo-E with the implication that a form of gene therapy involving the grafting of transfected keratinocytes is theoretically feasible. Stephen Sturley describes the use of mutant yeast strains for expressing and secreting human apolipoproteins. Peter Edwards also employed the yeast system; he cloned a human prenyl transferase by complementing a yeast mutant.

Three presentations are devoted to RNA metabolism. Donna Driscoll presents the post-transcriptional editing of apo-B mRNA. Jeff Ross and David Williams cover aspects of the regulation of mRNA degradation.

Post-translational processing of newly synthesized proteins is addressed by Reid Gilmore in his analysis of the mechanisms of protein translocation across the ER membrane. Vishwanath Lingappa and Roger Davis present novel aspects to the orientation of apo-B upon translocation across the ER. Chris Kaiser describes the use of yeast secretion mutants to characterize vesicles involved in transport between the ER and the Golgi. André Bensadoun discusses post-translational processing of lipoprotein lipase in relation to its cellular binding protein.

Reneé LeBoeuf and Sandra Schreyer describe mutations affecting HDL levels in mice and chickens, respectively. Lawrence Rudel pools together many studies exploring nutritional effects on apolipoprotein metabolism.

Several papers emphasize apolipoprotein structure. Leonard Banaszak presents the first crystal structure of an intact lipoprotein particle, lipovitellin. Hazel Holden presents the first crystal structure of an apolipoprotein. Jere Segrest conveys concepts relating to the structure and function of amphipathic helixes in apolipoproteins, particularly apo-AI. Stephen Meredith proposes that a segment of apo-E might have a π-helix structure, which has not yet been detected in any protein. Sissel Lund-Katz shows how ^{13}C-NMR studies of intact apo-B can be used to study the physical environment of lysine residues.

Finally, several papers integrate lipoprotein metabolism, growth control, and atherosclerosis. Jake Lusis, Alan Fogelman, and Urs Steinbrecher discuss modifications of LDL in relation to arterial wall metabolism. Richard Lawn discusses the biology of apo(a). Earl Ruley presents an unusual *in vitro* smooth muscle cell system displaying changes in lipid metabolism in response to the ras-oncogene. Dan Bowen-Pope provides an update on platelet-derived growth factor receptors. Brad Olwin presents the characterization of a new fibroblast growth factor receptor.

The eclectic array of papers clearly reflects the expansion of the atherosclerosis field into many new areas of biology.

An indispensable contributor to the success of the Steenbock Symposium was Ms. Joann Trodahl. We are all indebted to her for the care and thoughtfulness she devoted to the organization of the symposium and the preparation of these proceedings.

Participants

Aiello, Robert J.
Department of Biochemistry
University of Wisconsin-Madison
420 Henry Mall
Madison, WI 53706 USA

Aker, Kathryn A.
Parke-Davis
2800 Plymouth Road
Ann Arbor, MI 48105 USA

Attie, Alan D.
Department of Biochemistry
University of Wisconsin-Madison
420 Henry Mall
Madison, WI 53706 USA

Auerbach, Bruce J.
Parke-Davis
2800 Plymouth Road
Ann Arbor, MI 48105 USA

Banaszak, Leonard J.
Dept. of Biochemistry
4-225 Millard Hall
University of Minnesota
435 Delaware Street S.E.
Minneapolis, MN 55455 USA

Bensadoun, André
Div. of Nutritional Sciences
321 Savage Hall
Cornell University
Ithaca, NY 14853 USA

Binder, Roberta
Dept. of Pharmacological Sciences
Health Sciences Center
BHS T7-147
SUNY at Stony Brook
Stony Brook, NY 11794 USA

Borén, Jan
Department of Medical Biochemistry
University of Göteborg
Box 33031
S-400 33 Göteborg
SWEDEN

Bowen-Pope, Daniel
Department of Pathology
University of Washington, SM-30
Seattle, WA 98195 USA

Braddock, Demetrios T.
5470 South Hyde Park Blvd.
Apt. 1 South
Chicago, IL 60615 USA

Brown, Eric R.
Department of Biochemistry
Rush Univ. of Rush Presbyterian
St. Luke's Medical Center
Chicago, IL 60612 USA

Brown, Maryanne L.
Dept. of Medicine, P+S 10-509
Columbia University
630 West 168th Street
New York, NY 10032 USA

Budzinski, Ralph-Michael
Dr. Karl Thomae GmbH
Department of Biochemistry
Birkendorfer Str. 65
Biberach/Riss 1
FRG

Burrus, Laura W.
Department of Biochemistry
University of Wisconsin-Madison
420 Henry Mall
Madison, WI 53706 USA

Checovich, William
Dept. of Physiological Chemistry
4580 Medical Science Center
University of Wisconsin-Madison
Madison, WI 53706 USA

Chiang, Anna
3171 Sepulveda Blvd., #4
Los Angeles, CA 90034 USA

Cohen, Louis H.
Gaubius Institute TNO
P.O. Box 612
2300 AP Leiden
THE NETHERLANDS

Connelly, Philip W.
Lipid Research
St. Michael's Hospital, Rm. 102 WA
38 Shuter Street
Toronto, Ontario
CANADA M5B 1A6

Cooper, Scott
Department of Biochemistry
University of Wisconsin-Madison
420 Henry Mall
Madison, WI 53706 USA

Cornicelli, Joseph A.
Parke-Davis
2800 Plymouth Road
Ann Arbor, MI 48105 USA

Davis, Richard C.
VA Wadsworth Medical Center
Building 113, Room 312
Los Angeles, CA 90073 USA

Davis, Roger A.
Hepatobiliary Center, Box 158
Univ. of Colorado Health Science
Center
4200 E. 9th Avenue
Denver, CO 80262 USA

Devall, Larry J.
Parke-Davis
2800 Plymouth Road
Ann Arbor, MI 48105 USA

Dimond, Randall
Promega Corporation
2800 Woods Hollow Road
Madison, WI 53711-5399 USA

Dixon, Joseph L.
Department of Medicine
Columbia University
630 W. 168th Street
New York, NY 10032 USA

Donati, Robert J.
University of Chicago
5801 Ellis Avenue
Chicago, IL 60637 USA

Doolittle, Mark
Lipid Research
Bldg. 113, Rm. 312
VA Wadsworth Medical Center
Los Angeles, CA 90073 USA

Dory, Ladislav
Dept. of Pharmacology
University of Tennessee
100 Crowe Bldg.
874 Union Avenue
Memphis, TN 38163 USA

Driscoll, Donna
Southwest Foundation for Biomedical
Research
P.O. Box 28147
San Antonio, TX 78238 USA

Dueland, Svein
University of Colorado Health
Sciences Center
4200 E. 9th Avenue, Box B-158
Denver, CO 80262 USA

Edwards, Peter
Depts. Medicine & Chemistry
Univ. of California, Los Angeles
10833 LeConte
Los Angeles, CA 90064 USA

Ellsworth, Jeff L.
Research Institute
Palo Alto Medical Foundation
860 Bryant Street
Palo Alto, CA 94301 USA

Feinstein, Sheldon I.
Univ. of Pennsylvania School
of Medicine
1 John Morgan Building
36th Street and Hamilton Walk
Philadelphia, PA 19104-6068 USA

Fogelman, Alan M.
Division of Cardiology
UCLA School of Medicine
47-123 CHS
Los Angeles, CA 90024 USA

Forgez, Patricia
Dept. Pharmacology
SUNY at Stony Brook
Stony Brook, NY 11794 USA

Friedman, Alan D.
Department of Embryology
Carnegie Institution of Washington
115 West University Parkway
Baltimore, MD 21210 USA

Furukawa, Seiichi
c/o Henry Ginsberg
Department of Medicine P&S 9-501
Columbia University
630 West 168th Street
New York, NY 10032 USA

Gilmore, Reid
Department of Biochemistry
University of Massachusetts
Medical School
Worcester, MA 01655 USA

Glick, Jane M.
Dept. of Physiology &
Biochemistry
Medical College of Pennsylvania
3300 Henry Avenue
Philadelphia, PA 19129 USA

Gretch, Daniel
Department of Biochemistry
University of Wisconsin-Madison
420 Henry Mall
Madison, WI 53706 USA

Guilds, Linda S.
Parke-Davis
2800 Plymouth Road
Ann Arbor, MI 48105 USA

Hajjar, David P.
Cornell Medical School
Department of Pathology
1300 York Avenue
New York, NY 10021 USA

Hasler-Rapacz, Judith
Department of Genetics
Genetics Building
University of Wisconsin-Madison
Madison, WI 53706 USA

Hoeg, Jeffrey M.
12913 Stallion Court
Potomac, MD 20854 USA

Hofker, Marten H.
Department of Human Genetics
University of Leiden
P.O. Box 9503
Leiden
THE NETHERLANDS 2300 RA

Holden, Hazel
Department of Chemistry &
Enzyme Research
Institute for Enzyme Research
1710 University Avenue
Madison, WI 53705 USA

Hospattankar, Ashok V.
CIBA-GEIGY Corporation
556 Morris Avenue, Bldg. J-108
Summit, NJ 07901 USA

Huang, Fen
Promega Corporation
2800 Woods Hollow Road
Madison, WI 53711 USA

Hughes, Thomas E.
Department of Lipid and Lipoprotein
Metabolism
403/212, Sandoz Research Institute
59 Route 10
East Hanover, NJ 07936 USA

Jeenah, Mohamed
Dept. Medical Biochemistry
Univ. of Cape Town Medical School
Observatory 7925
SOUTH AFRICA

John, Michelle
Department of Biochemistry
University of Wisconsin-Madison
420 Henry Mall
Madison, WI 53706 USA

Kaiser, Chris
Div. Biochemistry & Molecular Biol.
Barker Hall
University of California, Berkeley
Berkeley, CA 94720 USA

Kaiser, Mary
Department of Biochemistry
University of Wisconsin-Madison
420 Henry Mall
Madison, WI 53706 USA

Kaner, Robert J.
Pulmonary Service
Department of Medicine
Sloan-Kettering Cancer Center
1275 York Avenue
New York, NY 10021 USA

Karathanasis, Sotirios K.
Children's Hospital
Department of Cardiology
300 Longwood Ave.
Boston, MA 02115 USA

Kirchgessner, Todd
Squibb Institute for Medical Research
P.O. Box 4000
Princeton, NJ 08540 USA

Kletzien, Rolf F.
Metabolic Diseases Research
7250-126-3
The Upjohn Company
Kalamazoo, MI 49001 USA

Koller, Beth
318 Genetics
University of Wisconsin-Madison
445 Henry Mall
Madison, WI 53706 USA

Kudla, Arthur J.
Department of Biochemistry
University of Wisconsin-Madison
420 Henry Mall
Madison, WI 53706 USA

Lawn, Richard
Genentech, Inc.
460 Point San Bruno Blvd.
South San Francisco, CA 94080 USA

LeBoeuf, Reneé C.
Department of Medicine
Div. Metabolism, Endocrinology, and Nutrition, DL-10
University of Washington
Seattle, WA 98195 USA

Leff, Todd
Rockefeller University
1230 York Avenue
New York, NY 10021 USA

Li, Yi-Shuan
Biotechnology Center
Rightmire Hall #220
Ohio State University
1060 Carmack Road
Columbus, OH 43210 USA

Lieder, Kafryn W.
Department of Biochemistry
University of Wisconsin-Madison
420 Henry Mall
Madison, WI 53706 USA

Lingappa, Vishwanath R.
Depts. Physiology & Medicine
Box 0444
Univ. of California-San Francisco
San Francisco, CA 94143 USA

Lowe, Scott W.
Department of Biology and Center for Cancer Research
Massachusetts Institute of Technology
Cambridge, MA 02139 USA

Lund-Katz, Sissel
Department of Physiology & Biochemistry
Medical College of Pennsylvania
3300 Henry Avenue
Philadelphia, PA 19129 USA

Lusis, Aldons J.
Department of Medicine & Microbiology
Division of Hematology-Oncology
Univ. of California, Los Angeles
Los Angeles, CA 90024 USA

Madore, Steven J.
Dept. of Pharmacological Sciences
Health Sciences Center
SUNY at Stony Brook
Stony Brook, NY 11794 USA

Maeda, Nobuyo
Department of Pathology
Brinkhous-Bullitt Bldg.
University of North Carolina
Chapel Hill, NC 27599 USA

Marotti, Keith R.
Molecular Biology Research
The Upjohn Company
301 Henrietta Street
Kalamazoo, MI 49007 USA

Martner, John E.
Department of Oncology
McArdle Laboratory for Cancer Research
University of Wisconsin-Madison
Madison, WI 53706 USA

Mellow, Ellen
Division of Cardiology
Department of Medicine
The New York Hospital-Cornell
Medical Center
525 E. 68th Street
New York, NY 10021 USA

Meredith, Steven
Department of Pathology
University of Chicago
Chicago, IL 60637 USA

Mitra, Sudha W.
Merck Sharp & Dohme Res. Labs
P.O. Box 2000 (80W-206)
Rahway, NJ 07065-0900 USA

Moberly, James B.
Pfizer Central Research
Eastern Point Road
Groton, CT 06340 USA

Naggert, Juergen K.
Children's Hospital
Oakland Research Institute
747 52nd Street
Oakland, CA 94609 USA

Neath, Sean-Xavier
Dept. of Pathology
Box 414
University of Chicago Hospitals
5841 S. Maryland Ave.
Chicago, IL 60637 USA

Nicosia, Monica
Department of Pharmacology
HSC SUNY at Stony Brook
Stony Brook, NY 11794 USA

Nishina, Patsy M.
Children's Hospital
Oakland Research Institute
747 52nd Street
Oakland, CA 94609 USA

Nevin, David N.
H4/554 Clinical Sciences Center
Department of Medicine
600 Highland Avenue
Madison, WI 53792 USA

O'Connell, William A.
Department of Pathology
Box 414
University of Chicago
5841 S. Maryland Ave.
Chicago, IL 60637 USA

Ohringer, Jack D.
Rush-Presbyterian-St. Luke's
Medical Center
Section of Digestive Diseases
Suite 256
1725 W. Harrison
Chicago, IL 60612 USA

Olson, Lisa M.
Department of Pathology
Box 414
The University of Chicago
5841 South Maryland Avenue
Chicago, IL 60637 USA

Olwin, Bradley
Department of Biochemistry
University of Wisconsin-Madison
420 Henry Mall
Madison, WI 53706 USA

Paigen, Beverly J.
Jackson Laboratory
600 Main Street
Bar Harbor, ME 04609 USA

Pape, Michael E.
Metabolic Diseases Research
7250-209-4
The Upjohn Company
Kalamazoo, MI 49001 USA

Pawson, Tony
Samuel Lunenfeld Res. Institute
Mount Sinai Hospital
600 University Avenue
Toronto, Ontario M5G 1X5
CANADA

Pech, Michael
Hoffmann-La Roche Ltd.
Pharmaceutical Research Department
CH-4002 Basel
SWITZERLAND

Peffley, Dennis M.
Department of Pharmacology
University of Tennessee
874 Union Avenue
Memphis, TN 38163 USA

Piedrahita, Jorge A.
Department of Pathology
University of North Carolina
Chapel Hill, NC 27599-7525 USA

Plump, Andrew
Box H29
1230 York Avenue
New York, NY 10021 USA

Polacek, Denise C.
Department of Pathology
Box 414
University of Chicago
5841 S. Maryland Avenue
Chicago, IL 60637 USA

Rabin, Michael S.
Massachusetts Inst. of Technology
E17-518
77 Massachusetts Ave.
Cambridge, MA 02139 USA

Rapacz, Jan
Department of Genetics
Genetics Building
University of Wisconsin-Madison
Madison, WI 53706 USA

Rawat, Mukul
Department of Medicine
Section of Endocrinology
Rush-Presbyterian St. Luke's
Medical Center
Chicago, IL 60612

Reardon-Alulis Catherine
Dept. of Pathology, Box 414
The University of Chicago
5841 South Maryland Avenue
Chicago, IL 60637 USA

Redgrave, Trevor G.
Dept. of Physiology
University of Western Australia
Nedlands
AUSTRALIA 6009

Reue, Karen
Wadsworth V.A. Medical Center
Bldg. 113, Rm. 312
Wilshire & Sawtelle Blvds.
Los Angeles, CA 90073 USA

Reyland, Mary E.
Dept. of Pharmacology
SUNY at Stony Brook
Stony Brook, NY 11794 USA

Rine, Jasper
Department of Biochemistry
Univ. of California-Berkeley
Berkeley, CA 94720 USA

Ringold, Gordon
Syntex Research, S3-1
3401 Hillview Avenue
Palo Alto, CA 94304 USA

Ross, Jeffrey
625 McArdle Cancer Research
University of Wisconsin-Madison
Madison, WI 53706 USA

Ross, Stuart A.
Dept. of Anatomy and Cardiovascular
Research Institute
University of California, San Francisco
San Francisco, CA 94143 USA

Rubin, Edward
Cell and Molecular Biology
Lawrence Berkeley Lab
Berkeley, CA 94720 USA

Rudel, Lawrence L.
Department of Comparative Medicine
Bowman Gray Medical School
Wake Forest University
300 S. Hawthorne Road
Winston-Salem, NC 27103 USA

Ruley, Earl
MIT Center for Cancer Research
77 Massachusetts Ave., E17-517
Cambridge, MA 02139 USA

Schneider, Wolfgang J.
Lipid & Lipoprotein Research Group
327 Heritage Medical Research Center
University of Alberta
Edmonton, Alberta
CANADA T6G 2C2

Schreyer, Sandra
204 Biochemistry Building
University of Wisconsin-Madison
420 Henry Mall
Madison, WI 53706 USA

Schultz, Paul
Parke-Davis
2800 Plymouth Road
Ann Arbor, MI 48105 USA

Segrest, Jere P.
Atherosclerosis Res. Unit
Univ. of Alabama in Birmingham
Volker Hall, Rm. G-018
Birmingham, AL 35294 USA

Sekerke, Catherine
Parke-Davis
2800 Plymouth Road
Ann Arbor, MI 48105 USA

Sensel, Martha
Department of Pharmacology
Health Science Center
SUNY at Stony Brook
Stony Brook, NY 11794-8651 USA

Shaw, Mary Kay
Parke-Davis
2800 Plymouth Road
Ann Arbor, MI 48105 USA

Smith, Jonathan
Rockefeller University
1230 York Avenue
New York, NY 10021 USA

Smith, Terry
Department of Pathology
University of North Carolina
Chapel Hill, NC 27599-7525 USA

Sobol, Mary
2800 Fish Hatchery Road
Madison, WI 53711 USA

Sorci-Thomas, Mary
Bowman Gray School of Medicine
Wake Forest University
300 S. Hawthorne Road
Winston-Salem, NC 27103 USA

Spangler, Elizabeth
Lawrence Berkeley Laboratory
Bldg. 74-157
1 Cyclotron Road
Berkeley, CA 94720 USA

Steinberg, Daniel
Department of Medicine, M-013D
Univ. of California, San Diego
La Jolla, CA 92093 USA

Steinbrecher, Urs
Department of Medicine
University of British Columbia
Vancouver, British Columbia
CANADA

Sturley, Stephen
Department of Biochemistry
University of Wisconsin-Madison
420 Henry Mall
Madison, WI 53706 USA

Sword, John T.
252 Food Research Institute
University of Wisconsin-Madison
1925 Willow Drive
Madison, WI 53706 USA

Taichman, Lorne
Dept. of Oral Biology & Pathology
School of Dental Medicine
State University of New York
Stony Brook, NY 11794-8702 USA

Tanabe, Steven M.
University of Chicago
5841 S. Maryland Ave.
Chicago, IL 60637 USA

Taylor, John M.
Gladstone Foundation Laboratories
Univ. of California, San Francisco
P.O. Box 40608
San Francisco, CA 94140 USA

Teng, Ba-Bie
Department of Medicine
GI Section
University of Chicago
5841 South Maryland Ave.
Chicago, IL 60037 USA

Thanassi, Jane
Bristol Myers Squibb Co.
5 Research Parkway
Wallingford, CT 06492 USA

Thompson, John F.
Department of Molecular Genetics
Pfizer Central Research
Groton, CT 06340 USA

Uelmen, Patricia J.
Department of Biochemistry
University of Wisconsin-Madison
420 Henry Mall
Madison, WI 53706 USA

VandeBerg, John L.
Department of Genetics
Southwest Foundation for
Biomedical Research
P.O. Box 28147
San Antonio, TX 78228-0147 USA

van der Westhuyzen, Deneys R.
Department of Medical Biochemistry
University of Cape Town Medical School
Observatory 7925
SOUTH AFRICA

Volin, Michael V.
Department of Pathology
Box 414
University of Chicago
5841 S. Maryland Avenue
Chicago, IL 60637 USA

Watson, John
Room 4590 Medical Sciences Center
University of Wisconsin-Madison
Madison, WI 53706 USA

Williams, David L.
Dept. of Pharmacological Sciences
Health Sciences Center
SUNY at Stony Brook
Stony Brook, NY 11794-8651 USA

Zuber, Michael
Department of Biochemistry
University of Wisconsin-Madison
420 Henry Mall
Madison, WI 53706 USA

TRANSCRIPTIONAL AND POST-TRANSCRIPTIONAL REGULATION

Independent Regulatory Elements Control Expression of the Human Apolipoprotein E Gene in the Liver and Kidney of Transgenic Mice[1]

W. Scott Simonet, Nathan Bucay, Stephen J. Lauer, Robert E. Pitas,* Karl H. Weisgraber,* and John M. Taylor†

*Gladstone Foundation Laboratories for Cardiovascular Disease, Cardiovascular Research Institute, Departments of † Physiology and *Pathology, University of California, San Francisco, California*

ABSTRACT

Human apolipoprotein (apo) E gene constructs with either 30, 5, or 2 kilobases of the 5′-flanking and 1.5 kilobases of the 3′-flanking regions were used to create transgenic mice. High levels of human apoE mRNA were present in the transgenic kidney, but none was detected in the liver, which is normally the major source of apoE. When a construct with 5 kilobases of the 5′- and 23 kilobases of the 3′-flanking regions was used, only trace levels of human apoE mRNA were detected in the kidney, whereas high levels were found in the liver. These results indicated that regulatory elements downstream of the human apoE gene interacted with the transcription initiation complex to stimulate gene expression in the liver while suppressing expression in the kidney. In each case, human apoE was secreted into the plasma. The source of human apoE in the transgenic kidney was the epithelial cells lining the proximal tubule and Bowman's capsule.

INTRODUCTION

Apolipoprotein (apo) E is a major structural component of several classes of mammalian lipoproteins, including chylomicron remnants, very low density lipoproteins, and high density lipoproteins (1). Human apoE is a single-chain protein of 299 amino acids (M_r=34,200) (2). It can have an additional 3-5% of its mass in a carbohydrate moiety attached to threonine 194 that can exist in multiply sialylated forms (3, 4). Human apoE is encoded by a 3597-nucleotide gene that has four exons and three introns and is located on chromosome 19 (5, 6). The apoCI gene is located 5.0 kilobases (kb) downstream of the apoE gene, in the same transcriptional orientation (7). An apoCI pseudogene is located 7.5 kb downstream of the apoCI gene (7).

The major source of circulating apoE is the hepatocyte (8-10). Specific cell types in several extrahepatic tissues, including brain, kidney, and spleen, are responsible for the remainder of the apoE that is found in the plasma and interstitial fluid. Apolipoprotein E is a major product of astrocytic glial cells in the central and peripheral nervous systems (11) and of terminally differentiated macrophages (12, 13). Lower amounts of apoE are produced by ovarian granulosa cells (14), growth-arrested smooth muscle cells (15), and specific epithelial cells in many tissues (10). This same distribution of sites of apoE synthesis is found in several different species, although there are interspecies differences

[1]Significant portions of this work were published in The *Journal of Biological Chemistry* (Simonet et al., *J. Biol. Chem.* 265:10809-10812, 1990).

© 1990 by Elsevier Science Publishing Co., Inc.
Molecular Biology of Atherosclerosis
A.D. Attie, Editor

in relative production levels. The expression of most other apolipoproteins is restricted primarily to the liver and intestine (8, 9).

Apolipoprotein E has a major role in the redistribution of cholesterol and other lipids between peripheral tissues and the liver. It mediates the cellular uptake of specific lipoproteins, especially chylomicron remnants and intermediate density lipoproteins, through an interaction with low density lipoprotein (LDL) receptors and distinct hepatic receptors (1). Naturally occurring apoE variants with single amino acid substitutions in the proposed receptor-binding domain (residues 140-160) exhibit decreased binding activity and are associated with type III hyperlipoproteinemia and accelerated atherosclerosis (1).

The function of the widespread extrahepatic apoE production may be to control the availability and redistribution of lipid for local metabolic requirements in a variety of tissues. For example, it has been shown that accumulated macrophage-derived apoE participates in remyelination during peripheral nerve regeneration (16).

To understand the role of apoE in extrahepatic lipid metabolism, a knowledge of the molecular signals that regulate apoE gene expression is required. An important first step would be the identification of tissue-specific control sequences associated with the gene. Since apoE appears to have a central role in linking extrahepatic lipid metabolism with that of the liver, the use of transgenic animals to examine the expression of modified constructs of the apoE gene is likely to be especially informative. In this study with transgenic mice, we have identified multiple regulatory elements that influence the tissue expression pattern of the human apoE gene.

RESULTS AND DISCUSSION

The location of tissue-specific regulatory elements that control expression of the human apoE gene was investigated through a detailed analysis of sequences flanking the gene. The DNA fragments intended for integration into the mouse genome were purified by CsCl gradient centrifugation, gel electrophoresis (17), phenol extraction, and ethanol precipitation and then diluted to 1 ng/ml in 5 mM Tris, pH 7.4, 0.2 mM EDTA. Single cell embryos from ICR x ICR-bred mice were microinjected with the DNA fragments as described (18). The embryos surviving microinjection were transferred to the oviducts of pseudopregnant ICR female mice. Offspring were weaned at 3 to 4 weeks of age, and DNA was prepared from a 1-cm portion of their tails as described (18). Transgenic founder animals (F0), which averaged 30% of the offspring derived from implanted embryos, were identified by Southern blot analysis (19), and they were mated with nontransgenic mice to generate transgenic F1 progeny. Serial dilutions of transgenic mouse DNA followed by Southern blot analysis indicated that the number of integrated copies of the transgene varied between 1 and 100 (data not shown). Additional Southern blot mapping confirmed the absence of any gross rearrangement in any of the gene constructs transferred to the transgenic mice. Approximately 30% of the founders were mosaic, and less than 50% of their F1 offspring carried the transgene. Therefore, the animals used for all RNA and protein analysis were transgenic F1 male mice between 6 and 10 weeks of age.

Initially, a series of human apoE gene constructs with various lengths of the 5′-flanking sequence were used to prepare transgenic mice. The constructs depicted in Figure 1 contained either 2.0 kb, 5.0 kb, or 30 kb of the 5′-flanking sequence and a constant 1.5 kb of the 3′-flanking sequence. The number of founder (F0) transgenic mice identified for each construct is indicated in the legend to Figure 1. Total cellular RNA was isolated from tissues of F1 transgenic progeny (20) and examined by RNase protection analysis with a human apoE ^{32}P-labeled antisense RNA probe. Human apoE mRNA in all the transgenic mice harboring 5′ deletion constructs was abundant in the kidney and present at low levels in testis (Fig. 1). CLE1, the construct containing 30 kb of the 5′-flanking sequence, also produced significant levels of human apoE mRNA in the skin and brain. Longer exposures of the autoradiograms for the two shorter constructs containing 5 kb or less of the 5′-flanking sequence detected low levels of human apoE mRNA in the brain (data not shown). Although cell-free transcription experiments using hepatic cell nuclear extracts have demonstrated that the apoE promoter contains strong transcriptional control sequences (21), no expression of these human apoE gene constructs was detected in the livers of these transgenic mice. The expression pattern of the human apoE transgenes contrasted markedly with that of the endogenous mouse apoE gene, which was expressed at high levels in the liver, at moderate levels in the skin and brain, and at low levels in other tissues.

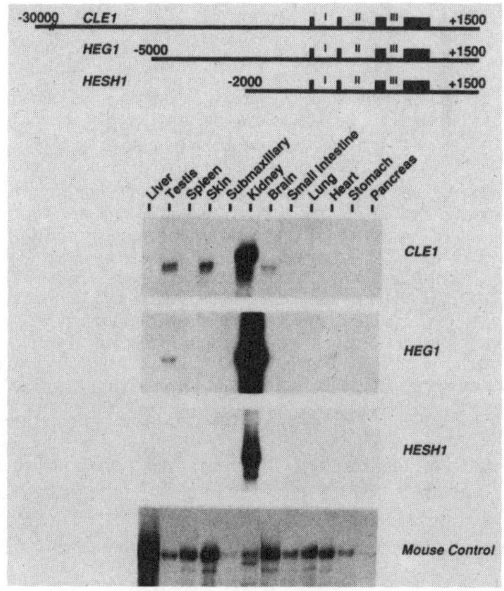

Figure 1. Expression of the human apolipoprotein E gene with different lengths of 5′-flanking sequence. The apoE construct CLE1 (22) consisted of recombinant cosmid DNA that included 30 kb of 5′-flanking sequence and 1.5 kb of 3′-flanking sequence. The portion of the cosmid vector sequence that included SV40 regulatory regions (23) was deleted before use in these studies. HEG1 was a 10-kb *Hin*dIII fragment isolated from the CLE1 cosmid. It included only the proximal 5.0 kb of 5′-flanking sequence but the same 1.5 kb of 3′-flanking sequence as in the cosmid. The 7.5-kb fragment making up the HESH1 construct was isolated from HEG1 by digestion with *Sph*I and *Hin*dIII. It contained 2.0 kb of 5′-flanking sequence and 1.5 kb of 3′-flanking sequence. Exons of the apoE gene are indicated by the solid boxes, and introns by Roman numerals. For the CLE1 construct, three independent transgenic founders (F0) were obtained from 25 animals that were screened (*i.e.*, 3 F0/25); for the HEG1 construct, 6 F0/9 animals; for the HESH1 construct, 4 F0/16 animals. Antisense RNA probes for either human or mouse apoE mRNA were transcribed using bacteriophage T3 RNA polymerase in the presence of [^{32}P]UTP from cDNA fragments that had been cloned in Bluescribe vectors (Stratagene, San Diego, CA). Ribonuclease protection analysis was performed as described previously (24). Human and mouse apoE mRNA protected 188 and 127 nucleotides of their respective probes. Protected fragments were analyzed by electrophoresis in 6% polyacrylamide gels containing 7 M urea, followed by autoradiography of dried gels. Transgenic and control mouse RNAs were analyzed with human and mouse probes in separate assays. Two to four independent lines of transgenic mice with different numbers of copies of the transgene were analyzed for each construct. No differences in mRNA tissue distribution were observed between lines containing the same construct. The top three autoradiograms show the pattern of expression of the human apoE gene in representative transgenic mice harboring each of the constructs depicted above. The lower autoradiogram shows the RNA expression pattern of a nontransgenic control mouse using the mouse antisense probe.

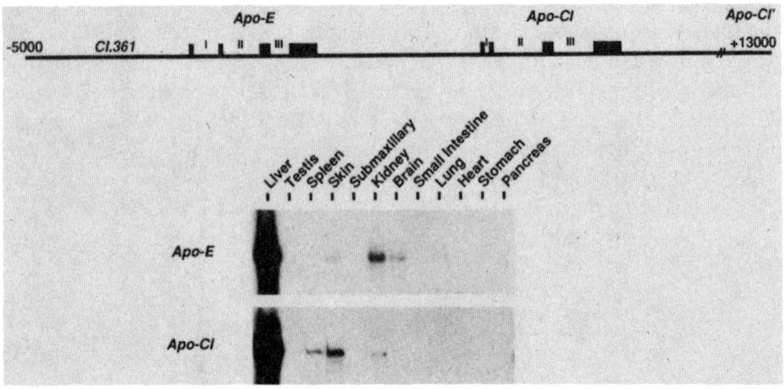

Figure 2. Expression of the human apolipoprotein E and C-I genes in a construct containing 23 kb of 3′-flanking sequence. The apoE construct, CI.361, was a recombinant cosmid that included 5 kb of proximal 5′-flanking sequence and 23 kb of 3′-flanking sequence around the apoE gene (5). This construct included the apoC-I gene, which was located 5 kb downstream of the apoE gene in the same transcriptional orientation, and an apoC-I pseudogene (apo-CI′), which was located 7.5 kb downstream from the normal apoC-I gene, also in the same transcriptional orientation. Exons of the apoE gene are indicated by the solid boxes, and introns by Roman numerals. For the CI.361 construct, 9 independent transgenic founders (F0) were obtained from 20 animals that were screened (*i.e.*, 9 F0/20). Ribonuclease protection analysis of transgenic mouse tissue RNA was performed as described in the legend to Fig. 1. Antisense RNA probes for human apoCI mRNA protected 288 nucleotides of its labeled probe. Although a probe for mouse apoC-I mRNA was unavailable, the human apoC-I probe showed limited cross-hybridization with mouse apoC-I mRNA, and it produced a protected fragment of about 20 base pairs, which served as an internal control for all apoC-I mRNA analysis (data not shown). Representative results showing the pattern of human apoE or human apoC-I gene expression in transgenic mice harboring the CI.361 construct depicted above are shown.

In marked contrast to the results with the 5′ deletion constructs, transgenic mice harboring the CI.361 construct (which has a 23-kb 3′-flanking sequence) expressed the human apoE gene at high levels in the liver (Fig. 2). Longer exposures of the autoradiograms showed trace levels of apoE mRNA in the testis, tail skin, and kidney (data not shown).

These results suggest that a strong regulatory sequence is located more than 1.5 kb downstream from the apoE gene and interacts with the transcription initiation complex to specify expression in the liver. In addition to a liver-specific element, there may be a silencer element located downstream of the apoE gene that decreases apoE gene transcription in the kidney and thus determines the final pattern of apoE gene expression. In the absence of these downstream sequences, a strong upstream control element drives expression of the apoE gene in the kidneys. The downstream elements may be located in the region between the apoE and the apoC-I gene. Such elements might play a role in regulating both genes. Although downstream regulatory elements are not unique to the apoE gene, the finding that the principal tissue-specific element necessary for apoE gene expression in the liver is located 3′ of the gene is unusual.

It is of interest to note that the apoA-I gene, linked closely to the genes for apoC-III and apoA-IV on chromosome 11 (25), requires a far distal element for expression in the intestine (26). However, the relative location of the intestine element with respect to this gene cluster is unclear. These findings with the apoE and apoA-I genes in transgenic mice suggest the possibility that common regulatory elements in each apolipoprotein gene cluster may determine expression in specific tissues.

Human apoE mRNA and plasma protein from the transgenic mice were examined to characterize the expression of the transgene. Northern blot analysis (27) (Fig. 3, left panel, lanes 1-7) showed that the human apoE mRNA produced in both the liver and kidney of the transgenic mice was of normal size and indistinguishable from the apoE mRNA of cultured human hepatoma cells and normal mouse tissues. Transgenic mice harboring the CI.361 genomic fragment also expressed human apoC-I mRNA in the liver, but no apoC-I mRNA was detectable in the kidney (Fig. 3, left panel, lanes 8-11).

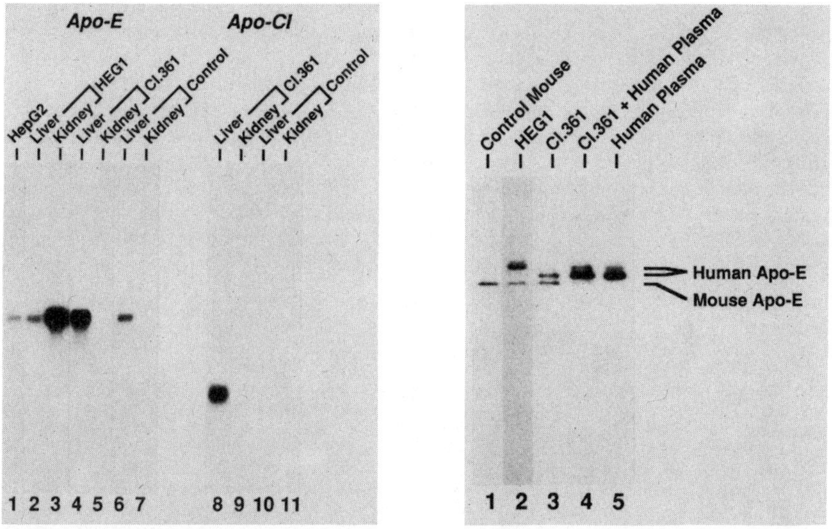

Figure 3. Analysis of human apoE mRNA and protein in transgenic mice. Left panel: Total RNAs (10 μg) from the liver and kidneys of transgenic mice and nontransgenic control mice, and from cultured HepG2 cells, were examined by Northern blot analysis (19, 27). After electrophoresis, RNAs were transferred to Gene Screen™ (DuPont, Wilmington, DE) and hybridized to a ^{32}P-labeled human apoE cDNA or ^{32}P-labeled human apoC-I cDNA. Because of partial nucleotide sequence homology, the human apoE cDNA cross-hybridized to the mouse apoE mRNA in Northern blot analyses. The human apoC-I cDNA did not cross-hybridize to mouse apoC-I mRNA. Right panel: Whole plasma from transgenic and nontransgenic mice was examined by Western blot analysis (28). Plasma was electrophoresed in a 7.5% polyacrylamide gel, transferred to Gene Screen™, incubated with a ^{125}I-labeled rabbit anti-human apoE IgG, and exposed on X-ray film. Lane 1, 1 μl of nontransgenic control mouse plasma; lane 2, 1 μl of HEG1 (kidney apoE expressing) transgenic mouse plasma; lane 3, 1 μl of CI.361 (liver apoE expressing) transgenic mouse plasma; lane 4, 0.5 μl of CI.361 plasma mixed with 0.5 μl of normal human plasma; lane 5, 1 μl of normal human plasma. The positions of different forms of human plasma apoE and of cross-reacting mouse apoE are indicated. Reproduced with permission from *The Journal of Biological Chemistry* (Simonet et al., *J. Biol. Chem.* 265:10809-10812, 1990).

Plasma was collected from the tails of F0 or F1 animals and examined by Western blot analysis (22) (Fig. 3, right panel). For plasma apoE analysis, a polyclonal antibody was employed that had a partial cross-reaction with mouse apoE, which was about 0.3 kDa smaller than human apoE. Most of the human apoE in the plasma of liver-expressing CI.361 transgenic mice migrated at a mobility similar to that of non-glycosylated human plasma apoE (Fig. 3, right panel, lanes 3, 4, and 5), which accounts for about 80% of circulating plasma apoE (3). In the plasma of the kidney-expressing HEG1 mouse, human apoE migrated with an electrophoretic mobility slower than that of normal human plasma apoE. Neuraminadase treatment did not alter the electrophoretic mobility of the human apoE produced by transgenic mouse kidney (data not shown). This latter finding suggests that sialic acid heterogeneity, which normally accounts for some polymorphism in human plasma apoE (1, 3, 4), was not responsible for the slow electrophoretic mobility of the human apoE produced by the transgenic kidney. A likely explanation for the differences in mobility is a difference in posttranslational processing of human apoE among mouse tissues, since differences in apoE processing in the tissues of other species, such as sulfation of rat cerebrospinal fluid apoE (29), have been reported (1, 16, 29).

The cellular distribution of apoE in the HEG1 transgenic mouse kidney was investigated by immunocytochemistry using human apoE antibodies. The results shown in Figure 4 indicate that human apoE was found in the epithelial cells that line Bowman's capsule and the proximal convoluted tubule. No human apoE was detectable in other tubular structures or in the medullary region of the kidney. These observations are consistent with a previous report that rat apoE synthesis in the kidney was limited to the epithelial cells of the proximal convoluted tubule (10). Thus, even when high levels of human apoE gene are expressed in the kidney, the cellular distribution of apoE protein production in this organ remains normal. Future studies will examine the mechanism of action of the downstream elements controlling kidney and liver expression and how the interaction of these elements with the apoE promoter may dictate the normal pattern of human apoE gene expression.

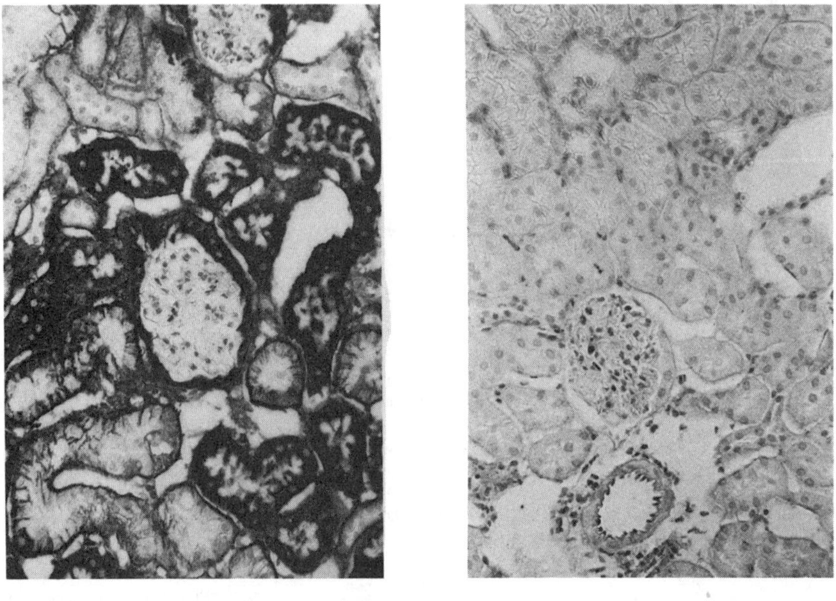

Figure 4. Immunocytochemistry of transgenic and control mouse kidneys. Transgenic and control mouse tissues were immersion-fixed for 4 h at 4°C in 4% formaldehyde (freshly prepared from paraformaldehyde) in 0.15 M phosphate buffer (pH 7.4) and cryoprotected by incubation overnight with 18% sucrose in phosphate-buffered saline. Small pieces of tissue were then quickly frozen in liquid nitrogen-cooled 2-methyl butane (11). Cryosections (10-μm) were dried onto gelatin-coated slides and treated with rabbit anti-human apoE IgG (0.5 μg/ml), followed by an immunoperoxidase detection assay (Vector Laboratories, ABC kit, Burlingame, CA) as described (16). The tissue was counterstained lightly with methyl green, and brightfield images were photographed. The left panel shows a micrographic cross-section of a kidney from a HEG1 transgenic mouse, and the right panel shows a cross-section of a kidney from a nontransgenic control mouse. Reproduced with permission from *The Journal of Biological Chemistry* (Simonet et al., *J. Biol. Chem.* 265:10809-10812, 1990).

REFERENCES

1. R.W. Mahley, Science 240, 622-630 (1988).
2. S.C. Rall, Jr., K.H. Weisgraber, and R.W. Mahley, J. Biol. Chem. 257, 4171-4178 (1982).
3. M.E. Wernette-Hammond, S.J. Lauer, A. Corsini, D. Walker, J.M. Taylor, and S.C. Rall, Jr., J. Biol. Chem. 264, 9094-9101 (1989).
4. V.I. Zannis and J.L. Breslow, Biochemistry 20, 1033-1041 (1981).
5. Y.K. Paik, D.J. Chang, C.A. Reardon, G.E. Davies, R.W. Mahley, and J.M. Taylor, Proc. Natl. Acad. Sci. USA 82, 3445-3449 (1985).
6. H.K. Das, J. McPherson, G.A. Bruns, S.K. Karathanasis, and J.L. Breslow, J. Biol. Chem. 260, 6240-6247 (1985).
7. S.J. Lauer, D.H. Walker, N.A. Elshourbagy, C.A. Reardon, B. Levy-Wilson, and J.M. Taylor, J. Biol. Chem. 263, 7277-7286 (1988).
8. N.A. Elshourbagy, W.S. Liao, R.W. Mahley, and J.M. Taylor, Proc. Natl. Acad. Sci. USA 82, 203-207 (1985).
9. T.C. Newman, P.A. Dawson, L.L. Rudel, and D.L. Williams, J. Biol. Chem. 260, 2452-2457 (1985).
10. C.T. Lin, Y. Xu, J.Y. Wu, and L. Chan, J. Clin. Invest. 78, 947-958 (1986).
11. J.K. Boyles, R.E. Pitas, E. Wilson, R.W. Mahley, and J.M. Taylor, J. Clin. Invest. 76, 1501-1513 (1985).
12. S.K. Basu, M.S. Brown, Y.K. Ho, R.J. Havel, and J.L. Goldstein, Proc. Natl. Acad. Sci. USA 78, 7545-7549 (1981).
13. Z. Werb and J.R. Chin, J. Biol. Chem. 258, 10642-10648 (1983).
14. D.M. Driscoll, J.R. Schreiber, V.M. Schmit, and G.S. Getz, J. Biol. Chem. 260, 9031-9038 (1985).
15. R.A. Majack, C.K. Castle, L.V. Goodman, K.H. Weisgraber, R.W. Mahley, E.M. Shooter, and P.J. Gebicke-Haerter, J. Cell Biol. 107, 1207-1213 (1988).
16. J.K. Boyles, C.D. Zoellner, L.J. Anderson, L.M. Kosik, R.E. Pitas, K.H. Weisgraber, D.Y. Hui, R.W. Mahley, P.J. Gebicke-Haerter, M.J. Ignatius, and E.M. Shooter, J. Clin. Invest. 83, 1015-1031 (1989).
17. T. Maniatis, E.F. Fritsch, and J. Sambrook, Molecular Cloning. A Laboratory Manual. Cold Spring Harbor Laboratory, Cold Spring Harbor, NY (1982).
18. R.L. Brinster, H.Y. Chen, M.E. Trumbauer, M.K. Yagle, and R.D. Palmiter, Proc. Natl. Acad. Sci. USA 82, 4438-4442 (1985).
19. G.M. Wahl, J.L. Meinkoth, and A.R. Kimmel, Methods Enzymol. 152, 572-581 (1987).
20. R.J. MacDonald, G.H. Swift, A.E. Przybyla, and J.M. Chirgwin, Methods Enzymol. 152, 219-227 (1987).
21. Y.-K. Paik, D.J. Chang, C.A. Reardon, D.W. Walker, E. Taxman, and J.M. Taylor, J. Biol. Chem. 263, 13340-13349 (1988).
22. C.A. Reardon, Y.F. Lau, Y.-K. Paik, K.H. Weisgraber, R.W. Mahley, and J.M. Taylor, J. Biol. Chem. 261, 9858-9864 (1986).
23. Y.F. Lau and Y.W. Kan, Proc. Natl. Acad. Sci. USA 80, 5225-5229 (1983).
24. M. Gilman, Current Protocols in Molecular Biology, F.M. Ausubel, ed. (Wiley & Sons, New York 1987).
25. N.A. Elshourbagy, D.W. Walker, M.S. Boguski, J.L. Gordon, and J.M. Taylor, J. Biol. Chem. 261, 1998-2002 (1986).
26. A. Walsh, Y. Ito, and J.L. Breslow, J. Biol. Chem. 264, 6488-6494 (1989).
27. R.C. Ogden and D.A. Adams, Methods Enzymol. 152, 61-87 (1987).
28. K.H. Weisgraber, S.C. Rall, Jr., R.W. Mahley, R.W. Milne, Y.L. Marcel, and J.T. Sparrow, J. Biol. Chem. 261, 2068-2076 (1986).
29. P.J. Gebicke-Haerter and E.M. Shooter, J. Neurochem. 53, 912-916 (1989).

Expression of Transfected Apolipoprotein E by Human Squamous Carcinoma Cells

Elizabeth S. Fenjves, Chana Fuchs, Jonathan A. Garlick, David L. Williams, and Lorne B. Taichman

School of Dental Medicine and School of Medicine, State University of New York at Stony Brook, Stony Brook, New York

ABSTRACT

A recombinant cDNA clone for human apolipoprotein E was used to transfect cultured squamous carcinoma cells. The transfected cells secrete apolipoprotein E into the culture media. When injected intradermally into athymic mice these cells form tumors, and human apolipoprotein E is detected in the serum of tumor-bearing mice. The cell line has been maintained for more than three years with no apparent change in its secretory capacity for apolipoprotein E. Transfected cells of epidermal origin may be useful for studying the expression and secretion of foreign genes.

Apolipoprotein E (apo E) plays an important role in cholesterol and triglyceride metabolism. Familial Hypercholesterolemia type III is a serious disorder of lipid metabolism associated with apo E2, an isotype not recognized by the hepatic receptors (Goldstein and Brown, 1983). There is evidence that amelioration of clinical signs may be obtained by replacing the abnormal apo E2 with the normal apo E3 isotype (Hui et al. 1984). Our lab is particularly interested in examining the potential of epidermally-derived cells for the secretion of transfected proteins (Fenjves et al. 1990). The question addressed in this study was whether transfer of apolipoprotein E3 gene into epidermally-derived cells would result in secretion of the encoded protein.

The introduction and expression of defined genes into somatic cells for the purpose of providing a needed gene product is currently being explored for gene replacement therapy. Most current research in this field has been focused on the use of marrow stem cells as a therapeutic vehicle. Another tissue being considered as a vehicle for gene therapy is the epidermis. Epidermis is composed primarily of a single cell type, the keratinocyte. Keratinocytes are easily obtained by biopsy and can be maintained in culture in semi-defined media (Rheinwald and Green, 1975). Their culture lifetime has been variably reported as between 50 to 150 doublings and addition of growth factors to the medium considerably extends

Published 1990 by Elsevier Science Publishing Co., Inc.
Molecular Biology of Atherosclerosis
A.D. Attie, Editor

this number (Rheinwald, 1975). In serum-containing medium, cultured keratinocytes form a partially keratinized epithelium (Holbrook and Hennings, 1983) consisting of replicating basal cells. In addition cultures of autologous epidermal keratinocytes have formed stable long term grafts with the re-expression of a fully keratinizing phenotype and differentiating suprabasal cells (Gallico et al. 1984). The aim of epithelial gene therapy is to provide a protein systemically by the application of genetically transformed keratinocyte grafts.

For the past several years we have been engaged in two projects related to epithelial gene therapy. The first addresses the question of synthesis, secretion, and fate of an epidermal protein, while the second deals with the expression of a foreign gene by keratinocytes. To determine if an epidermally secreted protein is absorbed by the circulation we have been studying apo E. Apo E is present on low density lipoproteins, high density lipoproteins and on chylomicrons. Unlike other apolipoproteins, apo E is produced in a variety of extrahepatic tissues in which it is thought to target lipoproteins for delivery to the liver or to redistribute cholesterol among peripheral tissues (Mahley and Innerarity, 1983). Apo E is also synthesized by normal epidermal keratinocytes in culture and secreted into the media with the correct post-translational modifications (Gordon et al. 1989). When cultured epidermal keratinocytes are grafted onto athymic mice, human apo E is detected in the sera of graft-bearing mice within four days of the procedure and for as long as the graft is present (Fenjves et al. 1989). Furthermore, when split-thickness skin is grafted onto athymic rats, serum apo E is detected in the vein draining the graft. These results show that apo E produced by keratinocytes in epidermis has a systemic distribution and suggest that other proteins produced and secreted by keratinocytes might have a similar fate.

To determine if a protein transfected into epidermally-derived cells would also reach the systemic circulation the CDNA for human apo E was cloned into a neomycin-containing retrovector pLJ (Cone and Muligan, 1984) to form pLJ-Apo. PLJ-Apo was then transfected into SCC9 cells (Rheinwald and Beckett, 1981), a line of keratinocytes derived from an oral squamous cell carcinoma. SCC9 cells share many features with epidermal cells from which they are derived. SCC9 cells contain mRNA for apo E (data not shown), but do not secrete detectable levels of the protein into the medium as shown both by immunoprecipitation (Fig. 1) and by an enzyme linked immunosorbent assay of the culture media (Table 1). In culture, SCC9 cells are phenotypically similar to keratinocytes but are blocked in their ability to undergo differentiation.

SCC9 cells transfected with the plasmid pLJ-Apo were selected by their ability to grow in the presence of the aminoglycoside G418, and then screened for apo E secretion. One clone, SCC9-3, was found to secrete 1.7 ng/h/10^6 cells whereas SCC9 wild type cells secreted no detectable apoE (Table I).

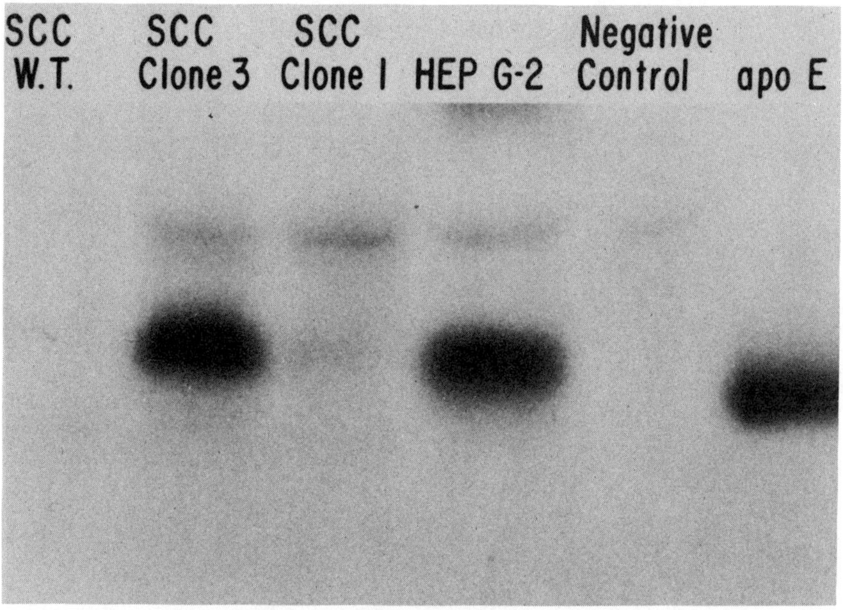

FIG. 1. Immunoprecipitation of human apo E secreted by transfected SCC9 cells. Aliquots of media from cells cultured for 4h in ^{35}S-methionine were immunoprecipitated with excess rabbit anti-human apoE as the primary antibody by the previously described procedure (Blue et al, 1983), and run on a 10% SDS- PAGE as described by Laemmli (1970). In this and all other figures SCC w.t. refers to the parental SCC9 cells, SCC 9-3 is the transfected SCC9 clone described in the text, SCC 9-1 is a transfected SCC9 clone that does not secrete apoE, HepG-2 is a hepatoma cell line which secretes apoE. Lane 5 is a negative control sample immunoprecipitated with pre-immune rabbit serum and Lane 6 is ^{14}C-labelled apoE.

TABLE I: Rate of Secretion of Apo E as Determined by Enzyme Linked Immunosorbent Assay (ELISA).

	CULTURE		ANIMALS
Cell Type	Conc.media ng/ml	Rate ng/hr/10^6 cells	Conc. serum ng/ml
SCC(wt)	0.07	undetectable	undetectable
SCC9-3	5.44	1.7	1.29
medium	0.044	undetectable	not done

Secretion of apo E in culture was measured by incubating cells in serum-free media for 12h and carrying out ELISAs as previously described (Gordon et al. 1989). Data is normalized for cell number. In nude mice, two to four weeks following intradermal injection of 10^6 cells, levels of apo E were measured in the sera of tumor-bearing animals.

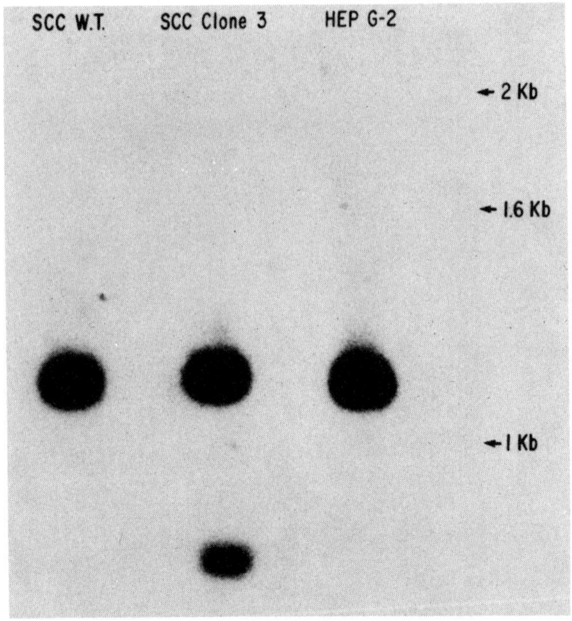

FIG. 2. Autoradiograph of a Southern blot prepared from 60 ug. of high molecular weight DNA from the various cell lines. DNA was cleaved with HinfI, BglII, subjected to electrophoresis on a 1% agarose gel, transferred to nitrocellulose and hybridized with ^{32}P-labelled pLJ-apo. An endogenous apo E band is seen in all 3 cell lines whereas integration of pLJ-Apo is evident only in the SCC9-3 line. Molecular weights are indicated.

To confirm that the SCC9-3 cell line had the apo E gene integrated, DNA was extracted and assayed for the presence of apo E cDNA band by Southern analysis (Fig.2). All cells showed the endogenous apo E DNA band, but only the SCC9-3 clone showed the integrated cloned cDNA band. From the intensity of the band we conclude that a single copy of PLJ Apo integrated per cell. When 10^6 SCC9-3 cells were injected intradermally into athymic mice, tumors were evident at the injection site within 10 days. Upon gross inspection the tumors measured 1cm x 0.4cm. The tumor mass was composed of cysts lined by a well differentiated stratified squamous epithelium and surrounded by a connective tissue pseudocapsule. When examined with immunofluorescence using a polyclonal antibody to human apo E, cells derived from the SCC9-3 tumor were clearly shown to contain human apo E (Fig. 3). As a control, tumors were formed in mice with the parental SCC9 cells as well as with SCC9 cells transfected with the pLJ vector alone. Upon histological examination, these did not show any positive immunofluorescent reaction to the polyclonal apoE antibody.

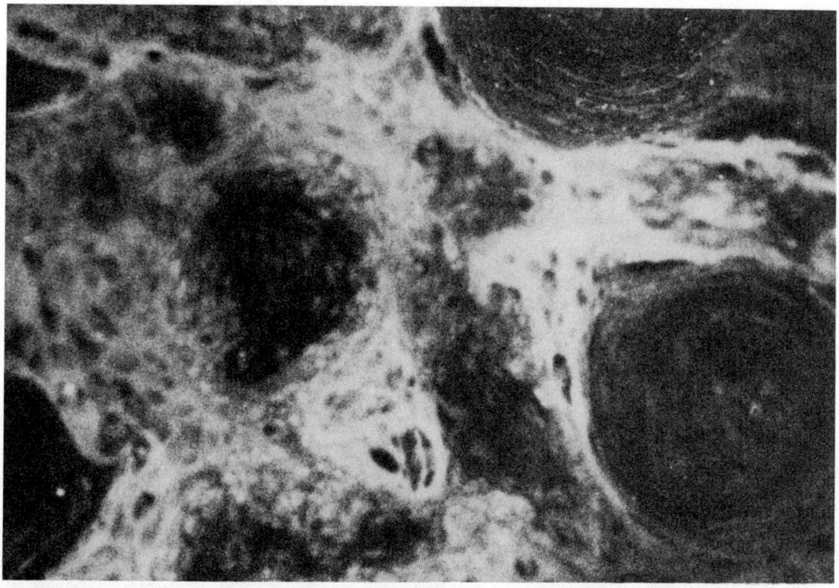

Fig. 3. Immunofluorescent microscopy of a cross section of the SCC9-3 tumor after incubation with rabbit anti-human apo E. Positive staining is seen in the dysplastic spinous cells (x75).

Sera from tumor-bearing mice were tested for the presence of human apo E using an ELISA assay. Apo E was detected in the sera of two mice bearing the SCC9-3 tumors but was undetectable in the sera of two mice bearing tumors derived from the nontransfected parental SCC9 cells (Table I). These results show that apo E produced by a gene introduced into SCC9 cells can be synthesized and secreted by the cells and subsequently detected in the serum of tumor bearing mice.

Numerous questions in addition to those related to synthetic and secretory capacity of epidermally-derived cells remain to be answered. For example, will an epidermis comprised of cells genetically engineered to produce a foreign protein continue to provide barrier and other functions? What is the behavior of genetically transformed cells in epidermis and are they stable or replaced?

We have demonstrated that a recombinant cloned apo E can be transfected into epidermally-derived cells and that the expressed protein has a systemic fate. This should prove to be an important step towards making epidermal gene therapy a possibility. The ability to induce synthesis and secretion of apo E might also be helpful in studying its role in epidermal cells.

ACKNOWLEDGEMENTS

These studies were funded by grants from the National Institutes of Health (DE 04511, HL 32868, DK 18171, DC 00203, HL 07891).

REFERENCES

Blue, M-L, Williams, D. L. Zucker, S. Ali Khan, S. and Blum, C. B. Apolipoprotein E synthesis in human kidney, adrenal gland, and liver. Proc. Natl. Acad. Sci. USA 80:283 (1983).

Cone, R.D. and Mulligan, R.C. High-efficiency gene transfer into mammalian cells: Generation of helper-free recombinant retrovirus with broad mammalian host range,Proc. Natl. Acad. Sci. USA 81:6349 (1984).

Fenjves, E. S., Gordon, D. A., Pershing, L. K., Williams, D. L. and Taichman, L. B. Systemic distribution of apolipoprotein E secreted by grafts of epidermal keratinocytes: Implication for epidermal function and gene therapy, Proc. Natl. Acad. Sci. USA 86:8803 (1989).

Fenjves, E.S., Lee, J.I., Garlick, J.A., Gordon, D.A., Williams, D.L. and Taichman, L.B. Prospects for epithelial gene therapy. Brookhaven Symposia in Biology 36, DNA damage and repair in human tissues, in press (1990).

Gallico, G., O'Connor N., Compton, C., Kehinde, I. and Green, H. Permanent coverage of large burn wounds with autologous cultured human epithelium. N. Engl. J. Med. 311:448 (1984).

Goldstein, J.L. and Brown. in: The Metabolic Basis of Inherited Disease (McGraw -Hill, New York) 5th. ed.,672 (1983)

Gordon, D. A., Fenjves, E. S., Williams, D. L., and Taichman, L. B. Synthesis and secretion of apolipoprotein E by cultured human keratinocytes. J. Invest. Dermatol. 92:96 (1989).

Holbrook, K. and Hennings, H. Phenotypic expression of epidermal cells in vitro: A review, J. Invest. Dermatol. 81:11s (1983).

Hui, D.Y., Innerarity, T.L. and Mahley, R.W. Defective hepatic lipoprotein receptor binding of beta-VLDL from type III Hyperlipoproteinemic patients, J.Biol.Chem. 258:860 (1983).

Laemmli, U. K. Cleavage of structural proteins during the assembly of the head of bacteriophage T4, Nature, 227:680 (1970).

Mahley, R. W. and Innerarity, T. L. Apolipoproteins: Structure and function. Biochim. Biophys. Acta. 737:197, (1983).

Rheinwald, J. G. Serial cultivation of normal human epidermal keratinocytes, Methods Cell Biol. 21A:229 (1975).

Rheinwald, J. G. and Beckett, M. Tumorigenic keratinocytes lines requiring anchorage and fibroblast support cultured from human squamous cell carcinomas. Cancer Res. 41:1657, (1981).

Rheinwald, J. G. and Green, H. Serial cultivation of strains of human epidermal keratinocytes: the formation of keratinizing colonies from single cells. Cell. 6:317 (1975).

Heterologous Expression of Apolipoproteins

Stephen L. Sturley,* D. G. Gretch,* M.R. Culbertson,†**
P. D. Friesen,*† N. E. Beckage,††1 and A. D. Attie*

Departments of Biochemistry, Molecular Biology,† Genetics,** and Entomology,†† University of Wisconsin-Madison, Madison, Wisconsin*

ABSTRACT.

Two expression systems are described that have the potential to facilitate the molecular analysis of the structure and function of apolipoprotein B (apo-B). *Saccharomyces cerevisiae* (yeast) has a genetically defined, vesicular secretion pathway and thus is an ideal host in which to study apolipoprotein function. The *Autographa californica/Spodoptera frugiperda* (baculovirus) system has the major advantage that large quantities of the protein of interest can be produced in a potentially active form, both in cell culture and live infected insect larvae. Human apolipoprotein E (apo-E) was initially expressed in both systems. Although apo-E was synthesised and glycosylated in yeast, it was secreted only when the host strain possessed a mutation conferring sterol uptake. Conversely, the baculovirus system secreted approximately 50 μg/ml of apo-E in a lipid-associated form. In addition, larvae of the tobacco hornworm (*Manduca sexta*) were infected with the baculovirus-apo-E expressing virus. Immunoreactive proteins of the predicted molecular weight were detected in the insect hemolymph. Yeast was used to express the putative receptor binding domains of porcine apo-B. These polypeptides were glycosylated to the predicted extent and secreted by all yeast strains under study.

INTRODUCTION.

Apolipoprotein E is an important component of several classes of mammalian plasma lipoproteins. It plays an integral role in lipoprotein catabolism via specific, high affinity interaction with cell surface receptors in hepatic and extrahepatic tissues [1]. Similarly, in its full length form, apolipoprotein B (apo-B100) mediates the specific catabolism of LDL via high affinity binding to the LDL receptor. The binding of both lipoproteins is thought to at least partially result from the electrostatic interaction of clustered basic residues on the ligand with acidic residues on the receptor. Apo-B100 or its intestinal truncated form (apo-B48) are essential components of very low density lipoprotein (VLDL) and low density lipoprotein (LDL) or chylomicrons, respectively [2]. They are required for the structural integrity and secretion of these particles from the liver or intestine.

Genetic variation in these lipoproteins is correlated with several defects in lipoprotein metabolism. Polymorphisms in apo-E have been strongly implicated as causative for some of these disorders by heterologous expression in *Escherichia coli* [3]. Several isoforms of apo-B have been identified and elucidated at the molecular level (Table 1). However, despite the well-characterised molecular nature of these alleles, the precise mechanism leading to the observed phenotype is either unknown or only inferred in the absence of an expression system for apo-B. For example, mutations that produce truncated forms of apo-B smaller than apo-B-48, result in an overall deficiency in apo-B containing lipoproteins (hypobetalipoproteinemia). Whether this results from a decrease in the synthesis or secretion of these forms of apo-B or from a different mechanism is unknown. Isoforms of apo-B that lack the C-terminal 11% and 20% of normal

[1] Current address: Department of Entomology, University of California, Riverside, CA 92521-0314.

© 1990 by Elsevier Science Publishing Co., Inc.
Molecular Biology of Atherosclerosis
A.D. Attie, Editor

apo-B (B-89 and B-80 respectively) also result in hypobetalipoproteinemia due to an increase in the affinity of these particles for the LDL receptor, resulting in LDL hypercatabolism. In contrast, hyperbetalipoproteinemia, a surfeit of apo-B containing lipoproteins, has been identified in two instances to result from defective catabolism and/or increased production of apo-B containing lipoproteins. In the only case of familial defective apolipoprotein B-100, a change of arginine to glutamine at residue 3500 of human apo-B produces an LDL particle that is virtually devoid of receptor binding activity [4]. In the porcine system, immunogenetically defined alleles of apo-B have been correlated with premature atherosclerosis, hypercholesterolemia and overproduction of an LDL particle with a 6-fold reduction in binding affinity for the LDL receptor [5]. In each of these cases the presumed receptor binding sites of apo-B were virtually indistinguishable from control alleles based on DNA sequence analysis.

TABLE I. Molecular defects in human apolipoprotein B mutant alleles. Amino acids are denoted by the single letter code. Sizes of the apo-B allelic products are indicated on a percentile scale (B-100 is therefore full length apo-B).

Syndrome	Protein Product	Mutation	Ref.
Hypobeta (Human)			
⇓synthesis			
	B-29	R1306 ⇒ STOP	[6]
	B-31	G1424 ⇒ VK-STOP	[7]
	B-37	N1728 ⇒ V-STOP	[8]
	B-39	H1795 ⇒ MWLVLT-STOP	[6]
	B-40	V1829 ⇒ C-STOP	[9]
	B-46	R2058 ⇒ STOP	[10]
	B-50	Q2252 ⇒ STOP	[11]
⇑catabolism			
	B-80	?	[12]
	B-89	E4043 ⇒ RQLLAC-STOP	[9]
	B-100	R4019 ⇒ W	[13]
Hyperbeta			
Human	B-100	R3500 ⇒ Q	[4]
Porcine (*lpb5.1*)	B-100	?	[5]

Human apo-E and apolipoprotein A1 have been stably expressed in mouse L and Chinese hamster ovary cells, respectively [14, 15, 16]. In each case the lipoprotein was secreted at low levels in a lipid-associated form and appeared to retain a degree of biological activity. Apo-E expression in *E. coli* was found to be toxic resulting in cell lysis and proteolysis of apo-E [17]. Despite this, apo-E was purified from total soluble bacterial cell proteins and was shown to be active in terms of its affinity for lipid and the LDL receptor. Recently, human apo-B has been expressed at low levels in a rat hepatoma cell line in a lipid-associated form resembling LDL [18]. Described here is the development of two alternate heterologous expression systems for apolipoproteins, yeast and insect baculovirus.

EXPRESSION OF APOLIPOPROTEINS USING THE BACULOVIRUS SYSTEM.

Numerous genes from various organisms have been expressed in insect cells infected with baculovirus expression vectors [19]. A major advantage of this invertebrate system over the majority of other hosts is the high level expression of recombinant proteins that is readily attained. Yields as high as 500 mg/liter of recombinant protein representing 50% of the total cell protein have been reported [20]. Unlike in bacteria, protein secretion by this host is mediated via a conventional vesicular process whereby many of the secondary modifications exhibited by mammalian proteins are performed. Furthermore, the production of lipoproteins by these hosts has been well characterised, particularly for the case of hemolymph lipoproteins from the larval form of the tobacco horn worm (*M. sexta* [21]). We have therefore utilised both insect tissue culture and larvae infected with a recombinant baculovirus containing the human apo-E cDNA to test the efficacy of this system for expression of human lipoproteins.

<u>Expression of Human Apo-E in Insect Tissue Culture.</u>

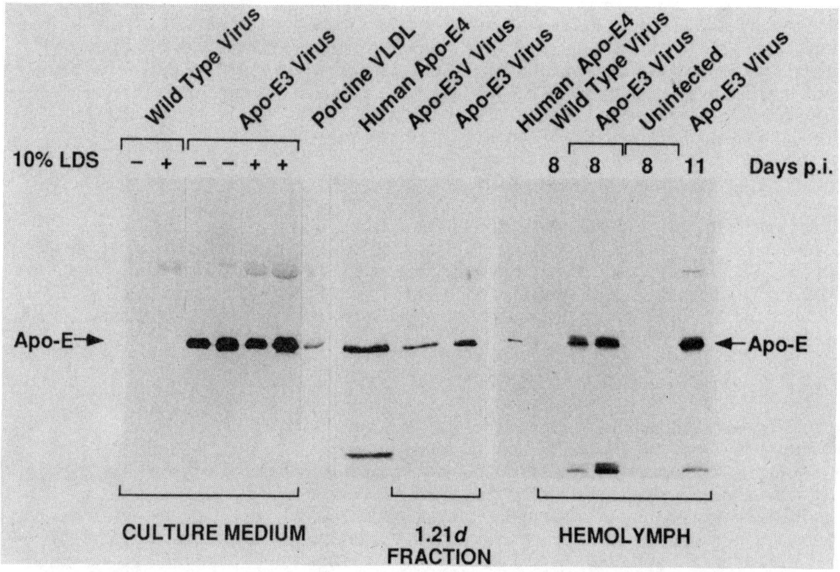

FIG. 1. Human apo-E expression in insect cells and larvae. Approximately 1 µl of tissue culture supernatant was resolved by SDS-PAGE and immunoblotting with 2 monoclonal antibodies to human apo-E. 12 mls of culture supernatants were subjected to density centrifugation for 48 hours. 5 µl of the top 1 ml fraction was then analysed by immunoblotting (1.21 *d* fraction). 1 µl of hemolymph from *M. sexta* larvae infected with recombinant and control viruses was also analysed by immunoblotting at various times after infection. Apo-E3V virus contains a cDNA to a variant of apo-E3 that is 77% defective in binding to the LDL receptor [3]. Human apo-E4 and porcine VLDL serve as molecular weight standards.

The human apo-E cDNA (a kind gift of John Taylor [22]) was fused to the powerful polyhedrin gene promoter in the baculovirus transfer vector pAcYM1 [23] at the unique *Bam*HI site by conventional methods. The resulting chimera was co-transfected with wild-type baculovirus into *S. frugiperda Sf*21 cells. Recombinant apo-E viral plaques were identified and plaque purified 3 times and used to infect Sf21 cells at a high multiplicity of infection [24]. Culture supernatants were collected at various times post-infection and analysed for the presence of apo-E by SDS polyacrylamide gel electrophoresis and 'western' immunoblotting with a pair of monoclonal antibodies (m1E and m13E, a kind gift from Linda Curtiss) to human apo-E.

As shown in Figure 1, a protein of approximately 34 kDa was uniquely present in culture supernatants from cells transfected with the recombinant baculovirus containing the apo-E gene. The presence of 10% lipoprotein deficient serum had no detectable effect on expression levels. By comparison to a standard of purified human apo-E4, it appeared that approximately 50 µg of apo-E was found per ml of culture supernatant per 10^6 cells. When culture supernatants expressing apo-E were spun to equilibrium at a density of 1.21 gm/l of sodium bromide, a protein of similar size and immunoreactivity to apo-E was found to concentrate in the top 1 ml fraction, indicating an association of apo-E with lipid under these culture conditions.

Expression of Human Apo-E in Insect Larvae.

Fourth instar larvae of *M. sexta* were injected with approximately 10^6 plaque forming units of the recombinant apo-E and control baculovirus derived from the infected tissue culture system described above. Hemolymph was collected from fifth instar infected larvae and analysed by SDS PAGE and immunoblotting. As shown in Figure 1, immunoreactive polypeptides of the correct molecular weight were only detected in the hemolymph of larvae infected with the apo-E recombinant virus. These proteins were detected at day 8 post-infection and increased in abundance at day 11. The heterogeneity in the immunoreactive polypeptides may represent differential glycosylation. Lower molecular weight species were presumably proteolytic breakdown products of apo-E.

Future Prospects.

As shown here, cultured insect cells and larvae infected with baculovirus carrying a cDNA to human apo-E readily express and secrete high levels of apo-E in a lipid-associated form. We are currently analysing the particles produced with respect to their lipid composition and LDL receptor binding ability. This system should provide a rapid source of high levels of apo-E. Furthermore, the baculovirus system offers the greatest potential for expressing human apolipoprotein B as a lipoprotein particle

EXPRESSION OF APOLIPOPROTEINS BY YEAST.

The advanced nature of yeast genetics and molecular biology [25], coupled with the ease of inexpensive scale-up production, make *S. cerevisiae* particularly attractive for the heterologous expression of mammalian proteins. In contrast to bacterial expression systems, yeast possesses a vesicular secretion pathway and performs many of the secondary modifications found in proteins from higher eukaryotes [26]. Although the major yeast sterol is ergosterol and not cholesterol, lipid metabolism in yeast is otherwise very similar to higher cells and is exceptionally well-defined genetically [27]. Furthermore, the sterol status of the yeast cell can be modulated by anaerobic growth or the utilization of cholesterol uptake mutants. We have therefore taken the approach of expressing human apo-E and domains of porcine apo-B in several genetic backgrounds. Yeast strains defective in the *PEP4* gene product lack active vacuolar hydrolases and therefore produce higher levels of more stable proteins [28]. A host lacking a wild-type *UPC2* gene displays the phenotype of a 30-fold increase in the uptake of sterol under aerobic growth conditions [29]. This strain was originally identified and kindly provided by Leo Parks. A repressible promoter from the structural gene for acid phosphatase (*PHO5*) was used in all cases to provide regulated high level expression [30].

Expression of Human Apo-E in *S. cerevisiae*.

The human apo-E cDNA gene was fused to the *PHO5* promoter at the unique *Eco*RI site of plasmid p1A1R1-15 and used to transform wild-type, *pep4* and *upc2* mutant host strains. Intracellular and concentrated secreted proteins from repressed (high phosphate growth conditions) and derepressed (low phosphate) transformants were analysed by SDS-PAGE and immunoblotting using monoclonal antibodies m1E and m13E. Immunoreactive proteins of 34 and 36 kDa were uniquely detected in intracellular preparations from derepressed *pep4* (Figure 2) and *upc2* (not shown) cultures. Since the predicted molecular weight of apo-E is approximately 34 kDa, the higher molecular weight form may result from increased glycosylation. Protein preparations from wild-type cultures showed considerable degradation compared to the *pep4* preparations. Surprisingly, wild-type and *pep4* yeast strains did not secrete detectable levels of apo-E, even when grown anaerobically in the presence of sterol. *upc2* mutants, by contrast, secreted relatively high levels of apo-E. This secretion was blocked by the inclusion of sterol (cholesterol and ergosterol) and fatty acid (oleic and palmitoleic acid) in the growth medium (Figure 2).

Further experiments indicated that in a *upc2* mutant strain, cholesterol uptake induces the secretion of apo-E, whereas oleic acid blocks the appearance of apo-E in the culture medium. This has led to the proposition that apo-E is directed to peroxisomes which proliferate in oleic acid grown yeast cells. We are currently testing this hypothesis.

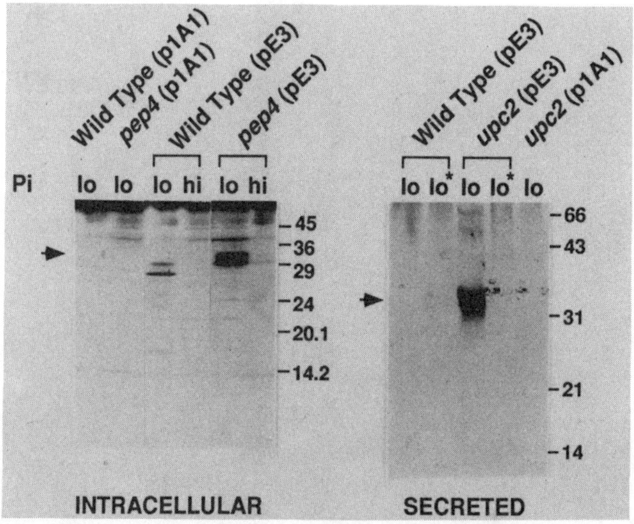

FIG.2. Apo-E expression in yeast. Harvested cells from repressed and derepressed cultures of the indicated strains were fractured with glass beads and solubilised with 0.1% Triton X100 (T-X100) [30]. Secreted proteins were concentrated by stirred cell ultrafiltration using Amicon PM10 membranes (molecular weight cut-off, 10 kDa). Proteins were analysed by SDS-PAGE and immunoblotting as described in Figure 1. Host strains (*pep4*, *upc2* and wild-type) are described in the text. p1A1 is a control plasmid lacking an apo-E insert. Molecular weight standards are as indicated. The inclusion of sterol and fatty acid in the growth medium is indicated by an asterisk (*).

Expression of Domains of Porcine Apo-B by *S. cerevisiae.*

Apolipoprotein E has been successfully expressed in mammalian tissue culture, bacteria, and now yeast and insect cells. However apo-B is probably more difficult to express due to its insolubility in an aqueous environment and its large size [31]. Bacterial expression systems may be unsuitable due to the apparent toxicity of certain domains of apo-B as was found for apo-E [17]. To investigate the potential of yeast as an expression system for porcine apo-B, we initially expressed and secreted domains implicated in receptor binding.

Human apo-B is a 4536 amino acid protein with a calculated molecular weight of 513 kDa [32]. There are 12 regions enriched in basic residues which fit a consensus sequence for receptor binding [33]. However, two pronounced clusters of basic amino acids (residues 3134-3157 and 3359-3367) are located in an 800 amino acid domain intimately associated with the LDL receptor during LDL binding (see Figure 3; [34]). In addition, the epitopes for monoclonal antibodies that inhibit binding of apo-B to the LDL receptor are located in this region [35]. One of these regions (residues 3359-3367) displays strong identity [36] in porcine and human apo-B to residues 142-150 of human apo-E, shown by mutagenic analysis to be essential for receptor binding. An additional region conserved between pig and human apo-B defines the epitope for the monoclonal antibody, MB47 (encompassing residue 3500). This domain has been implicated in receptor binding due to the identification of a familial defective human apo-B100 mutant with a single amino acid change in this region. MB47 also inhibits binding of apo-B to the LDL receptor. We describe here the use of *S. cerevisiae* to express the basic domains of porcine apo-B as a first step in defining the contribution of these regions to receptor binding.

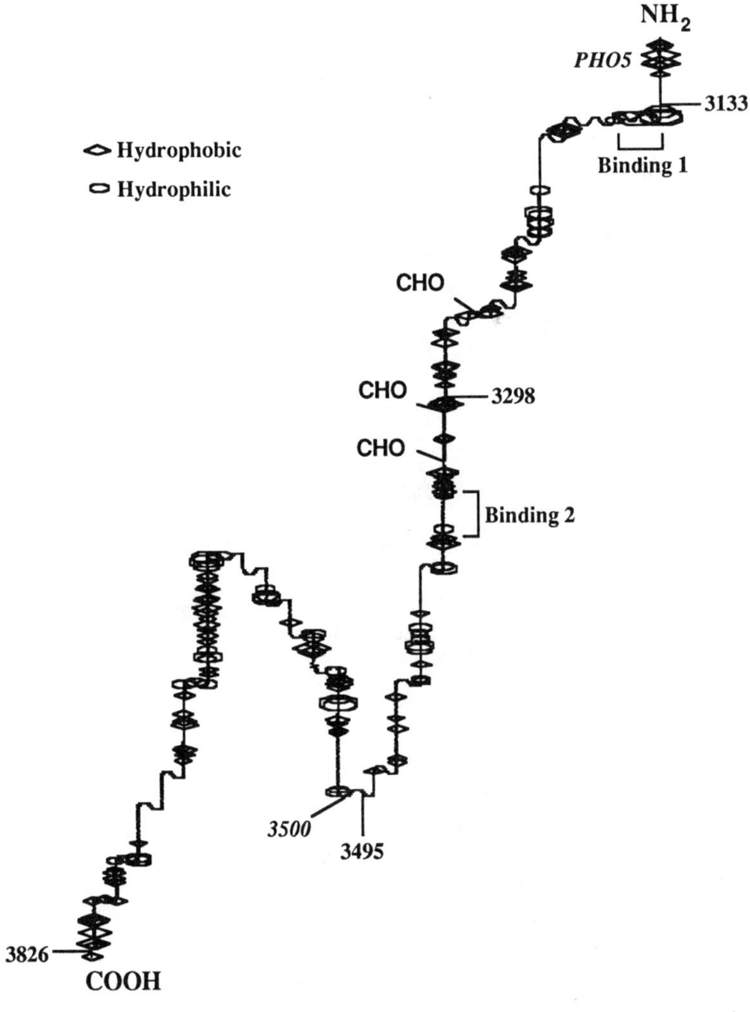

FIG. 3. The region of porcine apo-B expressed in yeast. A secondary structure prediction [37] for porcine apo-B between residues 3133 and 3826 [38] using a Genetics Computer Group (UW-Madison) algorithm. Indicated are regions of strong hydrophobicity and hydrophilicity [39] as well as the putative receptor binding sites of apo-B. *PHO5* indicates the presence of the *PHO5* signal peptide and *3500* is the position of a mutation in human apo-B associated with defective receptor binding. CHO indicates the predicted position of N-linked glycosylation.

The region of porcine apo-B expressed in these studies is shown in Figure 3. In all cases, the regions of interest were fused to the *PHO5* promoter and signal peptide to facilitate entry into the secretion pathway [40]. On the assumption that the region of apo-B most strongly conserved with apo-E (Binding 2) would be particularly relevant with respect to binding activity, we chose to express this domain in isolation (B_{72-77}, residues 3298-3495). It was then expressed in conjunction with the contiguous N-terminal basic region (Binding 1, B_{69-77}, residues 3133-3495) and separately with sequences surrounding Arg_{3500} (B_{72-84}, residues 3298-3826).

As shown in Figure 4, several protein species were produced by these constructs under derepressing growth conditions. Expression of the B_{72-77} domain of apo-B encompassing Binding site 2 would be predicted to produce a 24 kDa primary translation product. The presence of two predicted sites for N-linked glycosylation would produce a polypeptide of approximately 30 kDa. In intracellular, T-X100 soluble protein preparations from transformants of derepressed *pep4* mutant strains, unique polypeptides of these magnitudes were produced. As expected, they were considerably less stable in a wild-type host strain. Unlike the situation with apo-E expression in yeast, both forms of this protein were secreted by all host strains tested (not shown).

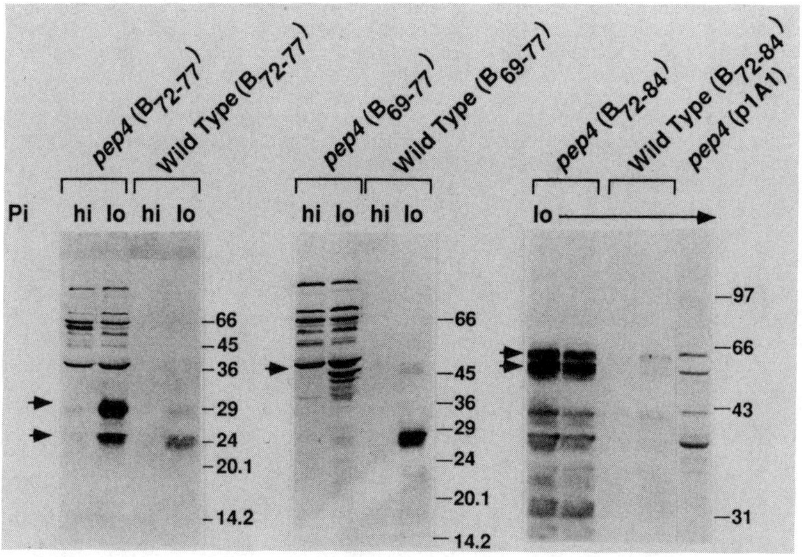

FIG. 4. Expression of porcine apo-B in yeast. T-X100 (B_{72-77}) and urea (B_{69-77} and B_{72-84}) soluble intracellular proteins from repressed (hi) and derepressed (lo) transformants were resolved by SDS-PAGE. Immunoreactive polypeptides were observed by immunoblotting with a polyclonal antibody to porcine LDL. Host strains (*pep4* and wild-type) are described in the text. p1A1 is a control plasmid lacking apo-B sequences. Molecular weight standards are as indicated.

Expression of porcine apo-B_{69-77} encompassing both putative binding sites (3133-3495) would be predicted to produce a polypeptide of approximately 42 kDa. The presence of 3 sites for N-linked glycosylation would increase the size of this region to about 49 kDa. As shown in Figure 4, proteins of this molecular weight were detected in a urea and T-X100 soluble intracellular fraction. The additional protein species presumably resulted from pauses in glycosylation or from proteolytic degradation. As was found for the $B_{72\text{-}77}$ region, this domain was considerably less stable in wild-type strains. The larger molecular weight forms (i.e. fully glycosylated) of this polypeptide were also secreted into the culture supernatant by wild-type and *pep4* hosts (not shown).

The expression of the putative receptor binding domains of apo-B in yeast was further extended to include sequences surrounding residue 3500. The region denoted $B_{72\text{-}84}$ in Figure 4 consists of Binding site 2 combined with residues through Arg_{3500} to amino-acid 3824. This domain has a predicted molecular weight of approximately 59 kDa and contains two sites for N-linked glycosylation. As shown, proteins of approximately 64 kDa were detected in urea and T-X100 soluble intracellular protein fraction. These polypeptides were most prevalent in derepressed preparations from *pep4* strains. As before, the lower molecular weight forms may represent non-glycosylated forms of this polypeptide. The higher molecular weight forms were also secreted by the strains studied here (not shown). Unlike the other peptides expressed in yeast (i.e.apo-$B_{72\text{-}77}$ and apo-$B_{69\text{-}77}$), this region of apo-B also cross-reacted with the monoclonal antibody MB47 (not shown) indicating the requirement of sequences C-terminal to residue 3495 for expression of this epitope. Since MB47 inhibits binding of LDL to the receptor, it is tempting to speculate that this region when expressed in yeast might function as a ligand for the receptor.

Future Prospects.

The failure of normal yeast strains to secrete human apolipoprotein E was a surprising result and led to the proposition of peroxisomal localisation of apo-E. If verified, this system may be particularly illuminating with regard to the mechanism and function of this intracellular targetting. Similarly the demonstration of secretion of the putative receptor binding domains of porcine apo-B by yeast has the potential to define the residues involved in binding to the receptor, and thus to elucidate the functional nature of apo-B polymorphisms in this region. In addition, expression of apo-B by yeast may ultimately provide a system in which to study the events leading to the synthesis of a lipoprotein particle.

CONCLUSIONS.

Two systems are described for the expression of apolipoproteins. Baculovirus mediated expression in insect cell culture and larvae produced high levels of recombinant human apo-E in a lipid-associated form. We are currently assessing this host for its ability to express apo-B. The use of *S. cerevisiae* as an expression system for apolipoproteins was rendered possible by the availability of a series of host mutations. This approach will both define the *cis* acting sequences required for activity of these apolipoproteins as well as indicate the requirement for host mediated factors. Considering the conservation of many biological processes between yeast and human, extrapolation from studies with this microrganism may be of relevance to lipoprotein biogenesis and function in mammals.

ACKNOWLEGEMENTS.

We are grateful for the kind provision of vectors, host strains and antibodies from Leo Parks, Beth Jones, Keith Bostian, John Taylor, Elaine Krul, Linda Curtiss and David Bishop. This work was supported by N.I.H. grant HL37251 and the Council for Tobacco research grant 2077. D.G.G. was supported by National Research Service Award 1 T32 GM08349-01 from N.I.G.M.S.

REFERENCES.

1. Mahley, R. W. Apolipoprotein E: cholesterol transport protein with expanding role in cell biology. Science. 240: 622, (1988).
2. Gibbons, G. F. Assembly and secretion of hepatic very-low-density lipoprotein. Biochem. J. 268: 1, (1990).
3. Lalazar, A., K. H. Weisgraber, S. C. Rall, H. Giladi, T. L. Innerarity, A. Z. Levanon, J. K. Boyles, B. Amit, M. Gorecki, R. W. Mahley and T. Vogel. Site-specific mutagenesis

of human apolipoprotein E: Receptor binding activity of variants with single amino acid substitutions. J. Biol. Chem. 263: 3542, (1988).

4. Innerarity, T. L., K. H. Weisgraber, K. S. Arnold, R. M. Mahley, R. M. Krauss, G. L. Vega and S. M. Grundy. Familial defective apolipoprotein B-100: Low density lipoproteins with abnormal receptor binding. Proc. Natl. Acad. Sci. USA. 84: 6919, (1987).
5. Rapacz, J., J. Hasler-Rapacz, K. M. Taylor, W. J. Checovich and A. D. Attie. Lipoprotein mutations in pigs are associated with elevated plasma cholesterol and atherosclerosis. Science. 234: 1573, (1986).
6. Collins, D. R., T. J. Knott, R. J. Pease, L. M. Powell, S. C. Wallis, S. Robertson, C. R. Pullinger, R. W. Milne, Y. L. Marcel, S. E. Humphries, P. J. Talmud, J. K. Lloyd, N. E. Miller, D. Muller and J. Scott. Truncated variants of apolipoprotein B cause hypobetalipoproteinaemia. Nucleic Acids Res. 16: 8361, (1988).
7. Young, S. G., S. T. Hubl, R. S. Smith, S. M. Snyder and J. F. Terdiman. Familial hypobetalipoproteinemia caused by a mutation in the apolipoprotein B gene that results in a truncated species of apolipoprotein B (B-31): A unique mutation that helps to define the portion of the apolipoprotein B molecule required for the formation of buoyant, triglyceride-rich lipoproteins. J Clin Invest. 85: 933, (1990).
8. Young, S. G., S. T. Northey and B. J. McCarthy. Low plasma cholesterol levels caused by a short deletion in the apolipoprotein B gene. Science. 241:591, (1988).
9. Talmud, P., U. L. King, E. Krul, G. Schonfeld and S. Humphries. The molecular basis of truncated forms of apolipoprotein B in a kindred with compound heterozygous hypobetalipoproteinemia . J Lipid Res. 30: 1773, (1989).
10. Young, S. G., S. T. Hubl, D. A. Chappell, R. S. Smith, F. Claiborne, S. M. Snyder and J. F. Terdiman. Familial hypobetalipoproteinemia associated with a mutant species of apolipoprotein B (B-46) . N Engl J Med. 320: 1604, (1989).
11. Hardman, D. A., C. R. Pullinger, J. P. Kane and M. J. Malloy. Molecular defect in normotriglyceridemic abetalipoproteinemia. Circulation, supplement II. 80: II-466, (1989).
12. Gabelli, C., G. Baggio, C. Bilato, S. Martini, L. Previato, Y. Marcel, A. Corsini and G. Crepaldi. Identification of a new apoB variant associated with hypobetalipoproteinemia. Circulation, supplement II. 80: II-276, (1989).
13. Ladias, J., P. J. Kwiterovich, H. H. Smith, M. Miller, P. S. Bachorik, T. Forte, A. J. Lusis and S. E. Antonarakis. Apolipoprotein B-100 Hopkins (arginine4019 - tryptophan). A new apolipoprotein B-100 variant in a family with premature atherosclerosis and hyperapobetalipopro einemia . Jama. 262: 1980, (1989).
14. Reardon, C. A., Y.-F. Lau, Y.-K. Paik, K. H. Weisgraber, R. W. Mahley and J. M. Taylor. Expression of the human apolipoprotein E gene in cultured mammalian cells. J. Biol. Chem. 261: 9858, (1986).
15. Ruiz-Opazo, N. and V. I. Zannis. Expression of the human apolipoprotein A-1 gene in rat myogenic L6E9 cells. J. Biol. Chem. 263: 1739, (1988).
16. Mallory, J. B., P. J. Kushner, A. A. Protter, C. L. Cofer, V. L. Appleby, K. Lau, J. W. Schilling and J.-L. Vigne. Expression and characterization of human apolipoprotein A-I in Chinese hamster ovary cells. J. Biol. Chem. 262: 4241, (1987).
17. Vogel, T., K. H. Weisgraber, M. I. Zeevi, H. Ben-Artzi, A. Z. Levanon, S. C. Rall, T. L. Innerarity, D. Y. Hui, J. M. Taylor, D. Kanner, Z. Yavin, B. Amit, H. Aviv, M. Gorecki and R. W. Mahley. Human apolipoprotein E expression in *Escherichia coli*: Structural and functional identity of the bacterially produced protein with plasma apolipoprotein E. Proc. Natl. Acad. Sci. USA. 82: 8696, (1985).
18. Blackhart, B. D., Z. Yao and B. J. McCarthy. An expression system for human apolipoprotein B100 in a rat hepatoma cell line. J. Biol. Chem. 265: 8358, (1990).
19. Luckow, V. A. and M. D. Summers. Trends in the development of Baculovirus expression vectors. Bio/technology. 6: 47, (1988).
20. Smith, G. E., G. Ju, B. L. Ericson, J. Moschera, H.-W. Lahm, R. Chizzonite and M. D. Summers. Modification and secretion of human interleukin 2 produced in insect cells by a baculovirus expression vector. Proc. Natl. Acad. Sci. USA. 82: 8404, (1985).
21. Law, J. H. and M. A. Wells. Insects as biochemical models. J. Biol. Chem. 264: 16335, (1989).

22. McLean, J. W., N. A. Elshourbagy, D. J. Chang, R. W. Mahley and J. M. Taylor. Human apolipoprotein E mRNA cDNA cloning and nucleotide sequencing of a new variant. J. Biol. Chem. 259: 6498, (1984).
23. Matsuura, Y., R. D. Possee, H. A. Overton and D. H. L. Bishop. Baculovirus expression vectors: The requirements for high level expression of proteins, including glycoproteins. J. Gen. Virol. 68: 1233, (1987).
24. Summers, M. D. and G. E. Smith. "A manual of methods for baculovirus vectors and insect cell culture procedures." 1988 Texas Agricultural Experimental Station. Texas.
25. Struhl, K. The new yeast genetics. Nature. 305: 391, (1983).
26. Nevalainen, L. T. and M. Makarow. Intracellular transport in interphase and mitotic yeast cells. Eur. J. Biochem. 178: 39, (1988).
27. Parks, L. W., C. D. Bottema, R. J. Rodriguez and T. A. Lewis. Yeast sterols: yeast mutants as tools for the study of sterol metabolism. Methods Enzymol. 111: 333, (1985).
28. Woolford, C. A., L. B. Daniels, F. J. Park, E. W. Jones, J. Van Arsdell and M. A. Innis. The *pep4* gene encodes a aspartyl protease implicated in the posttranslational regulation of *Saccharomyces cerevisiae* vacuolar hydrolases. Mol. Cell. Biol. 6: 2500, (1986).
29. Lewis, T. L., G. A. Keesler, G. P. Fenner and L. W. Parks. Pleiotropic mutations in *Saccharomyces cerevisiae* affecting sterol uptake and metabolism. Yeast. 4: 93, (1988).
30. Sturley, S. L., Q. Elliot, J. LeVitre, D. J. Tipper and K. A. Bostian. Mapping of functional domains within the *Saccharomyces cerevisiae* type 1 killer preprotoxin. EMBO J. 5: 3381, (1986).
31. Yang, C., Z.-W. Gu, S. Weng, T. W. Kim, S.-H. Chen, H. J. Pownall, P. M. Sharp, S.-W. Liu, W.-H. Li, A. M. Gotto and L. Chan. Structure of apolipoprotein B-100 of human low density lipoproteins. Arteriosclerosis. 9: 96, (1989).
32. Ludwig, E. H., B. D. Blackhart, V. R. Pierotti, L. Caiati, C. Fortier, T. Knott, J. Scott, R. W. Mahley, B. Levy-Wilson and B. J. McCarthy. DNA sequence of the Human apolipoprotein B gene. DNA. 6: 363, (1987).
33. Hospattankar, A. V., S. L. Law, K. Lackner and H. B. Brewer. Identification of low density lipoprotein receptor binding domains of human apolipoprotein B-100: A proposed consensus LDL receptor binding sequence of apo B100. Biochem. Biophys. Res. Comm. 139: 1078, (1986).
34. Milne, R., R. J. Théolis, R. Maurice, R. J. Pease, P. K. Weech, E. Rassart, J. C. Fruchart, J. Scott and Y. L. Marcel. The use of monoclonal antibodies to localize the low density lipoprotein receptor-binding domain of apolipoprotein B . J. Biol. Chem. 264: 19754, (1989).
35. Pease, R. J., M. R.W., W. K. Jessup, A. Law, P. Provost, J.-C. Fruchart, R. T. Dean, Y. L. Marcel and J. Scott. Use of Bacterial expression cloning to localize the epitopes for a series of monoclonal antibodies against apolipoprotein B100. J. Biol. Chem. 265: 553, (1990).
36. Ebert, D. L., N. Maeda, S. W. Lowe, J. Hasler-Rapacz, J. Rapacz and A. D. Attie. Primary structure comparison of the proposed low density lipoprotein (LDL) receptor binding domain of human and pig apolipoprotein B: implications for LDL receptor interactions. J. Lipid Res. 29: 1501, (1988).
37. Chou, P. Y. and G. D. Fasman. Prediction of the secondary structure of proteins from their amino acid sequence. Adv. in Enzymol. 47: 45, (1978).
38. Maeda, N., D. L. Ebert, T. M. Doers, M. Newman, J. Hasler-Rapacz, A. D. Attie, J. Rapacz and O. Smithies. Molecular genetics of the apoliprotein B gene in pigs in relation to atherosclerosis. Gene. 70: 213, (1988).
39. Kyte, J. and R. F. Doolittle. A simple method for displaying the hydropathic character of a protein. J. Mol. Biol. 157: 105, (1982).
40. Monod, M., R. Haguenauer-Tsapis, I. Rauseo-Koenig and A. Hinnen. Functional analysis of the signal -sequence processing site of yeast acid phosphatase. Eur. J. Biochem. 182: 213, (1989).

Prenyltransferases: From Yeast to Man

Matthew N. Ashby, David H. Spear, and Peter A. Edwards

Division of Cardiology, Department of Medicine, and Department of Biological Chemistry, UCLA School of Medicine, Los Angeles, California

INTRODUCTION

Isoprene biosynthesis in eukaryotes involves a complex and diverging pathway resulting in the synthesis of a variety of sterol and nonsterol products. The basic building block in isoprenoid biosynthesis is the five carbon compound isopentenyl pyrophosphate (IPP) derived from acetate. IPP participates in a series of head-to-tail (1'-4) condensation reactions with an elongating allylic prenyl pyrophosphate to form various polyprenyl pyrophosphates. These polyprenyl groups then serve as donors or intermediates in the synthesis of numerous products (see Figure 1).

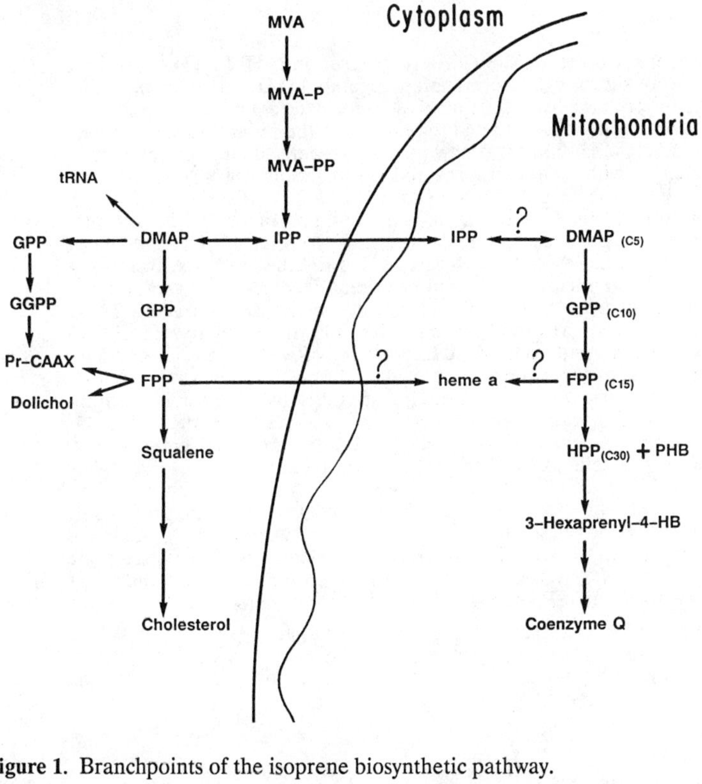

Figure 1. Branchpoints of the isoprene biosynthetic pathway.

© 1990 by Elsevier Science Publishing Co., Inc.
Molecular Biology of Atherosclerosis
A.D. Attie, Editor

Products of isoprene biosynthesis include sterols, dolichols, and the polyprenyl substituents of coenzyme Q, heme a, and certain proteins containing the carboxy-terminal sequence -CAAX (where C, cysteine; A, aliphatic; X, any amino acid). Interestingly, the branched pathways leading to the synthesis of sterols, dolichol and coenzyme Q each contain a prenyltransferase catalyzing 1'-4 condensation reactions. While heme a (Weinstein, *et al.*, 1986), ras (Hancock *et al.*, 1989; Schafer *et al.*, 1989), lamin B (Farnsworth *et al.*, 1989) and the yeast a-factor (Anderegg *et al.*, 1988) have been shown to be modified by a fifteen-carbon farnesyl group, the prenyltransferase responsible for the synthesis of this prenyl group remains obscure. Additionally, a large number of proteins have been found to be modified by a twenty-carbon geranylgeranyl group which suggests one or more additional prenyltransferase enzymes exist in mammals (Rilling *et al.*, 1990; Farnsworth *et al.*, 1990). Although a family of prenyltransferase enzymes exist, very little is known about the specific enzymes that participate in the synthesis of non-sterol isoprenoid compounds.

Farnesyl pyrophosphate synthetase (FPS) is a well studied enzyme of sterol biosynthesis which catalyzes the 1'-4 condensation of two molecules of isopentenyl pyrophosphate with dimethylallyl pyrophosphate to form the fifteen-carbon farnesyl pyrophosphate (Poulter and Rilling, 1981). The regulation of FPS and its location in the isoprene biosynthetic pathway are important since both the substrates and products of FPS participate in the various branched pathways leading to the synthesis of isoprenoid products. Thus, large perturbations in FPS activity could alter the flux of isoprenoid compounds down the various branches of the pathway.

REGULATION OF FPS

In previous studies HMG-CoA reductase and HMG-CoA synthase mRNA levels were shown to be coordinately regulated (Mehrabian *et al.*, 1986). Subsequently, differential hybridization was used in attempts to isolate other genes that were coordinately regulated together with the reductase and synthase genes. These studies identified two new genes that were induced in rat liver by diets supplemented with cholestyramine and mevinolin, and were repressed by dietary cholesterol. These genes were shown to be FPS (Clarke *et al.*, 1987; Ashby and Edwards, 1989) and the low-density-lipoprotein (LDL) receptor (Wilkin, Martin and Edwards, unpublished data). FPS, HMG-CoA reductase and HMG-CoA synthase mRNA levels and protein synthesis were also coordinately regulated in cultured human hepatoma HepG2 cells in response to the addition of 25-hydroxycholesterol and mevalonic acid (Rosser *et al.*, 1989). The protein stability of HMG-CoA reductase, but not FPS or HMG-CoA synthase, was affected by addition of LDL to the cells (*ibid*). These latter results indicated that the coordinate regulation was at the level of enzyme synthesis, possibly at the transcriptional level, but not at the level of protein stability. Other studies showed that the developmental profile of the three mRNAs in rats and humans were very similar (Levin et al., 1989) and that the three proteins were all localized to cells in the periportal region of rat liver (Li *et al.*, 1988; Singer *et al.*, 1984; Edwards and Krisans, unpublished data). The reason for the enhanced expression of the three cholesterogenic enzymes, and presumably enhanced cholesterol synthesis, in a few liver cells in the periportal region is intriguing but unknown. It will be of interest to determine whether these same cells have high rates of bile acid biosynthesis, and hence result in altered levels of reductase, synthase and FPS due to cellular cholesterol depletion.

Taken together, all these studies indicated that the mRNA levels of HMG-CoA reductase, HMG-CoA synthase and FPS were regulated by a similar mechanism(s) that might involve a common cis acting element(s) in the promoters of the three genes.

Attempts to isolate the gene for FPS were complicated by the presence of multiple genomic loci that hybridized to the rat FPS cDNA (Clarke *et al.*, 1987; Heinzmann *et al.*, 1989). Current evidence indicates that only one locus encodes a functional gene (unpublished data). This one gene appears to contain two promoters; one promoter functions only in the testis, while the other promoter is functional in all tissues (Teruya *et al.*, 1990). The functional rat FPS gene spans approximately 12 Kb and contains 8 exons (Spear *et al.*, submitted). Various FPS promoter-CAT (chloramphenicol acetyl transferase) hybrid genes have been constructed and transfected into HepG2 cells. Assay for CAT activity in the transfected cells has led to the proposal that a 320 bp FPS promoter fragment contains all the information required for regulation of CAT by added sterols. This 320 bp fragment contains two sterol-regulatory-element (SRE-1) sequences (*ibid*). Such SRE-1 sequences have been shown to be involved in the sterol-mediated regulation of HMG-CoA reductase, HMG-CoA synthase and the LDL receptor (Goldstein and Brown, 1990).

Taken together, these studies demonstrate that four genes involved in cellular cholesterol homeostasis, namely HMG-CoA synthase, HMG-CoA reductase, FPS and the LDL receptor, are coordinately regulated by cellular sterols and/or derivatives of mevalonic acid as a result of one or more *cis*-acting SRE-1 sequences in the promoter of these genes.

The next important steps are to determine which proteins are involved in the regulation of transcription, to determine the mechanism by which such proteins exert their effect and to determine the nature of the physiological sterol or nonsterol derivative of mevalonic acid that is involved in these regulatory events.

HOMOLOGY OF FPS WITH OTHER PRENYL SYNTHETASES: IMPLIED LINEAGE

As mentioned above a family of prenyltransferase, or more specifically, prenyl synthetase enzymes, exist, each catalyzing the same 1'-4 condensation reaction for the synthesis of a variety of sterol and nonsterol products.

We were interested in isolating a second prenyl synthetase for the purpose of identifying a conserved active site sequence(s) which would be critical to the 1'-4 condensation reaction and thus, common in all prenyl synthetase enzymes. Northern blot experiments of human RNA probed with the rat liver FPS cDNA as well as preliminary sequence comparisons with the human FPS cDNA indicated that FPS was highly conserved throughout the sequence between species. Therefore, inter-species FPS sequence differences were not great enough to identify highly conserved (enzymatically involved) regions in which we were interested. Cross-hybridization experiments to look for related prenyl synthetase sequences both on Northern and Western blots indicated that apparently these other enzymes did not share enough sequence identity to detect, and therefore isolate, by hybridization techniques. While the divergence (or lack of convergence) of other prenyl synthetase enzymes with FPS was too great to facilitate their isolation by methods based on sequence similarities, we thought that once isolated, comparative analyses of FPS with another prenyl synthetase would reveal critical domains if they did in fact exist.

In coenzyme Q biosynthesis isopentenyl pyrophosphate (IPP) is transported into the mitochondria where it serves as a substrate for a membrane-associated polyprenyl synthetase enzyme (see Figure 1). The length of the polyprenyl pyrophosphate product is determined in a species-specific

DOMAIN 1 (HOMOALLYLIC SITE)

```
HPS Yeast[a]      V E M I H T A S L L H D D V I D H S D T R R G
FPS Rat[b]        V E L L Q A F F L V L D D I M D S S Y T R R G
 "  Human[c]      V E L L Q A F F L V A D D I M D S S L T R R G
 "  Yeast[d]      I E L L Q A Y F L V A D D M M D K S I T R R G
IPP Isomerase[e]  L M N E N C I V L D W D D N A I G A G T K K V
```

DOMAIN 2 (ALLYLIC SITE)

```
HPS   Yeast[a]    L G I C F Q L V D D M L D F I V S G K D L G K
FPS   Rat[b]      M G E F F Q I Q D D Y L D L F G D P S V T G K
 "    Human[c]    M G E F F Q I Q D D Y L D L F G D P S V T G K
 "    Yeast[d]    L G E Y F Q I Q D D Y L D C F G T P E Q I G K
MOD5  Yeast[f]    P E P L F Q R L D D R V D D M L E R G A L Q E

MOD5  Yeast[f]    P E P L F Q R L D D R V D D M L E R G A L Q E
ipt   TiBo542[g]  K G T I R L Y L D D R P L V K G I I T A K Q A
 "    TiT37[h]    K G T S R L Y L D D R P L V K G I I A A K Q A
 "    TiAch5[i]   K G T T R L Y L D D R P L V E G I I A A K Q A
 "    pCK1[j]     Q S T R R I Y L D N R R I S E G V I S A E E A
```

[a]Ashby and Edwards (1990)
[b]Clarke *et al.* (1987)
[c]Sheares *et al.* (1989); Wilkin *et al.* (1990)
[d]Anderson *et al.* (1989a)
[e]Anderson *et al.* (1989b)
[f]Najarian *et al.* (1987)
[g]Strabala *et al.* (1989)
[h]Goldberg *et al.* (1984)
[i]Heidelkamp *et al.* (1983)
[j]Powell and Morris (1986)

Figure 2. Alignment of the amino acid sequences from several proteins which utilize allylic and homoallylic prenyl pyrophosphates as substrates. The aspartate motif direct repeats present in Domains 1 and 2 of the prenyl synthetase sequences is shown in **boldface**.

manner. Once synthesized the polyisoprenoid group is added onto the C4 position of p-hydroxybenzoate, a precursor of coenzyme Q. The length of the polyprenyl chain dictates the coenzyme Q homolog present in a particular species (for review see Olson and Rudney, 1983). The yeast *Saccharomyces cerevisiae* possesses an enzyme hexaprenyl pyrophosphate synthetase (HPS) which is involved in the synthesis of coenzyme Q_6. Tzagoloff *et al.* (1975, 1990) isolated a set of nine different complementation groups of yeast coenzyme Q mutants. Presumably these strains are deficient in specific steps of coenzyme Q biosynthesis. We measured the activities of HPS and the subsequent enzyme PHB:polyprenyltransferase in the individual complementation groups and found two strains deficient in either of these enzyme activities (Ashby and Edwards, 1990). The strain deficient in HPS activity, C296 (designated coq1) was complemented by the plasmid pG3/T1. Analyses of the yeast genomic DNA contained in this plasmid revealed the presence of a 1,419 base-pair open reading frame and was shown to encode the structural gene for HPS. Comparison of the amino acid sequences of HPS from yeast with the FPS sequence from rat indicated approximately 20 percent amino acid identity and unveiled the presence of three highly conserved domains (*ibid*).

Domains 1 and 2 are located internally in the FPS and HPS polypeptides and contain a direct repeat of an aspartate-rich motif (see Figure 2). Domain 3 is located at the extreme carboxy-termini of the polypeptide sequences and is characterized by a basic and hydrophilic terminus. The aspartate-rich consensus sequence, (ILV)xDDxxD, present in Domains 1 and 2 was entered into the NBRF protein data base to search for related sequences. With the exception of the FPS sequence from rat (Clarke *et al.*, 1987), human (Sheares *et al.*, 1989; Wilkin *et al.*, 1990) and yeast (Anderson *et al.*, 1989) and the yeast HPS sequence (Ashby and Edwards, 1990) the consensus sequence was not present twice in any other proteins within the database. The most apparent interpretation of the presence of Domains 1 and 2 is that they are functionally active in the catalytic site of prenyl synthetase enzymes, most likely acting as binding sites for the allylic and homoallylic substrates. We have further proposed that Domains 1 and 2 facilitate the binding of the elongating allylic pyrophosphate and homoallylic pyrophosphate (IPP) substrates by forming magnesium salt bridges from the carboxylate groups of the aspartic acids to the pyrophosphate moieties of the prenyl substrates (Ashby and Edwards, 1990; Figure 3). This type of interaction is consistent with the observation by King and Rilling (1977) that the allylic and homoallylic substrates of FPS bind as their respective magnesium salts. Additionally, Gotoh *et al.* (1988) studying substrate binding in purified pig liver FPS, suggested that the magnesium cation of the IPP-Mg complex is captured by the IPP (homoallylic) binding site of the enzyme during the 1'-4 condensation reaction.

If Domains 1 and 2 do indeed comprise the allylic and homoallylic binding sites then we could predict that they may be present in other enzymes, not necessarily involved in the prenyltransferase reaction, which bind to IPP or an allylic prenyl pyrophosphate substrate. A candidate for an IPP binding enzyme is IPP isomerase which converts IPP to the allylic prenyl group dimethylallyl pyrophosphate (Poulter and Rilling, 1981; Anderson *et al.*, 1989b). Figure 2 shows that IPP isomerase does share a reasonable sequence identity with Domain 1 including two of the three aspartates. Several other amino acids represent conservative substitutions such as at the carboxyl end of Domain 1 where the tripeptide Arg-Arg-Gly (invariant in the four prenyl synthetase sequences) is replaced by Lys-Lys-Val in IPP isomerase.

Figure 2 also shows alignment of several prenylating enzymes with Domain 2. *MOD5* is a yeast gene encoding a prenylating enzyme which transfers dimethylallyl pyrophosphate to certain tRNAs (Dihanich *et al.*, 1987; Najarian *et al.*, 1987). The Ti plasmid of *Agrobacterium tumefaciens* encodes several enzymes involved in auxin and cytokinin biosynthesis. One of these include the *ipt* gene encoding isopentenyl transferase which transfers a dimethylallyl group onto adenosine monophosphate in cytokinin biosynthesis (Akiyoshi *et al.*, 1984). The predicted amino acid sequences from three *ipt* genes isolated from the Ti plasmids of different strains of *Agrobacterium tumefaciens* has been reported (Strabala *et al.*, 1989; Goldberg *et al.*, 1984; Heidelkamp *et al.*, 1983) and is included the alignment in Figure 2. The counterpart to the *ipt* gene is present in *Pseudomonas* on the plasmid pCK1 (Powell and Morris, 1986) and is also included in Figure 2.

The alignment of the *MOD5* gene product with the prenyl synthetase amino acid sequences in Figure 2 shows considerable sequence identity with Domain 2. Five of the amino acids are identical, including the three aspartates. In addition, the *MOD5* protein shows considerable sequence identity with the bacterial *ipt* gene products. Interestingly, while the *MOD5* protein shows significant similarities with both the prenyl synthetases and with the bacterial *ipt* proteins, the latter two groups are not apparently similar other than the two aspartic acids. Therefore, *MOD5* appears to "bridge the gap" between the eukaryotic prenyl synthetase enzymes and the prokaryotic *ipt* proteins.

Taken together these sequence alignments strongly suggest that Domain 1 represents the homoallylic (IPP) binding site while Domain 2 represents the allylic prenyl pyrophosphate binding site. If Domains 1 and 2 are conserved in other prenyl synthetases, we would predict that it will be possible to isolate other cDNAs using the Polymerase Chain Reaction with degenerate primers to these

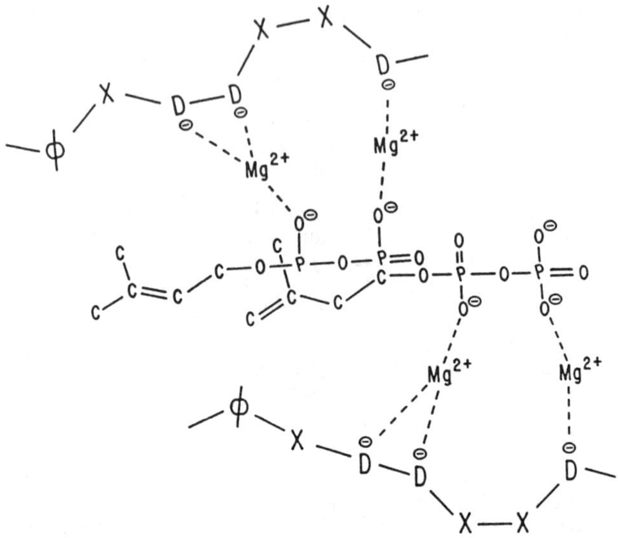

Figure 3. Proposed model for the formation of magnesium salt bridges between Domains 1 and 2 and the homoallylic and allylic prenyl substrates, respectively.

domains. Preliminary results indicate that this approach may be successful as a means of cloning this family of related enzymes.

REFERENCES

Akiyoshi, D. E., Klee, H., Amasino, R. M., Nester, E. W. and Gordon, M. P. (1984) *Proc. Natl. Acad. Sci USA* **81**, 5994-5998

Anderson, M. S., Yarger, J. G., Burck, C. L. and Poulter, C. D. (1989) *J. Biol. Chem.* **264**, 19176-19184

Anderson, M. S., Muehlbacher, M., Street, I. P., Proffitt, J., and Poulter, C. D. (1989) *J. Biol. Chem.* **264**, 19169-19175

Ashby, M. N., and Edwards, P. A. (1989) *J. Biol. Chem.* **264**. 635-640

Ashby, M. N., and Edwards, P. A. (1990) *J. Biol. Chem.* in press

Clarke, C. F., Tanaka, R. D., Svenson, K., Wamsley, M., Fogelman, A. M., and Edwards, P. A. (1987) *Mol. Cell. Biol.* **7**, 3138-3146

Dihanich, M. E., Jajarian, D., Clark, R., Gillman, E. C., Martin, N. C., and Hopper, A. K. (1987) *Mol. Cell. Biol.* **7**, 177-184

Farnsworth, C. C., Wolda, S. L., Gelb, M. H., and Glomset, J. A. (1989) *J. Biol. Chem.* **264**, 20422-20429

Farnsworth, C. C., Gelb, M. H., and Glomset, J. A. (1990) *Science* **247**, 320-322

Goldberg, S. B., Flick, J. S. and Rogers, S. G. (1984) *Nucleic Acids Res.* **12**, 4665-4677

Goldstein, J. L., and Brown, M. S. (1990) *Nature* **343**, 425-430

Gotoh, T., Koyama, T., and Ogura, K. (1988) *Biochem. Biophys. Res. Comm.* **156**, 396-402

Hancock, J. F., Magee, A. I., Childs, J. E., and Marshall, C. J. (1989) *Cell* **57**, 1167-1177

Heinzmann, C., Clarke, C. F., Klisak, I., Mohandas, T., Sparkes, R. S., Edwards, P. A., and Lusis, A. J. (1989) *Genomics* **5**, 493-500

King Jr., H. L., and Rilling, H. C. (1977) *Biochemistry* **16**, 3815-3819

Levin, M. S., Pitt, A. J. A., Schwartz, A. L., Edwards, P. A., and Gordon, J. I. (1989) *Biochim. Biophys. Acta* **1003**, 293-300

Li. A. C., Tanaka, R. D., Callaway, K., Fogelman, A. M., and Edwards, P. A. (1988) *J. Lipid Res.* **29**, 781-796

Mehrabian, M., Callaway, K. A., Clarke, C. F., Tanaka, R. D., Greenspan, M., Lusis, A. J., Sparkes, R. S., Mohandas, T., Edmond, J., Fogelman, A. M., and Edwards, P. A. (1986) *J. Biol. Chem.* **261**, 16249-16255

Najarian, D., Dihanich, M. E., Martin, N. C., and Hopper, A. K. (1987) *Mol. Cell. Biol.* **7**, 185-191

Olson, R. E., and Rudney, H. (1983) *Vitam. Horm.* **40**, 1-43

Poulter, D. C., and Rilling, H. C. (1981) *in* Biosynthesis of Isoprenoid Compounds (Porter, J. W., and Spurgeon, S. L., eds) Vol. 1, pp 162-202, Wiley & Sons, New York

Powell, G. K., and Morris, R. O. (1986) *Nucleic Acids Res.* **14**, 2555-2563

Rilling, H. C., Breunger, E., Epstein, W. W., and Crain, P. F. (1990) *Science* **247**, 318-320

Rosser, D. S. E., Ashby, M. N., Ellis, J. L., and Edwards, P. A. (1983) *J. Biol. Chem.* **264**, 12653-12656

Schafer, W. R., Kim, R., Sterne, R., Thorner, J., Kim, S., and Rine, J. (1989) *Science* **245**, 379-385

Sheares, B. T., White, S. S., Molowa, D. T., Chan, K., Ding, V. D. H., Kroon, P. A., Bostedor, R. G., and Karkas, J. D. (1989) *Biochemistry* **28**, 8129-8135

Singer, I. I., Kawka, D. W., Kazazis, D. M., Alberts, A. W., Chen, J. S., Huff, J. W., and Ness, G. C. (1984) *Proc. Natl. Acad. Sci. USA* **81**, 5556-5560

Spear, D. H., Kutsunai, S. Y., Correll, C. C., and Edwards, P. A. (1990) *J. Biol. Chem.* submitted

Strabala, T. J., Bednarek, S. Y., Bertoni, G., and Amasino, R. M. (1989) *Mol. Gen. Genet.* **216**, 388-394

Teruya, J., Kutsunai, S. Y., Spear, D. H., Edwards, P. A., and Clarke, C. F. (1990) *Mol. Cell. Biol.* **10**, 2315-2326

Tzagoloff, A., Akai, A., and Needleman, R. B. (1975) *J. Biol. Chem.* **250**, 8228-8235

Tzagoloff, A., and Dieckmann, C. L. (1990) *Microbiol. Rev.* in press

Weinstein, J. D., Branchaud, R., Beale, S. I., Bement, W. J., and Sinclair, P. R. (1986) *Arch. Biochem. Biophys.* **245**, 44-50

Wilkin, D. J., Kutsunai, S. Y., and Edwards, P. A. (1990) *J. Biol. Chem.* **265**, 4607-4614

Analysis of Intermediates in Protein Translocation across the Endoplasmic Reticulum

Reid Gilmore, Paula Collins, and Tim Connolly

Department of Biochemistry, University of Massachusetts Medical School, Worcester, Massachusetts

ABSTRACT

Protein translocation across mammalian rough endoplasmic reticulum (RER) has been investigated by characterizing intermediates that accumulate when the transport process is interrupted by deletion or modification of an essential component. Several components of the translocation apparatus have previously been identified by this approach including: the signal recognition particle (SRP), the SRP receptor, the signal sequence receptor (SSR) and signal peptidase. In addition, this strategy was used to demonstrate that translocation requires both adenine and guanine ribonucleotide triphosphates. We have examined the role of GTP in translocation by a molecular characterization of intermediates that accumulate after incubation of SRP-ribosome-nascent chain complexes with microsomal membranes. These studies demonstrated that the SRP receptor is a GTP binding protein. Intermediates in nascent chain translocation can be obtained by in vitro translation of truncated mRNA molecules. Partially translocated nascent chains of 100 amino acid residues or less are remarkably insensitive to protease digestion after detergent solubilization of the membrane. An association between the nascent polypeptide and the translocation apparatus apparently persists after detergent solubilization of the membrane and this continued association probably accounts for the protease insensitivity of low molecular weight nascent polypeptides.

INTRODUCTION

The transport of a protein to its correct site of function within a eukaryotic cell represents an essential event in gene expression. All proteins located within intracellular organelles, with the exception of those mitochondrial and chloroplast proteins that are encoded by the organellar genome, must be transported across at least one membrane bilayer either during or shortly after biosynthesis. Membrane proteins must be integrated into the correct cellular membrane in the proper topological orientation to be functional. Protein translocation and sorting mechanisms

© 1990 by Elsevier Science Publishing Co., Inc.
Molecular Biology of Atherosclerosis
A.D. Attie, Editor

have evolved in eukaryotic cells to selectively translocate proteins to their correct cellular location while at the same time maintaining the permeability barrier of intracellular membranes [1]. Mislocalization of proteins is deleterious to the organism.

The rough endoplasmic reticulum is the site of synthesis for a significant proportion of cellular proteins including secretory proteins, lysosomal proteins and the lumenal proteins of the endoplasmic reticulum, Golgi apparatus and endosome [2]. The majority of integral membrane proteins are also synthesized on the endoplasmic reticulum, including proteins destined for the plasma membrane, lysosome, nuclear envelope and the endocytotic and exocytotic membrane systems [2]. The selective translocation of proteins across an intracellular membrane occurs through the combination of a sorting reaction and a transport reaction. Proteins destined to be translocated across the endoplasmic reticulum are selected during synthesis from among all polypeptides that are translated within the cytoplasm by virtue of containing an endoplasmic reticulum specific signal sequence. These sorted proteins are then delivered or "targeted" to the endoplasmic reticulum membrane. Transport of the polypeptide across the membrane is then proposed to occur at a specific translocation competent site which has been termed the translocon [3].

RECOGNITION OF SIGNAL SEQUENCES

Signal sequences that specify translocation across, or integration into, the endoplasmic reticulum are located at or near the amino terminus of the polypeptide. Secreted and lumenal proteins almost always contain cleavable signal sequences while integral membrane proteins may retain a non-cleavable signal sequence as a transmembrane spanning segment (as reviewed in [2, 4]). Cleavable signal sequences from numerous proteins have been compared to identify sequence motifs of functional significance [5, 6]. A highly conserved signal sequence was not identified. Instead, these studies revealed that the typical 15-25 amino acid residue signal sequence contains the following structural features: (a) a basic amino terminal region, (b) a central core of hydrophobic amino acids and (c) a C terminal region that specifies cleavage by the enzyme signal peptidase [5, 6]. Of these three regions, the central hydrophobic core has subsequently been shown to be the most important determinant as a sorting signal for translocation across the endoplasmic reticulum.

Our current understanding of protein translocation across mammalian endoplasmic reticulum has been obtained through the use of in vitro systems which monitor specific events during nascent chain synthesis and transport. These in vitro systems consist of a translation system derived from rabbit reticulocytes [7] or wheat germ [8], microsomal membrane vesicles isolated from canine pancreas [9], and a mRNA that encodes a secretory or integral membrane protein.

Proteins that catalyzed the translocation process were first detected in experiments where microsomal membranes were inactivated by protease digestion [10] or high salt extraction [11]. A protein essential for translocation competence was shown to be released from microsomal membrane vesicles by high ionic strength [11], and this protein was subsequently purified as a heteroligomeric protein complex consisting of six polypeptides with molecular weights of 72, 68, 54, 19, 14 and 9 kD [12]. Elegant studies soon demonstrated that the protein complex binds with high affinity to ribosomes translating nascent secretory proteins, and in so doing, causes a site-specific elongation arrest of translation after synthesis of roughly 70 residues of the polypeptide [13, 14, 15]. Based upon these observations, and the finding that the complex also contains the 7S small cytoplasmic RNA [16], this translocation factor was named the signal recognition particle (SRP). At physiological ionic strength, SRP is distributed between free, membrane bound and ribosome bound forms [17].

The 7S RNA is essential for the activity of SRP [16], and it appears to provide a framework upon which the protein subunits of SRP are assembled into three structurally and functionally distinct domains [18, 19]. SRP particles have been disassembled into protein and RNA components and then reconstituted into active particles [20]. Deletion or modification of the protein subunits has allowed Siegel and Walter to define the functional activity of each of the three domains of SRP [19, 21, 22]. A heterodimer consisting of the 9 and 14 kD polypeptides binds to the Alu-like region of the 7S RNA to comprise the elongation arrest domain of SRP [18, 21, 22]. Although an elongation arrest of nascent chain synthesis by SRP is not essential for protein translocation [21, 23], a decreased protein synthetic rate caused by SRP may prevent premature folding of nascent chains in the cytoplasm. The 54 kD subunit of SRP was shown to bind to the signal sequence shortly after it merges from the ribosome, as shown by crosslinking of the 54 kD subunit to nascent chains containing photoactivatable amino acid analogues [24, 25]. The 54 kD subunit together with the 19 kD protein correspond to a signal sequence recognition domain [19]. The remaining two protein subunits of SRP form a heterodimer that comprises what has been termed the translocation promotion domain of SRP [19].

TARGETING OF SRP-RIBOSOME COMPLEXES TO THE RER

Ribosomes translating a secretory protein bind to microsomal membranes in a SRP-dependent reaction [13]. We shall refer to SRP-elongation arrested ribosomes synthesizing a protein with an endoplasmic reticulum-specific signal sequence as SRP-ribosome complexes. After targeting of the SRP-ribosome complex to the membrane, translation of the nascent polypeptide resumes [14] and the protein is translocated into the lumen of the membrane vesicle. Further research demonstrated that microsomal membranes contain a receptor for SRP-ribosome complexes that has the ability to reverse the SRP-induced elongation arrest of protein synthesis [26]. A protein with this activity was purified from detergent extracts of microsomal membranes and named the SRP receptor based upon its affinity for SRP [27]. A 60 kD protease-derived fragment from the SRP receptor had actually been purified several years before [28, 29] as the cytoplasmically exposed domain of a 72 kD protease sensitive translocation factor [30]. Thus, these two separate lines of research identified a receptor for SRP, which is known either as the SRP receptor [27] or as the docking protein [31]. The SRP receptor is a heterodimer composed of a 69 kD α subunit (SRα) and a 30 kD β subunit (SRβ) [32]. Limited proteolysis of microsomal membranes followed by a high salt extraction can be used to separate the 60 kD fragment of the α subunit from the remainder of the SRP receptor. Neither portion of the receptor retains an affinity for SRP when tested alone [33, 34], yet recombination of the the two fragments restores translocation competence to microsomal membrane vesicles [26, 31]. One possible explanation for this observation has been provided by sequence analysis of the SRα cDNA clone [33]. The sequence of SRα contains several regions with a high density of charged amino acids near the protease cleavage site. This highly charged portion of SRα was proposed to interact with SRP based upon homology to sequences found in nucleic acid binding proteins [33].

SRP and the SRP receptor function in concert to target ribosomes to the rough endoplasmic reticulum. The targeting reaction does not require ongoing protein synthesis [34] and it can occur after a significant portion of the nascent polypeptide chain has been synthesized [35, 36]. The membrane content of the SRP receptor is approximately 5 fold lower than that of membrane bound ribosomes [27, 32]. Thus, it seemed unlikely that SRP and the SRP receptor would also function as a ribosome binding site on the endoplasmic reticulum membrane. Additional research showed that SRP was displaced from the ribosome upon interaction of the SRP-ribosome complex with either the purified SRP receptor or microsomal membranes [37]. Furthermore, no affinity between the SRP receptor and the ribosome was detected [37]. These studies indicated that SRP and the SRP receptor act transiently during ribosome targeting to the membrane. Additional proteins of the endoplasmic reticulum are presumably responsible for the continued association of the ribosome with the membrane during nascent chain transport.

GTP-DEPENDENCE OF PROTEIN TRANSLOCATION

A potential requirement for ribonucleotide triphosphates in translocation of proteins across the RER could not be investigated without modification of the in vitro assay systems used prior to 1985. Protein synthesis requires both ATP and GTP, and translocation of proteins across the RER was believed to be an obligatory cotranslational reaction. Targeting of SRP-ribosome complexes to microsomal membranes does not require continued protein synthesis [34]. These latter experiments used low molecular weight nascent chains that were of insufficient length to traverse the bilayer. Could larger nascent chains be completely translocated across the membrane in the absence of continued protein synthesis? Several laboratories showed that translation of mRNAs that were truncated within the protein coding region allowed the assembly of ribosomes bearing a discrete sized nascent chain [38, 39, 40]. Following synthesis of the nascent polypeptide, cycloheximide was added to block further protein synthesis prior to the addition of microsomal membrane vesicles. These ribosome-tethered secretory or membrane proteins were shown to be translocated across, or integrated into the membrane in the absence of continued protein synthesis provided that ATP was present [38, 39, 40]. Initially, these results were interpreted as proof for an ATP hydrolysis-coupled transport site. Further experiments have suggested an alternate interpretation. Partially folded polypeptides appear to be converted into transport competent substrates by an ATP-dependent unfolding reaction [41]. Proteins belonging to the 70 kD heat shock family are proposed to unfold, or prevent premature folding of, nascent chains prior to transport across mammalian [41] and yeast [42, 43] endoplasmic reticulum.

A similar strategy led to the detection of a requirement for GTP in translocation across the endoplasmic reticulum [44]. SRP-ribosome complexes bearing a nascent preprolactin chain were incubated with microsomal membranes either in the absence or presence of ribonucleotide triphosphates. Neither GTP nor ATP were required for targeting of SRP-ribosome complexes to the membrane. Several criteria were initially detected which indicated that a subsequent nascent chain insertion reaction required GTP. In the absence GTP, the nascent chains could be removed by extraction with either high salt or EDTA [44]. Nascent chains targeted in the absence of GTP remained sensitive to externally added protease and were incompetent for translocation upon addition of puromycin [44]. In contrast, targeting of SRP-ribosome complexes to the membrane in the presence of GTP alone allowed the production of a functional intermediate in nascent chain transport. The observation that most clearly distinguished the GTP requirement from the ATP hydrolysis requirement discussed above was the finding that 10 μM guanylyl-5-imidodiphosphate could replace GTP to allow insertion of nascent chains into the membrane [44]. Thus, guanine ribonucleotides, but not ribonucleotide hydrolysis, is essential for assembly of a functional ribosome-membrane junction. Entirely analogous results were obtained when the integration of membrane proteins was investigated [45, 46]. Taken together, these results indicated that an essential component of the translocation apparatus was a GTP binding protein.

Several lines of evidence eventually indicated that the SRP receptor was the GTP-dependent translocation component [47]. An amino acid sequence comparison of GTP binding proteins allowed the identification of three sequence elements that comprise a guanine nucleotide binding site [48]. Amino acid segments of between 40 and 80 residues separate three sequence elements that were shown by X-ray crystallography of EF-Tu [49] and H ras p21 [50] to correspond to loops at the ends of adjacent parallel β strands. The sequence elements GXXXXGK and DXXG are the binding sites for the phosphoryl group and chelated Mg^{++} ion of GTP. The asparagine and aspartate residues within the third sequence element (NKXD) are in direct contact with the keto and amino group of the guanine ring, while the lysine residue was shown to be part of a hydrophobic binding pocket [49]. Canine [33] and human [51] SRα cDNA clones have been isolated and sequenced. The amino acid sequence of SRα contains sequence elements which are similar, but not

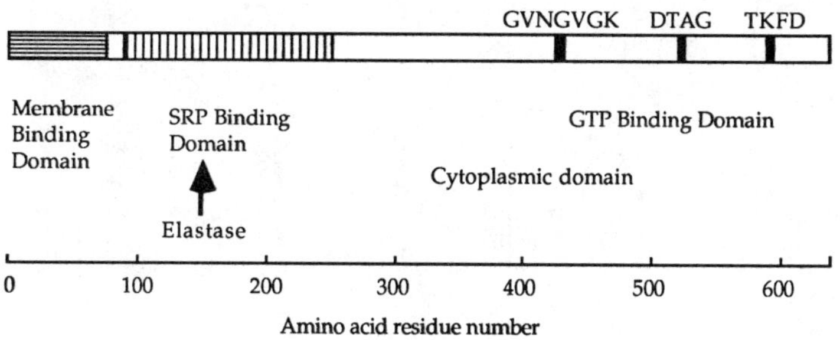

Figure 1. Location of a potential GTP binding site in the α subunit of the SRP receptor.

identical, to the consensus sequence elements present in other GTP binding proteins (Figure 1). The region of the α subunit proposed to be a GTP binding domain [47] was recently shown to be homologous to a portion of the 54 kD subunit of SRP [52, 53]. The diagram in Figure 1 indicates the location of the proposed SRP binding region [33] of SRα near the the elastase cleavage site. Elastase or trypsin severs the protein between the putative GTP binding domain and the membrane binding domain.

Biochemical data was also obtained which indicated that the α subunit of the SRP receptor was a GTP binding protein. Direct photoaffinity labeling of SRP receptor preparations with GTP resulted in radiolabeling of both SRα and SRβ [47]. Radiolabeling of both subunits was sensitive to competition by unlabeled GTP and GDP and to a lesser extent by ATP. Additional evidence suggesting that SRα binds GTP was obtained by probing nitrocellulose blots of the receptor after resolution of the subunits by polyacrylamide gel electrophoresis in SDS. SRα but not SRβ bound GTP after electrophoresis under denaturing conditions. While many low molecular weight GTP binding proteins are detected by this procedure [54, 55], members of the G protein family apparently do not renature after transfer to the nitrocellulose membrane. Therefore, this experiment does not eliminate the β subunit as a possible GTP binding protein.

Functional evidence indicating that SRP receptor is a GTP binding protein is summarized in Figure 2. This model is a compilation of current evidence and a great deal of speculation concerning the role of GTP in protein translocation across the endoplasmic reticulum. The three domains of the SRP particle are depicted in Fig. 2A. Binding of SRP to a ribosome synthesizing a protein with a signal sequence (2B) is via the 54 kD subunit of SRP. The SRP-ribosome complex (2C) is

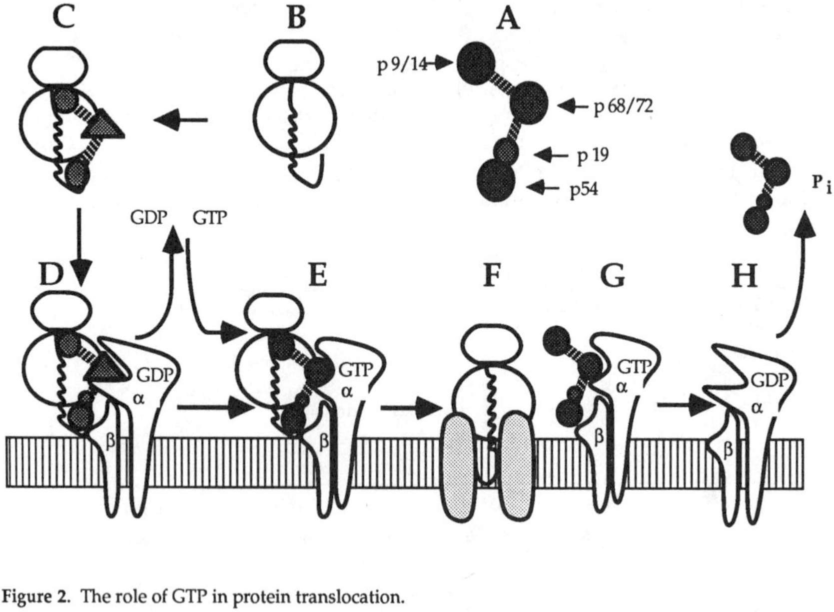

Figure 2. The role of GTP in protein translocation.

targeted to the membrane bound SRP receptor in a GTP-independent reaction to yield the high salt or EDTA extractable intermediate (2D). Formation of intermediate 2D is not inhibited by the presence of GDP nor influenced by preincubation of membranes with nonhydrolyzable GTP analogues (Connolly and Gilmore, unpublished observations). The interaction between SRP receptor and SRP may be mediated by the p68/72 domain of SRP [19]. The addition of GTP or a nonhydrolyzable GTP analogue leads to nascent chain insertion (2F). The functional evidence indicating that the SRP receptor was the relevant GTP binding protein was obtained by a molecular characterization of translocation intermediates that accumulate in the absence (2D) or presence of GTP (2F). Digestion with proteinase K can be used to distinguish between intermediates 2B, 2C and 2F [56]. SRP partially shields nascent chains from proteolytic digestion in the SRP-ribosome complex (2C), while membrane inserted chains (2F) are extremely protease resistant [56]. In the absence of GTP (2D), newly targeted nascent chains showed a protease digestion profile that was indistinguishable from intermediate 2C [47]. The continued presence of SRP in intermediate 2D was confirmed by preparing SRP-ribosome complexes containing radioiodinated SRP. Sucrose gradient analysis demonstrated that the ^{125}I labeled-SRP remained ribosome bound in the absence of GTP [47]. Purified preparations of SRP receptor can displace ^{125}I labeled-SRP from ribosomes only in the presence of GTP [47]. Based upon these functional results we proposed that the SRP receptor is a GTP binding protein. As noted above, the identification of the α subunit as the GTP binding subunit remains tentative. A possible function for the putative GTP binding site in SRP 54 has not been indicated by experimental evidence obtained to date. In our in vitro system, SRP is present during synthesis of the nascent chain, where it has ample opportunity to bind GTP. Bernstein et al. [52] have suggested that the GTP binding site in SRP 54 may function to control the fidelity of signal sequence recognition. GDP is a competitive inhibitor of the production of intermediate 2F [44], suggesting that intermediate 2D contains bound GDP. We suggest that the SRP-ribosome complex catalyzes a GDP-GTP exchange reaction involving the receptor to yield intermediate 2E. Based upon analogies to other GTP binding proteins [57], we proposed that the GTP-bound form of the SRP receptor has an increased affinity for an additional ligand, which may correspond to the 54 kD subunit of SRP [47]. This increase in binding affinity may be mechanistically coupled to displacement of the signal sequence from SRP to yield intermediates 2F and 2G. The association between the nascent chain and integral membrane proteins depicted in intermediate 2F will be discussed in a later section of this article. We postulate that SRP will remain bound to the receptor (2G) until GTP is hydrolyzed. After GTP hydrolysis, SRP will dissociate from the receptor and return to the cytoplasm for participation in subsequent rounds of ribosome targeting (2H). These latter proposals are based upon analogies to other GTP binding proteins [57]. Several important aspects of this model obviously will remain as mere speculation until further evidence is obtained. We are currently investigating whether nonhydrolyzable GTP analogues interfere with recycling of SRP and SRP receptor.

NASCENT CHAIN TRANSPORT

A central question concerning nascent chain transport across the RER is whether transport is a protein mediated or phospholipid mediated process. Early models for protein translocation postulated the existence of a protein pore or tunnel through which the nascent chain was threaded [9, 58]. Alternative proposals based primarily on thermodynamic considerations indicate that spontaneous transfer of a protein through a lipid bilayer in an alpha helical conformation is possible [59]. Several lines of experimental evidence now provide support for a protein mediated transport process. Partially translocated nascent chains can be extracted from microsomal membrane vesicles by protein denaturants, but not by high salt or EDTA solutions [34]. Although these results suggested that the nascent chain is in contact with protein instead of phospholipid, they did not provide information about the identity or properties of the putative transport proteins. The first identification of a protein involved in nascent chain transport was provided by a crosslinking approach. Partially translocated nascent chains containing a photoactivatable amino acid analogue were crosslinked to a 35 kD integral membrane glycoprotein [60]. In the initial experiments, the photoactivatable amino acid residues were located within the signal sequence, hence the protein was named the signal sequence receptor (SSR) [60]. Subsequent crosslinking experiments by other investigators demonstrated that contact between the nascent chain and a 39 kD glycoprotein is maintained at all stages of nascent chain transport [61].

Based upon the preceding observations we decided to use proteolysis as a probe to monitor the conformation of proteins undergoing transport across the RER. Are proteins transported in a extended conformation, or are partially folded protein domains transported in a discontinuous or segmental fashion as recently proposed [62]? To address this question, we have taken advantage of the fact that translation of truncated mRNAs yields nascent chains which remain tethered to the ribosome via peptidyl-tRNA [38, 40, 44]. By translating a series of truncated mRNAs derived from a single protein in the presence of SRP and microsomal membranes, we were able to generate a series of partially translocated nascent chains that correspond to sequential intermediates in the transport of the protein (Figure 3). The presence of SRP during translation of the mRNAs insured that the various translocation intermediates discussed below represent different final stages in a single cotranslational transport pathway.

Proteinase K was used as a probe to detect cytoplasmically and lumenally exposed segments of nascent polypeptides undergoing transport across microsomal membranes. Cytoplasmically exposed segments of the nascent chain were detected by protease digestion of intact microsomal membrane vesicles. Partially translocated nascent chains derived from both preprolactin and VSV G protein were substantially more resistant to proteolytic digestion than nascent chains synthesized in the absence of SRP and microsomal membranes. Protection of the translocation intermediate from externally added protease was greatest when the nascent chain did not exceed 100 amino acid residues in length. We propose that close contact between the ribosome and the membrane surface limits access of the protease to the nascent polypeptide during early stages of transport. Larger translocation intermediates (i.e. pG-200) were more sensitive to digestion by externally added protease, suggesting that a portion of the nascent chain may be exposed upon the cytoplasmic side of the membrane at late stages of the transport reaction (Figure 3). Nascent chain transport may not be directly coupled to elongation of the polypeptide, even when translocation is conducted in a cotranslational mode.

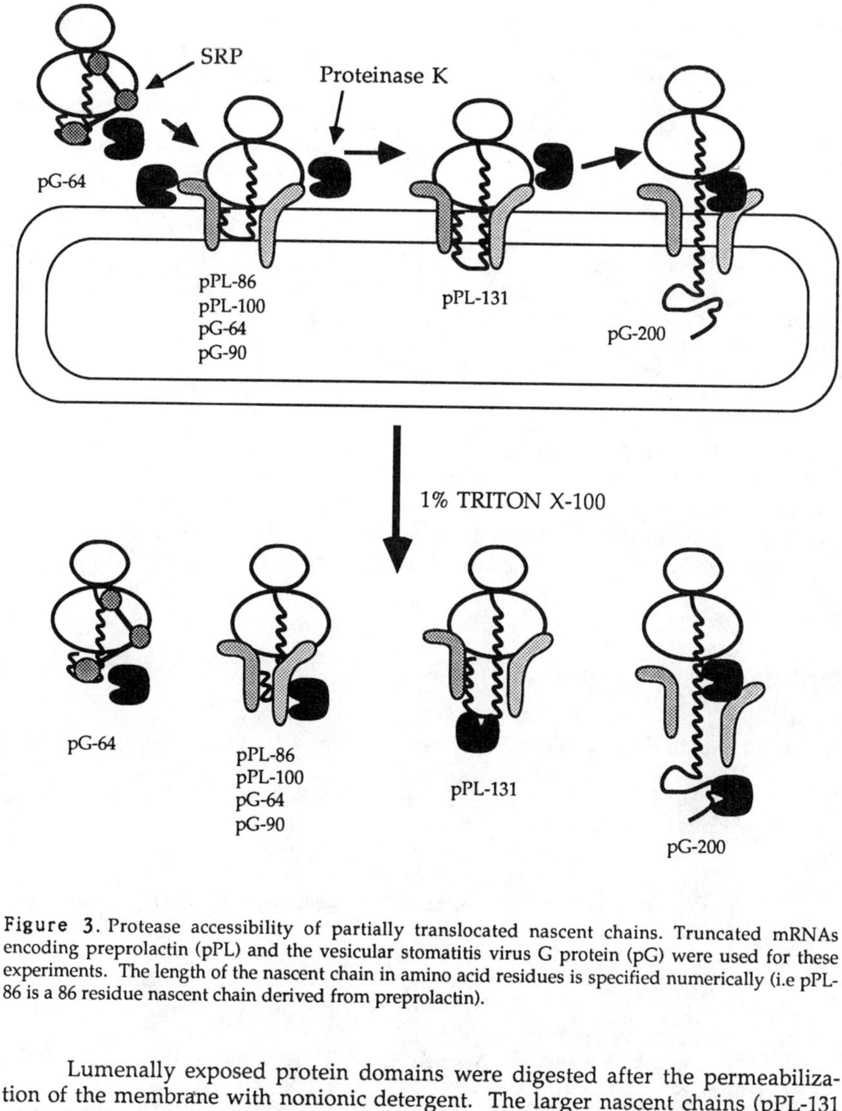

Figure 3. Protease accessibility of partially translocated nascent chains. Truncated mRNAs encoding preprolactin (pPL) and the vesicular stomatitis virus G protein (pG) were used for these experiments. The length of the nascent chain in amino acid residues is specified numerically (i.e pPL-86 is a 86 residue nascent chain derived from preprolactin).

Lumenally exposed protein domains were digested after the permeabilization of the membrane with nonionic detergent. The larger nascent chains (pPL-131 and pG-200) were readily digested after permeabilization of the membrane, indicating that portions of these polypeptides were now exposed within the lumen of the membrane vesicle. Surprisingly, nascent chains of 100 amino acids or less did not display a detergent-enhanced sensitivity to protease digestion (Figure 3). Based upon these results, we concluded that the membrane bound components of the translocation apparatus in combination with the ribosome can shield roughly 100 amino acid residues of a nascent chain [56]. Protection of a polypeptide segment of this size may suggest that transport is initiated by the insertion of a hairpin loop of polypeptide into the membrane [59]. Lumenally exposed domains of translocation components (e.g. signal peptidase) may also shield portions of the nascent chain from protease digestion. We are now attempting to identify integral membrane proteins that are responsible for protecting low molecular weight nascent chains from protease digestion. The signal sequence receptor [60, 61] is perhaps the most reasonable candidate for such a protein.

CONCLUSIONS

Research during the past ten years has provided considerable information concerning the sorting and targeting phases of the protein translocation reaction. The majority of proteins transported across the endoplasmic reticulum are delivered to the membrane through the combined action of SRP and the SRP receptor. Interesting exceptions to this generalization have also been discovered. Low molecular weight proteins such as prepromelittin can be targeted to the membrane in an SRP and SRP receptor-independent reaction [63, 64, 65]. Insight into the transport phase of the translocation reaction is being slowly gained. Several laboratories have recently reported methods which allow reconstitution of translocation activity from detergent solubilized extracts of microsomal membranes [66, 67, 68]. These reconstitution methods will provide investigators with methods to identify and characterize the polypeptides which catalyze nascent chain transport.

REFERENCES

1. G. Blobel, Proc. Nat. Acad. Sci. USA 77, 1496-1500 (1980).
2. D. D. Sabatini, G. Kreibich, T. Morimoto, and M. Adesnick, J. Cell Biol. 92, 1-22 (1982).
3. P. Walter, and V. R. Lingappa, Ann. Rev. Cell Biol. 2, 499-516. (1986).
4. W. Wickner, and H. Lodish, Science 230, 400-407 (1985).
5. G. von Heijne, Eur. J. Biochem. 133, 17-21 (1983).
6. G. von Heijne, Nuc. Acids Res. 14, 4683-4690 (1986).
7. H. R. B. Pelham, and R. J. Jackson, Eur. J. Biochem. 67, 247-256 (1976).
8. A. H. Erickson, and G. Blobel, Met. Enzymol. 96, 38-50 (1983).
9. G. Blobel, and B. Dobberstein, J. Cell Biol. 67, 852-862 (1975).
10. P. Walter, R. C. Jackson, M. M. Marcus, V. R. Lingappa, and G. Blobel, Proc. Natl. Acad. Sci. USA 76, 1795-1799 (1979).
11. G. Warren, and B. Dobberstein, Nature 273, 569-571 (1978).
12. P. Walter, and G. Blobel, Proc. Natl. Acad. Sci. USA 77, 7112-7116 (1980).
13. P. Walter, and G. Blobel, J. Cell Biol. 91, 551-556 (1981).
14. P. Walter, and G. Blobel, J. Cell Biol. 91, 557-561 (1981).
15. P. Walter, I. Ibrahimi, and G. Blobel, J. Cell Biol. 91, 545-550 (1981).
16. P. Walter, and G. Blobel, Nature 299, 691-698 (1982).
17. P. Walter, and G. Blobel, J. Cell Biol. 97, 1693-1699 (1983).
18. V. Siegel, and P. Walter, Proc. Natl. Acad. Sci. USA 85, 1801-1805 (1988).
19. V. Siegel, and P. Walter, Cell 52, 39-49 (1988).
20. P. Walter, and G. Blobel, Cell 34, 525-533 (1983).
21. V. Siegel, and P. Walter, J. Cell Biol. 100, 519-528 (1985).
22. V. Siegel, and P. Walter, Nature 320, 81-84 (1986).
23. D. I. Meyer, EMBO J. 4, 2031-2033 (1985).

24. T. V. Kurzchalia, M. Wiedmann, A. S. Girshovich, E. S. Bochkareva, H. Bielka, and T. A. Rapoport, Nature 320, 634-636 (1986).
25. U. C. Krieg, P. Walter, and A. E. Johnson, Proc. Natl. Acad. Sci. USA 83, 8604-8608 (1986).
26. R. Gilmore, G. Blobel, and P. Walter, J. Cell Biol. 95, 463-469 (1982).
27. R. Gilmore, P. Walter, and G. Blobel, J. Cell Biol. 95, 470-477 (1982).
28. D. I. Meyer, and B. Dobberstein, J. Cell Biol. 87, 498-502 (1980).
29. D. I. Meyer, and B. Dobberstein, J. Cell Biol. 87, 503-508 (1980).
30. D. I. Meyer, D. Louvard, and B. Dobberstein, J. Cell Biol. 92, 579-583 (1982).
31. D. I. Meyer, E. Krause, and B. Dobberstein, Nature 297, 647-650 (1982).
32. S. Tajima, L. Lauffer, V. L. Rath, and P. Walter, J. Cell Biol. 103, 1167-1178(1986).
33. L. Lauffer, P. D. Garcia, R. N. Harkins, L. Coussens, A. Ullrich, and P. Walter, Nature 318, 334-338 (1985).
34. R. Gilmore, and G. Blobel, Cell 42, 497-505 (1985).
35. K. J. Ainger, and D. I. Meyer, EMBO J. 5, 951-955 (1986).
36. V. Siegel, and P. Walter, EMBO J. 7, 1769-1775 (1988).
37. R. Gilmore, and G. Blobel, Cell 35, 677-685 (1983).
38. E. Perara, R. E. Rothman, and V. R. Lingappa, Science 232, 348-352 (1986).
39. M. Mueckler, and H. F. Lodish, Cell 44, 629-637 (1986).
40. M. Mueckler, and H. F. Lodish, Nature 322, 549-552 (1986).
41. R. Zimmermann, M. Sagstetter, M. Lewis, and H. Pelham, EMBO J. 7, 2875-2880 (1988).
42. W. J. Chirico, M. G. Waters, and G. Blobel, Nature 322, 805-810 (1988).
43. R. J. Deshaies, B. D. Koch, M. Werner-Washburne, E. A. Craig, and R. Schekman, Nature 332, 800-805 (1988).
44. T. Connolly, and R. Gilmore, J. Cell Biol. 103, 2253-2261 (1986).
45. K. Hoffman, and R. Gilmore, J. Biol. Chem. 263, 4381-4385 (1988).
46. C. Wilson, T. Connolly, T. Morrison, and R. Gilmore, J. Cell Biol. 107, 69-77 (1988).
47. T. Connolly, and R. Gilmore, Cell 57, 599-610 (1989).
48. T. E. Dever, M. J. Glynias, and W. C. Merrick, Proc. Natl. Acad. Sci. USA 84, 1814-1818 (1987).
49. T. F. M. la Cour, J. Nyborg, S. Thirup, and B. F. C. Clark, EMBO J. 4, 2385-2388 (1985).
50. A. M. deVos, L. Tong, M. V. Milburn, P. Matias, J. Jancarik, S. Noguchi, S.Nishimura, K. Miura, E. Ohtsuka, and S.-H. Kim, Science 239, 888-893 (1988).
51. M. Hortsch, S. Labeit, and D. I. Meyer, Nucleic Acids Res. 16, 361-362 (1988).
52. H. Bernstein, M. Poritz, K. Strub, P. Hoben, S. Brenner, and P. Walter, Nature 340, 482-486 (1989).
53. K. Romish, J. Webb, J. Herz, S. Prehn, R. Frank, M. Vingron, and B. Dobberstein, Nature 340, 478-482 (1989).
54. E. G. Lapetina, and B. R. Reep, Proc. Natl. Acad. Sci. USA 85, 2261-2265 (1987).
55. B. Goud, A. Saiminen, N. C. Walworth, and P. J. Novick, Cell 53, 753-768 (1988).
56. T. Connolly, P. Collins, and R. Gilmore, J. Cell Biol. 108, 299-307 (1989).
57. H. Bourne, Cell 53, 669-671 (1988).
58. G. Blobel, and B. Dobberstein, J. Cell Biol. 67, 835-851 (1975).
59. D. M. Engelman, and T. A. Steitz, Cell 23, 411-422 (1981).
60. M. Wiedmann, T. V. Kurzchalia, E. Hartmann, and T. A. Rapoport, Nature 328, 830-833 (1987).

61. U. C. Krieg, A. E. Johnson, and P. Walter, J. Cell Biol. 109, 2033-2043 (1989).
62. S. J. Singer, P. A. Maher, and M. P. Yaffe, Proc. Natl. Acad. Sci. USA 84, 1015-1019 (1987).
63. R. Zimmermann, and C. Mollay, J. Biol. Chem. 261, 12889-12895 (1986).
64. G. Schlenstedt, and R. Zimmermann, EMBO J. 6, 699-703 (1987).
65. G. Muller, and R. Zimmermann, EMBO J. 6, 2099-2107 (1987).
66. C. Nicchitta, and G. Blobel, 60, 259-269 (1990).
67. Y. Yu, Y. Zhang, D. Sabatini, and G. Kreibich, Proc Natl Acad Sci USA 86, 9931-9935 (1989).
68. D. L. Zimmerman, and P. Walter, J. Biol. Chem. 265, 4048-4053 (1990).

Molecular Genetic Analysis of Vesicle Formation and Fusion in Protein Transport from the Endoplasmic Reticulum

Chris A. Kaiser and Randy Schekman

Division of Biochemistry and Molecular Biology, University of California, Berkeley, California

ABSTRACT

The process of protein transport from the endoplasmic reticulum is studied using conditional secretion-defective mutations identified in the yeast *Saccharomyces cerevisiae*. In a subset of mutants blocked early in the secretory pathway a vesicular intermediate in protein transport accumulates. The early *SEC* genes are thus grouped into either vesicle-forming functions or vesicle-fusion functions. Two of the genes required for vesicle fusion have mammalian counterparts. The products of *SEC18* and *SEC17* can functionally replace NSF and SNAP, factors required for vesicle fusion in transport between cisterna of the mammalian Golgi. Thus both the morphological and molecular properties of the protein transport pathway are remarkably similar in yeast and mammals.

INTRODUCTION

Secreted proteins follow a well defined pathway as they pass from their site of synthesis in the cytoplasm to the cell surface. Each of the membrane-bounded organelles of the secretory pathway acts as a conduit for the flow of secretory proteins to the cell surface while keeping a unique biochemical and morphological identity. The guiding principle to explain how proteins move between organelles was articulated by Palade who postulated that each step in the transport pathway is mediated by cargo-carrying vesicles that bud from one membrane-bounded compartment and then fuse with the next [1]. This mechanism would require that the flow of proteins through the secretory pathway be controlled at at least two points in each vesicle-mediated step. First, secretory proteins in transit would be sorted from the proteins that reside in each organelle. This molecular sorting event could occur prior to or during vesicle budding. Second, the transport vesicles once formed must have determinants that guarantee that they fuse with and release their contents into the appropriate acceptor organelle.

We anticipate that the specificity inherent in both vesicle budding and fusion will ultimately be dictated by precise protein-protein interactions and an understanding of these processes will hinge on the identification of the proteins involved. Two general approaches have been used to identify gene products involved in vesicle transport. Rothman and colleagues have used biochemical methods to reconstitute vesicular transport between Golgi cisterna in vitro [2]. Additional cell-free assays have since been developed to study transport between the ER and Golgi in yeast and mammals [3,4,5]. The mammalian Golgi assay was used to purify two protein factors, known as NSF and SNAP, that are required for fusion of vesicles with the Golgi membrane. The number of additional proteins that can be isolated by this approach will be limited by the availability of precise biochemical assays for substeps of the overall transport reaction.

The other approach is to identify genes whose products are required for protein transport in vivo by mutations in the yeast *Saccharomyces cerevisiae*. Secretion defects are studied by the use of temperature conditional mutations since protein secretion is an essential cellular process and mutations in secretion functions are lethal. We have focused our attention

© 1990 by Elsevier Science Publishing Co., Inc.
Molecular Biology of Atherosclerosis
A.D. Attie, Editor

on nine genes identified by mutations that block the secretory pathway at the point of transport between the ER and the Golgi [6,7]. At the nonpermissive temperature, these mutants accumulate excess ER-like membrane structures filled with core-glycosylated forms of secretory and vacuolar proteins [5,8,9,10]. These genes may encode proteins that are structural elements of the transport vesicles themselves or that act transiently in the assembly or disassembly of transport vesicles.

Mutations in genes whose products are required at multiple stages of the secretory pathway should exhibit a phenotype that corresponds to the earliest step in the pathway at which the gene product is required. Transport from the ER is the first vesicle mediated step in the secretory pathway and functions required for all vesicle mediated steps should principally exhibit a defect at this step. Therefore the class of ER-blocked *sec* mutants could include both general functions involved at all vesicle transport steps as well as functions only required for transport from the ER.

In this paper we present a combined morphological and genetic analysis of the early *SEC* genes. This analysis confirms the expectation that transport between the ER and Golgi is vesicle-mediated and characterizes the transport intermediate as a population of vesicles 50 nm in diameter. In addition, our work provides a more detailed classification of the early *SEC* genes into either vesicle forming functions or vesicle fusion functions. Confirmation for our assignment of function comes from the finding that two genes shown here to be required for vesicle fusion in vivo are the yeast homologs of mammalian proteins required for vesicle fusion in vitro [11,12].

RESULTS AND DISCUSSION

Small vesicles accumulate in a subclass of sec mutants

It is particularly difficult to identify the membrane-bounded organelles that comprise the secretory pathway in *S. cerevisiae* since these organelles are not as prominent as they are in many mammalian cell types. Two factors probably contribute to the low steady state abundance of secretory organelles in yeast. First, yeast have a limited capacity for secretion compared to those mammalian cell types dedicated to the production of secretory proteins. Second, the proteins that are secreted by yeast are exported rapidly with a transit time of about five minutes [7] instead of the much longer transit times that are typical of mammalian cells. Therefore yeast secretory organelles are most readily studied in *sec* mutants since the imposition of a *sec* mutant block in the pathway will cause copious quantities of the organelles to accumulate before the point of the block.

To identify membrane structures that could be intermediates in protein transport from the ER to the Golgi apparatus we looked for differences in the membrane morphology produced by mutations in genes required for transport of secretory proteins from the ER. Each of nine mutant strains (*sec12, sec13, sec16, sec17, sec18, sec20, sec21, sec22, sec23*) was grown at the permissive (17° C) then shifted to the nonpermissive temperature (37° C). Cells were fixed rapidly with glutaraldehyde, postfixed with potassium permanganate and prepared for electron microscopy . As found previously [6], all of the mutants had accumulated ER membranes after one hour at 37°C and in the three mutant strains *sec17, sec18*, and *sec22* small membrane-bounded vesicles had proliferated (Fig 1).

Quantitative comparison of the different *sec* mutants was achieved by counting vesicles in random cell sections and normalizing the number to cell volume. The nine mutants were grouped into two general classes. The number of small vesicles (smaller than 80 nm in diameter) in wild type cells was used as a standard for comparison, although not all such vesicles in a wild type cell can be assumed to be derived from the ER. Class I mutants *sec12, sec13, sec16,* and *sec23* contained approximately the same number of vesicles as wild type. Class II mutants *sec17, sec18,* and *sec22* contained about five times the number of vesicles as wild type (Fig 2). Two mutants, *sec20 and sec21*, contained an intermediate number of vesicles.

Class II mutants accumulate about 3,000 vesicles per cell body. A significant fraction of the total cellular membrane is thus incorporated into these vesicles as the total surface area of 3,000 spheres 50 nm in diameter is equivalent to about one third the area of the plasma membrane.

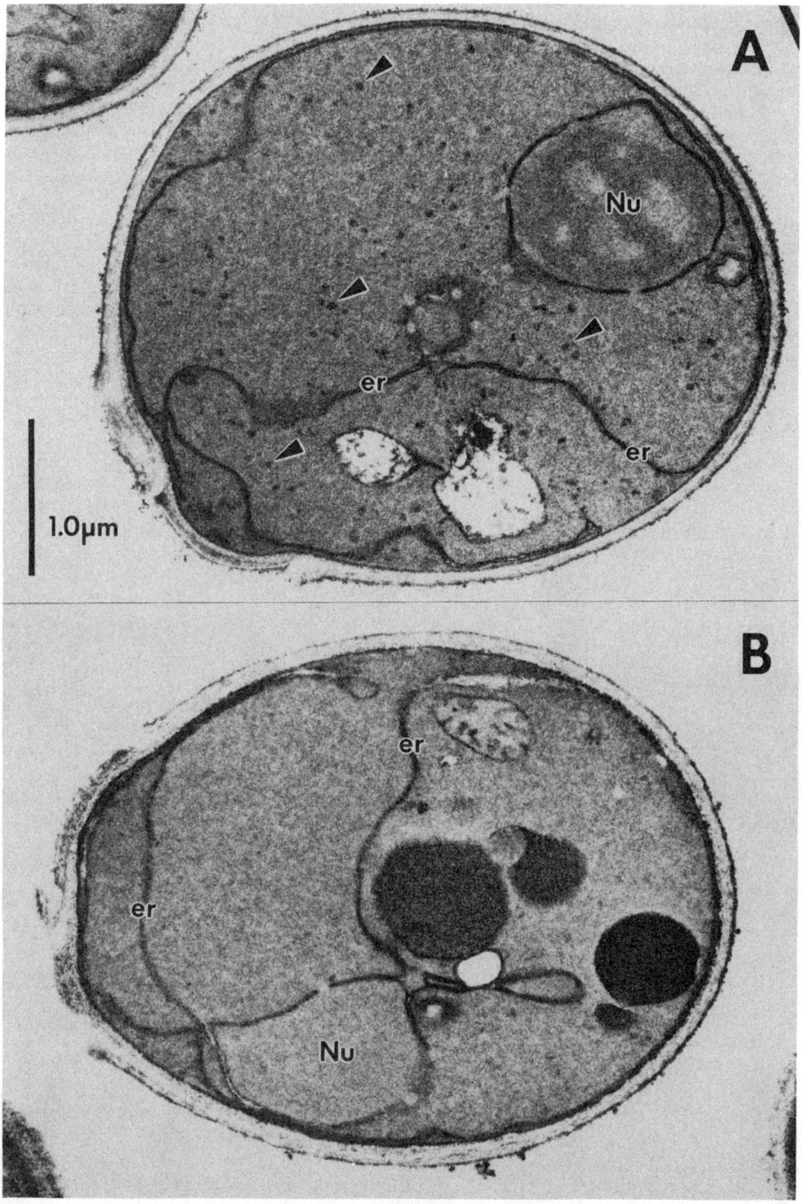

Figure 1. Thin section electron micrographs of yeast cells fixed with potassium permanganate. (A) *sec17-1* grown at 17°C then for 1 hr at 37°C showing accumulation of ER and 50 nm vesicles. (B) *sec12-4* grown at 24°C then for 1hr at 37°C. showing accumulation of ER only. Nu: nucleus. er: endoplasmic reticulum. Arrows in A point to representative 50 nm vesicles

Epistatic relationship between the two mutant classes

Accumulation of 50 nm vesicles in the class II mutants at the nonpermissive temperature suggested that the vesicles represent an intermediate stage in the transport pathway between the ER and the Golgi apparatus and that the products of the class II genes are required for the consumption of the vesicles. In this view, the class I genes could be required for vesicle formation. To address the order of function of the *SEC* genes, we performed epistasis tests by counting vesicles in doubly mutant strains with a mutation from both class I and class II. Double-mutants were constructed by genetic crosses and vesicles were counted in cells incubated one hour at 37° C prior to fixation. All of the double mutants contained about the same density of vesicles as the respective class I single mutants (Fig 2). The vesicles that accumulate at the nonpermissive temperature in the class II mutants must therefore depend on the function of the class I genes for their formation. That the 50 nm vesicles depended on at least four genes (class I) for formation and at least three genes (class II) for their consumption implied that transport from the ER results from the sequential action of the class I genes producing 50 nm vesicles followed by the action of the class II genes to consume this vesicle intermediate.

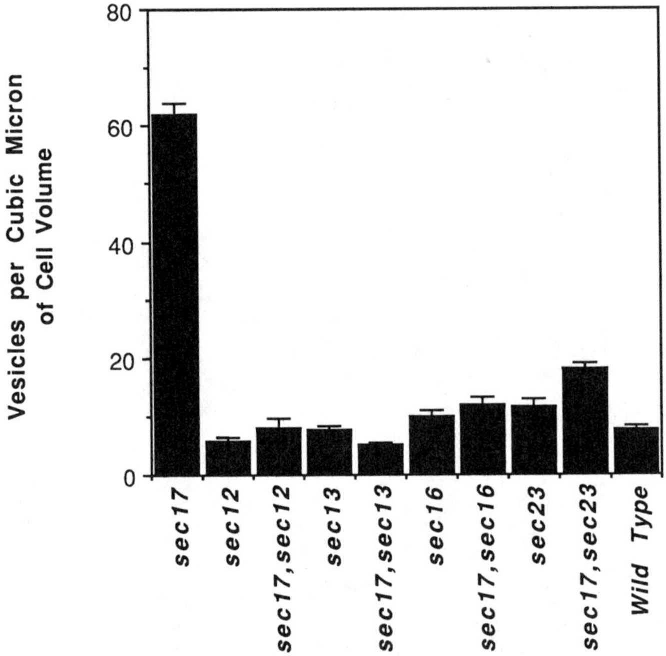

Figure 2 The influence of *sec* mutations on accumulation of 50 nm vesicles in sec17 mutant strains. Numbers of vesicles counted in electron micrographs are expressed as the density of vesicles per cell volume. Double mutants epistasis tests with *sec18* and *sec22* gave similar results. The mean vesicle densities for at least 32 cell sections for each strain are given with error bars indicating the standard error of the mean.

Genetic interactions among sec mutations

Independent evidence for two groups of mutants acting at distinct stages of the transport pathway between the ER and the Golgi apparatus was provided by interactions between *sec* mutations. While constructing doubly mutant strains, we found that certain combinations of *sec* mutations produced inviability at 24°C, which is ordinarily a permissive growth temperature for all of the *sec* mutant alleles (Table 1). The crosses between mutants in each of the nine genes under examination gave two different outcomes. In most cases, more than 95% of the spores were viable and the double mutants grew well at 24°C. All of the strains used in the morphological epistasis tests were from crosses of this type. For a few of the crosses, about one fourth of the spores did not produce visible colonies after five days at 24° C (Table 1). Analysis of the viable meiotic products from these crosses by complementation tests showed that the inviable spores were double mutants. The combination of *sec17* and *sec18* was lethal and five of the six possible pairwise combinations of the four genes *sec12*, *sec13*, *sec16*, and *sec23* were inviable. These groups exactly coincided with the two classes of mutations defined by vesicle accumulation (Fig 3). The specificity of interactions between sec genes suggests close functional connections within subsets of the class I and class II genes.

Table 1. Growth of Double Mutants at 24°C

	sec13-1	*sec16-1*	*sec17-1*	*sec18-1*	*sec20-1*	*sec21-1*	*sec22-1*	*sec23-1*
sec12-1	-	-	+	+	+	+	+	+
sec13-1		-	+	+	+	+	+	-
sec16-1			+	+	+	+	+	-
sec17-1				-	+	+	+	+
sec18-1					+	+	+	+
sec20-1						+	+	+
sec21-1							+	+
sec22-3								+

- Double mutant does not form a visible colony after five days at 24°C
+ Double mutant grows as well as wild type at 24°C

This phenomenon of mutations in different genes producing lethality when in combination is known as synthetic lethality and can be an indication of functional interaction between gene products [13]. The synthetic lethality produced by certain combinations of *sec* mutations can be interpreted in the following way. The inviability of particular combinations of *sec* mutations at 24°C implies that mutations in each of the genes, *SEC12*, *SEC13*, *SEC16*, *SEC17*, *SEC18* and *SEC23*, produce partial defects at 24°C. Although these defects are not sufficient on their own to affect cell growth overtly, particular combinations of mutations in one cell can lead to extreme growth defects. One explanation for the apparent synergism between some *sec* mutations would be that each mutation causes cells to be sickly at 24°C because of a partial defect in protein secretion or membrane organization. In certain double mutants, these defects would add to one another to the point of lethality. This explanation based on additive effects of general sickness is not supported by our data. Consider the four genes *SEC16*, *SEC23*, *SEC17* and *SEC18*. For all alleles tested, the combinations *sec17 sec18* and *sec16 sec23* grow very slowly or are dead at 24°C. If these synergistic effects were simply the result of addition of general growth defects then some or all of the other four pairwise combinations of these genes should similarly produce inviability. The other gene combinations such as *sec17 sec16* and *sec18 sec23* are healthy at 24°C. Thus, the synthetic lethality of mutant combinations is quite specific for certain gene combinations indicating specific functional relationships between *SEC17* and *SEC18* and among the four genes *SEC12, SEC13, SEC16* and *SEC23*. The combined genetic and morphological data imply that the products of *SEC12*, *SEC13*, *SEC16*, and *SEC23* cooperate in the formation of transport vesicles and that the products of *SEC17* and *SEC18* cooperate to execute vesicle fusion.

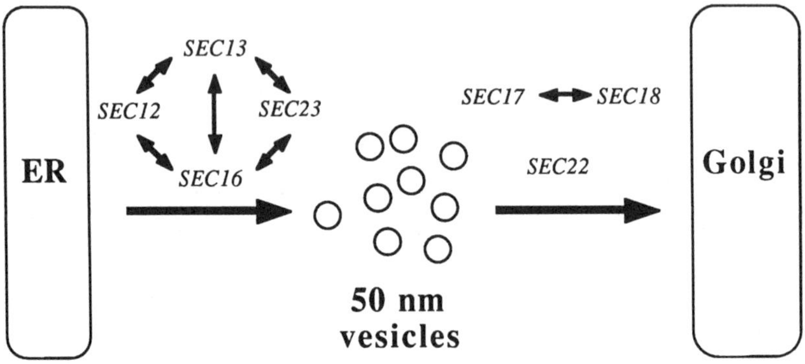

Figure 3. Role of early *SEC* genes in either the formation or consumption of a vesicular intermediate in transport between the ER and Golgi apparatus. Genes whose temperature sensitive mutant alleles exhibit synthetic lethal interactions are connected by arrows.

Functions required for vesicle fusion are conserved.

Protein transport between the cisterna of the mammalian Golgi apparatus is mediated by transport vesicles of about the same size as the vesicles accumulated in yeast class II mutants [14]. Fusion of Golgi-derived vesicles with their target membranes has been reconstituted *in vitro* [2] and proceeds in two distinct stages [15]. The two stages are defined by successive chemical blocks in the fusion process. The first block, imposed by the nucleotide analog GTPγS, causes coated transport vesicles to accumulate [15, 16]. These vesicle coats are neither morphologically nor immunologically related to clathrin coats [14]. Uncoated vesicles are accumulated at the second stage if the transport factor, NEM-sensitive fusion protein (NSF), is inactivated by treatment with an alkylating agent [17]. NSF was purified by its ability to restore transport activity to N-ethylmaleimide treated membranes [18]. The cloned hampster gene for NSF shows high amino acid sequence similarity to yeast Sec18p. Further, the yeast protein can functionally replace the mammalian protein since yeast cytosol can provide NSF activity to mammalian membranes in a manner dependent on the presence of the wild type *SEC18* gene product [11].

The mammalian SNAPs (Soluble NSF Attachment Proteins) were identified as proteins that bring about the association of NSF with Golgi membranes [19]. The SNAP proteins were purified by their ability to restore transport activity to membranes that were washed with high salt [20]. Under the appropriate conditions, yeast cytosol will restore activity to salt washed mammalian membranes. The SNAP activity in yeast extract is sensitive to *sec17* mutations and is corrected by addition of purified SNAP indicating that Sec17p is the yeast homolog of SNAP [2]. The homology between Sec17p and SNAP has now been confirmed by comparison of the *SEC17* gene sequence [Kaiser and Schekman unpublished observations] and a partial peptide sequence of SNAPα [Clary and Rothman personal communication].

These findings imply that NSF/Sec18p and SNAP/Sec17p are vesicle fusion functions that are conserved on two levels. First, the sequence similarities and functional interchangability of the yeast and mammalian proteins show high evolutionary conservation. Second, Sec17p and Sec18p act in ER to Golgi transport in yeast and can function in transport between stacks of the mammalian Golgi in vitro indicating that fundamentally the same molecular mechanism may be employed in transport from the ER to the Golgi and between the individual Golgi stacks. Since *SEC17* and *SEC18* appear to be general fusion functions acting at multiple steps of the pathway, other proteins must impose specificity on the fusion process to insure that vesicles derived from the ER fuse with the appropriate acceptor organelle.

Analysis of the biochemical interaction between NSF and SNAP shows saturable membrane binding of both proteins and indicates that these proteins form a roughly stoichiometric complex on the membrane [19]. The synthetic lethal interaction between temperature sensitive *sec17* and *sec18* mutations can now be understood in the following way. At 25°C a functional complex will form if either Sec17p or Sec18p is mutant but the complex will not form if both proteins are mutant. These findings give hope that the other synthetic lethal interactions between genes required for vesicle formation will also have as their basis simple physical interactions between their respective gene products.

Table 2. Properties of SEC gene products proposed to function in transport vesicle fusion.

Gene	Molecular weight	Genetic interaction	Location	Function or Homolog
SEC18	84 kD	SEC17	peripheral membrane	NSF
SEC17	34 kD	SEC18	peripheral membrane	SNAP
SEC22	unknown	none	unknown	unknown

SEC genes required for vesicle formation.

The process of vesicle budding is likely to be driven by the assembly of a regular protein scaffold that molds the vesicle membrane. An obvious candidate for such a protein would be clathrin which is assembled as a membrane bound coat on the cytoplasmic face of coated pits and endocytic vesicles. However, clathrin is unlikely to have a role in the formation of 50 nm vesicles studied here since genetic data shows clathrin not to be required for ER to Golgi transport [21] and as mentioned above, the related Golgi-derived vesicles have protein coats that do not contain clathrin. A possible function of some or all of the *SEC* genes that appear to be required for vesicle formation would be as structural components of a novel kind of vesicle coat.

Preliminary characterization of these gene products show that they are associated with intracellular membranes consistent with a role as vesicle components. Sec12p is an integral membrane glycoprotein [22], Sec13p and Sec23p appear to be cytoplasmic by their intrinsically hydrophilic amino acid sequences and cell fractionation studies show that both proteins are peripherally associated with a cell membrane [23 and Kaiser and Schekman unpublished data], Sec16p is a hydrophilic protein whose location is not yet known [Kaiser and Schekman unpublished data].

The genetic and morphological data indicate that Sec12p, Sec13p, Sec16p and Sec23p act in the process of vesicle budding or some ER function that precedes the vesicle forming step and that these gene products may function cooperatively as a multisubunit complex. These proteins could be structural components of the 50 nm vesicles or they could be components of the ER membrane that act transiently in vesicle assembly.

Table 3. Properties of SEC gene products proposed to function in transport vesicle formation.

Gene	Molecular weight	Genetic interaction	Location	Function or Homolog
SEC12	70 kD	SEC13, SEC16, SAR1	integral membrane	unknown
SEC13	34 kD	SEC12, SEC16, SEC23	peripheral membrane	unknown
SEC16	~190 kD	SEC12, SEC13 SEC23, SAR1	unknown	unknown
SEC23	85 kD	SEC13, SEC16	peripheral membrane	unknown

REFERENCES

1. G. Palade, Science **189**, 347-358 (1975).
2. W. E. Balch, W. G. Dunphy, W. A. Braell and J. E. Rothman, Cell **39**, 405-416 (1984).
3. D. Baker, L. Hicke, M. Rexach, M. Schleyer and R.Schekman, Cell **54**, 335-344 (1988).
4. H. Ruohola, A. K. Kabcenell and S. Ferro-Novick, J. Cell Biol. **107**, 1465-1476 (1988).
5. C. J. M. Beckers, D. S. Keller and W. E. Balch, Nature **339**, 397-398 (1989).
6. P. Novick, C. Field and R. Schekman, Cell **21**, 205-215 (1980).
7. P. Novick, S. Ferro and R. Schekman, Cell **25**, 461-469 (1981).
8. B. Esmon, P. Novick and R. Schekman, Cell **25**, 451-460 (1981).
9. T. Stevens, B. Esmon and R. Schekman, Cell **30**, 439-448 (1982).
10. D. Julius, R. Schekman and J. Thorner, Cell **36**, 309-318 (1984).
11. D. W. Wilson, C. A. Wilcox, G. C. Flynn, E. Chen, W.-J. Kuang, W. J. Henzel, M. R. Block, A. Ullrich and J. E. Rothman, Nature **339**, 355-359 (1989).
12. D. O. Clary, I. C. Griff and J. E. Rothman, Cell **61**, 709-721 (1990).
13. T. C. Huffaker, M. A. Hoyt and D. Botstein, Ann. Rev. Genet. **21**, 259-284 (1987).
14. L. Orci, B. S. Glick and J. E. Rothman, Cell **46**, 171-184 (1986).
15. L. Orci, V. Malhotra, M. Amherdt, T. Serafini and J. E. Rothman, Cell **56**, 357-368 (1989).
16. P. Melançon, B. S. Glick, V. Malhotra, P. J. Weidman, T. Serafini, M. L. Gleason, L. Orci and J. E. Rothman, Cell **51**, 1053-1062 (1987).
17. V. Malhotra, L. Orci, B. S. Glick, M. R. Block and J. E. Rothman, Cell **54**, 221-227 (1988).
18. M. R. Block, B. S. Glick, D. A. Wilcox, F. T. Wieland and J. E. Rothman, Proc. Nat. Acad. Sci. **85**, 7852-7856 (1988).
19. P. J. Weidman, P. Melançon, M. R. Block and J. E. Rothman, J. Cell Biol. **108**, 1589-1596 (1989).
20. D. O. Clary and J. E. Rothman, J. Biol. Chem. **265**, 10109-10117 (1990).
21. G. Payne and R. Schekman, Science **230**, 1009-1014 (1985).
22. A. Nakano, D. Brada and R. Schekman, J. Cell Biol. **107**, 851-863 (1988).
23. L. Hicke and R. Schekman, EMBO J. **8**, 1677-1684 (1989).

Organ-Specific Variations on the Mechanism of Protein Topogenesis: Two Examples from Brain and Liver

Vishwanath R. Lingappa,*† Charles D. Lopez,*†† and
Steven L. Chuck*†**

Departments of Physiology, Medicine,† Microbiology,** and the Graduate Program in Endocrinology,††
University of California, San Francisco, California*

ABSTRACT

Recent data suggests that the early events in protein secretion and transmembrane integration at the endoplasmic reticulum, long believed to occur constitutively, may sometimes be regulated. Based on these findings, arguments in favor of receptor-mediated transmembrane integration are advanced. These events are proposed to occur in an organ-specific fashion in some cases during ontogeny, in other cases during phylogeny. Their implications for physiology and medicine are considered.

INTRODUCTION

Conventional Protein Biogenesis

The biogenesis of newly synthesized secretory and and integral membrane proteins involves a number of compartmentalized cellular processes. The early events include targetting to and translocation across or into the membrane of the endoplasmic reticulum (ER). Subsequent events in the secretory pathway include trafficking to and through the Golgi apparatus, the Trans Golgi Network and then either the plasma membrane (via secretory vesicles and granules) or the lysosomal membrane. Whereas the nascent chain crosses the ER membrane directly in the early stages of the secretory pathway, the later transport events are mediated by fission and fusion of the membrane vesicles bearing the newly synthesized protein. Assembly into multi-subunit complexes and acquisition of various covalent post-translational modifications occur subsequent to appearance of the chain in the lumen of the ER. In at least some cases, specific modifications serve as recognition markers to distinguish protein fates (e.g. phosphomannosylation of lysosomal enzymes diverts them from the secretory pathway [51]).

Discrete sequences within the newly synthesized protein appear to direct many of these topology-determining processes [1]. Thus, signal sequences have been implicated in targetting and translocation, and stop transfer sequences in termination of chain translocation during integral transmembrane protein biogenesis at the ER membrane [45]. At least some, and perhaps all, of these so-called "topogenic" sequences are believed to engage proteinaceous machinery in or around the appropriate cellular membranes to effect a particular step in biogenesis. A major problem in eukaryotic cell biology has been to identify the different classes of topogenic sequences and their cognate receptors, and determine how they work. At present, several proteins have been identified or implicated as receptors for some of the early events of biogenesis. The role of signal recognition particle (SRP) and its receptor (SRP receptor) have been intensively studied [2, 3, 4, 5] Similarly, various proteins including a Signal Sequence Receptor (SSR), signal peptidase and HSP 78 have been implicated in directing translocation [6, 7, 8]. A combination of genetic and biochemical approaches in yeast has identified a number of gene products involved in these processes [46, 47].

© 1990 by Elsevier Science Publishing Co., Inc.
Molecular Biology of Atherosclerosis
A.D. Attie, Editor

While specific receptor proteins for stop transfer remain to be identified, indirect evidence suggests that they exist [9]. An appealing view is that the integration of membrane proteins can be divided into two steps. Initially, a receptor-mediated event terminates the translocation of a chain on its way into the ER lumen via a specialized translocation channel. Subsequently, dissembly of the channel and reformation of an intact bilayer establishes thermodynamically favorable conditions for passive integration of the hydrophobic protein domain into the bilayer. Evidence suggesting that the channel is aqueous supports this two-step view of transmembrane integration [10]. Otherwise, it is hard to imagine how a hydrophobic transmembrane domain could stop in an aqueous channel in the absence of the thermodynamic driving force provided by hydrophobic interactions with membrane lipids. Such a two-step receptor-mediated model of transmembrane integration has some unexpected implications for organ-specific variation on the mechanism of protein biogenesis, as will be discussed.

A striking feature revealed thus far is the remarkable *conservation* of the signals which direct the early events in protein biogenesis. That is, signal and stop transfer sequences appear interchangeable between tissues and across wide species barriers. This observation suggests that a universal set of events are involved in the biogenesis of all secretory or integral membrane proteins, although the details of their molecular mechanism remain, in large measure, unknown. Remarkably, inspite of this apparent functional conservation, the primary amino acid sequence of signal and stop transfer sequences are quite divergent [11]. Moreover, the rules by which common structural features can be identified are relatively uninformative [12]. While some data has emphasized the degeneracy of signal sequences implying that the functional interactions are therefore relatively non-specific [13] other studies suggest that the sequence divergence represents evolution of signal sequences for optimal translocation of their particular passenger sequences [14]. These latter studies have demonstrated that even subtle changes in the passenger sequence will result in significant loss of efficiency of translocation. Moreover this loss of translocation efficiency can be due to alterations in any of several signal-receptor interactions [14]. By implication, the crucial features for signal-receptor interaction remain to be identified and understood.

Unconventional Protein Biogenesis

Regulation is a recognized feature of the later steps in the secretory pathway (e.g. in the case of constitutive versus stimulus-triggered pathways of protein secretion), but until recently has not been recognized in the early steps of targetting, translocation and integration into the membrane of the ER. Instead, these early events have been viewed as "constitutive" features of protein biogenesis dictated solely by the presence or absence of functional topogenic sequences within the nascent chain. Thus, while biological control of gene expression has been studied intensively at the transcriptional [15], translational [16] and post-translational [17] levels, the possibility of *co-translational* regulation of protein phenotype by control of receptor interactions of targetting, translocation or integration at the ER membrane have not been investigated. Recent data, to be discussed below, suggests that indeed, at least some of these early co-translational events of protein biogenesis can also be regulated. These data raise the possibility of *organ-specific variations* of the general mechanisms of protein biogenesis. Such variations can explain paradoxical features of certain specialized proteins which are not easily encompassed by the conventional concepts of the early events of protein biogenesis. This notion is an appealing way of reconciling the fact that different proteins are likely to face different problems in biogenesis and might solve them by engaging different components of the common translocation machinery or by engaging common components in different ways. The studies discussed here present two possible examples of organ-specific variation of translocation. The first example, the prion protein (PrP) may be a biosynthetic variation that occurs with development, that is, true regulation of protein topogenesis. The second example, apolipoprotein B, may be an example of a variation selected through evolution. In that case, the variation results in dissociation of the normally coupled events of stop transfer and transmembrane integration, in order to accomodate the unusual physical properties of a lipid-carrying soluble protein chain.

An Experimental Approach

Much of our current understanding of targetting, translocation and transmembrane integration in the ER derives from studies in cell-free systems (figure 1). These systems have allowed manipulation of topogenic sequences, "passenger" protein domains (i.e. the regions of the protein which are substrates for the targetting, translocation and integration events to be directed), as well as the protein machinery in the ER membrane that carries out the event dictated by a topogenic sequence. Several sources are commonly used to generate the components needed to reconstitute mRNA translation and subsequent newly synthesized protein translocation in such systems. In particular, two sources are commonly used to generate cytosolic lysates containing ribosomes and soluble factors, namely wheat germ [18, 19] and rabbit reticulocytes [20, 21]. Both of these systems are remarkably active in protein synthesis when provided either a native mRNA or cell-free transcription product (of a cloned cDNA engineered behind appropriate nucleotide sequences for transcription and translation), together with amino acids and energy substrates necessary for translation and translocation [22, 23]. If at least one of the amino acids added is radiolabelled (e.g. ^{35}S methionine), the newly synthesized products can be specifically detected and studied by SDS-PAGE. The addition of microsomal membranes derived from the ER allows these newly synthesized proteins the opportunity to translocate to the vesicle lumen, the equivalent of the lumen of the ER in vivo [24, 25]. Typically these membranes are prepared from dog pancreas, but similar ER containing fractions from a variety of other tissues and species have been demonstrated to function in this manner.

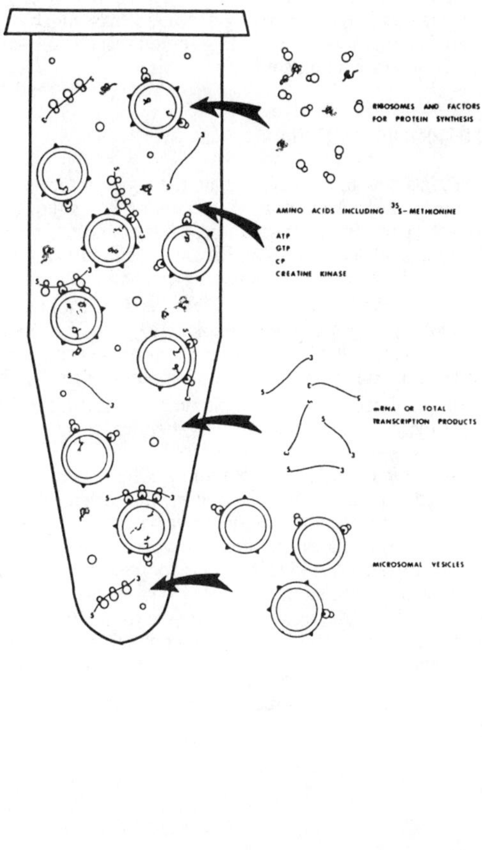

Figure 1.

In such a system, three distinct methods are commonly used to assay translocation across the endoplasmic reticulum. First, the translation products can be digested with exogenously added proteases after completion of synthesis [24]. Newly synthesized (i.e. radiolabelled) chains within the lumen of the added membrane vesicles will be protected from digestion. Solubilization of the membrane with low concentrations of non-ionic detergents should render the protease protected products accessible to digestion, and controls for the formation of protease resistant conformations. The proteolysis assay can be adapted to the study of transmembrane proteins if antibodies are available to distinguish translocated epitopes from those exposed to the cytosol, resulting in a shift to lower molecular weight during post-translational proteolysis.

A second assay of protein topology derives from the fact that certain post-translational modifications (e.g. N-linked glycosylation) are believed to occur exclulsively in the ER luminal space and hence are powerful markers for translocation of protein domains [26].

Finally, treatment of the microsomal membrane-containing translation reaction by extraction with sodium carbonate at pH 11.5 is a procedure designed to distinguish proteins integrated into the bilayer from those which are soluble or peripherally associated with the membrane [27].

Using these assays in conjunction with a panel of antisera to defined epitopes, it is possible to determine the topology of the newly-synthesized protein of interest. The results of such an analysis can be compared to the topology generated in living cells either by expression in cultured mammalian cells or by microinjection of Xenopus oocytes [28]. By applying molecular genetic approaches to engineering of passenger protein and topogenic sequence domains, features of the coding region responsible for particular aspects of topology can be identified and studied.

BIOGENESIS OF THE PRION PROTEIN

The prion protein (PrP) is a developmentally regulated glycoprotein of brain whose normal function is unknown [29]. An abnormal isoform of PrP is the only known component of the infectious particle causing scrapie, a transmissible, degenerative neurologic disease of animals related to similar diseases in humans (for example, Creutzfeld-Jacob Disease and Gerstmann-Straussler syndrome). Because the normal (PrP^{C}) and scrapie-associated (PrP^{Sc}) isoforms of PrP are identical in amino acid sequence and post-translational modifications some other explanation must be sought for their apparent functional distinction (i.e. the latter but not the former seems to cause scrapie). Our studies were initially designed to investigate the hypothesis that the difference between PrP^{C} and PrP^{Sc} involved regulated pathways of biogenesis resulting in different topology (and hence functions) for these proteins of seemingly identical structure.

We found that expression of cloned hamster PrP in the wheat germ cell-free translation system supplemented with dog pancreas microsomal membranes resulted in the polypeptide achieving a transmembrane disposition, as predicted by hydropathy analysis of the PrP coding sequence (see figure 2a) [30]. Surprisingly however, a very different topology predominated when PrP was translated in rabbit reticulocyte lysates (RRL) supplemented with the same dog pancreas microsomal membranes [31]. In this system, over 60% of all chains appeared to be secreted into the lumenal space (see figure 2b), with the remainder displaying a transmembrane disposition identical to that which predominated in WG . Previously, no such discrepancy in topology of a newly synthesized protein has been observed between the WG and RRL cell-free systems supplemented with dog pancreas microsomal membranes.

It should be noted that PrP is member of the class of proteins which contain a phosphatidylinositol-glycan linkage added after cleavage of a sequence at the carboxy terminus [49, 50]. It appears that both membrane associated and completely translocated forms of PrP as well as both PrP^{C} and PrP^{Sc} isoforms from brain contain the carboxy terminal phosphatidylinositol linkage which is cleavable by a phosphatidylinositol-linked phospholipase C. Thus, both the transmembrane and secretory forms discussed here are thus likely to contain this linkage. Nevertheless, the term "secretory" will be used to to describe the form of PrP whose translocation has not been terminated at the transmembrane regions TM1 and TM2 in order to simplify the discussion. However, this convention should not be taken to imply the lack of a phosphatidylinositol linkage to the membrane.

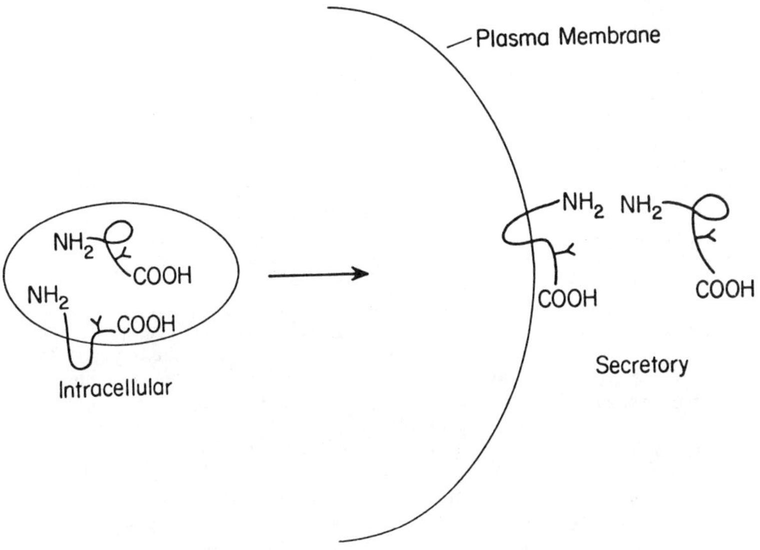

Figure 2

To understand why nascent PrP was predominantly in a transmembrane topology in WG but not in RRL, several experimental approaches were taken. First, mutagenesis of the PrP chain was used to identify domains crucial for stop transfer at the first predicted transmembrane region (TM1). From these studies two regions were implicated in determining a transmembrane topology for PrP [32]. Not surprisingly, the transmembrane regions themselves were necessary for transmembrane topology. Remarkably, however an additional region, comprising the 16 codons which immediately preceed the first transmembrane region (predicted by hydropathy analysis) appears to be required for transmembrane topology. These 16 codons (henceforth termed Stop Transfer Effector or STE sequence) comprised a lysine rich, non-hydrophobic domain. Mutants lacking STE but which leave the hydrophobic domain entirely intact, failed to stop and were completely translocated across the bilayer. A spatial relationship between STE and TM1 was suggested by the demonstration that engineering a 117 codon "spacer" between these sequences. disrupted transmembrane topology as efficiently as deletion of either sequence. Moreover, when STE was engineered adjacent to the codons for a hydrophobic domain normally completely translocated across the ER membrane, the resulting chimera was expressed as a protein stopping at the normally translocated hydrophobic domain both in cell-free systems and in Xenopus oocytes. These results suggested that STE was engaging a receptor in the microsomal membrane resulting in stop transfer and subsequent integration at the adjacent hydrophobic domain.

We then demonstrated that STE-TM1 would predictably confer a transmembrane topology at TM1 when engineered into heterologous secretory and transmembrane protein coding regions and expressed in WG. In contrast, expression of these chimeric proteins in RRL failed to stop transfer at TM1 [33]. Thus, the stop transfer activity conferred to heterologous chimeras by STE and TM1 was distinctive in its system preference (e.g. WG versus RRL) as is the case for wild type PrP. These results were not only consistent with regulation of stop transfer by receptor interactions with STE, alone or in conjunction with TM1, but also suggested that multiple interactions were involved.

Mixing experiments were also performed to determine whether trans-acting factors in one system conferred that system's topologic behavior to the other system. Our results suggest a cytosolic factor present in RRL which appears to mask the ability of STE-TM1 to direct transmembrane topology, resulting instead, in a molecule which is completely translocated.

How do these cytosolic and membrane factors work? One possibility is that the cytosolic factor is a "foldase" directing nascent PrP into a pathway of protein folding that masks STE thereby preventing engagement of the membrane factor (see figure 3). In the absence of the interaction with the cytosolic factor, nascent PrP engages the receptor in the membrane, stops and is integrated --unless the hydrophobic domain has been deleted, in which case translocation machinery is re-engaged. Alternatively, a co-translational modification of the chain directed by the cytosolic factor might achieve the same goal. Studies are currently in progress to purify and characterize this cytosolic factor in the RRL cytosol as well as the putative receptor in the ER membrane whose interaction with STE or TMI is altered or abolished by the preceding action of the cytosolic factor. Regardless of the precise mechanism by which these factors work, an important principle is suggested by these studies. Namely, that a particular chain (in this case PrP) can engage machinery in the cytosol and membrane in a fashion which subjects stop transfer to regulation (in this case by the presence or absence of a cytosolic activity). Thus, stop transfer --and perhaps topogenic sequence-receptor interactions more generally, are not necessarily just constitutive events dictated by the coding information of the protein to be translated. Rather, topogenesis can be regulated to confer alternate fates and hence, functional phenotypes, to a single protein coding region. In this way the coding potential of the genome and the ability of an organism to respond rapidly and precisely to changes in its environment is greatly expanded. It should be noted that these studies are suggestive of the receptor-mediated view of stop transfer described above and suggest that it may involve numerous and complex levels of control both cytosolic (e.g. action of the factor in RRL) and intra-membrane (e.g. STE-membrane interaction). Another implication of these studies grows out of a consideration of the unusual biology of PrP. Although our studies have involved the ostensibly "normal" isoform of PrP, it is tempting to speculate that this protein's unusual biogenesis is somehow related to its bizarre biology.

The debate over the pathogenesis of scrapie has generally been framed in terms of either a virus [34] or a novel infectious agent which lacks nucleic acid [35] as the etiologic agent of the disease. However, we wish to propose another hypothesis, namely that scrapie is a disorder of aberrant expression of a an endogenous gene whose regulation is quite unusual. The properties of this gene product and its mode of regulation mimic key features of an infectious disease. Nevertheless, we suggest that it may be more fruitful to formulate the problem of scrapie differently. The key features of our alternative hypothesis on scrapie pathogenesis are that:

i) A crucial "normal" function for PrP is to trigger cell death at key points in development of the nervous system. This is a plausible notion not only because neuronal death appears to be the final consequence of PrP "inoculation" in scrapie [35] but also because PrP in normal animals appears to be deveopmentally expressed in early post-natal life, a time of tremendous cell death necessary for ontogeny and remodelling of the mature central nervous system [36] .

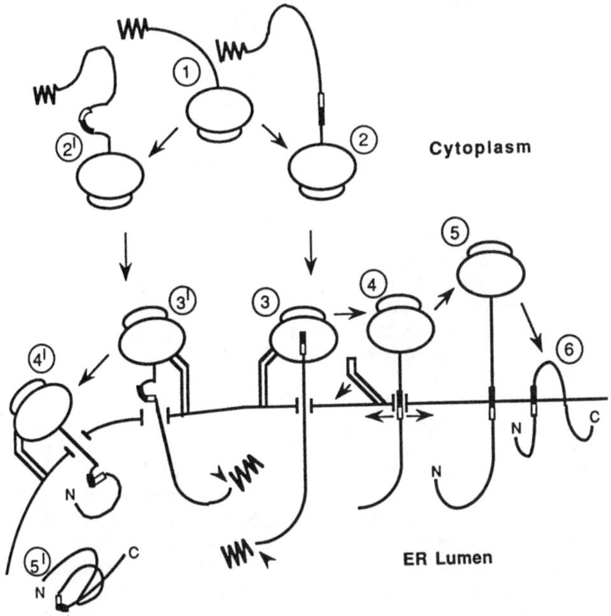

Figure 3.

PATHOGENESIS OF SCRAPIE

ii) Some members of the gene or gene family encoding both PrP and its receptor proteins are highly conserved through animal evolution in both function and regulation. Sequence data revealing 90% conservation of amino acids of PrP outside of the signal sequence between human and rodent PrP are consistent with this hypothesis [37] .

iii) Like conventional infectious agents, but unlike most endogenous genes, regulation of PrP synthesis involves *positive* rather than *negative* feedback control.

These features would enable an *exogenous* PrP to engage the machinery intended for use by *endogenous* genes should they be activated. Once engaged, the machinery triggers activation of endogenous PrP expression. Thus, it appears as if the exogenous PrP is "replicating" when in fact it is endogenous PrP that is being expressed in response to the exogenous stimulus. Strain and species-specific characteristics of scrapie transmission between animals may relate to either a) subtle changes in affinity of exogenous PrP for receptors and hence ability to activate the endogenous machinery or b) the response of the immune system to exogenous PrP thereby affecting whether or not it ever achieves access to receptor-bearing cells. Thus, for example, two alleles of PrP differing by two point mutations are associated with a dramatic change in incubation time for development of scrapie in mice [48, 52].

If PrP is a gene for programmed cell death the third assumption seems plausible because homeostasis must be maintained at other than the cellular level --since the action triggered culminates in cell death, an irreversible event incompatible with a "steady state". If homeostasis is maintained at the tissue, organ, or organismal level, then positive feedback control is a nice way of insuring that a cell that has been signalled to die does not linger on, but rather, proceeds to death forthwith. Thus, PrP has an extraordinary regulation because it functions in a feedback loop more complex than that of conventional hormones and effectors. In this regard it is not surprising that PrP is a developmentally regulated glycoprotein of brain, since ontogeny of the nervous system probably represents one of the most complex products of development and evolution, requiring the use of "every trick in the book" of regulatory control.

What is the role of the unusual biogenesis of PrP in this model? It is tempting to speculate that the transmembrane form is the effector of neuronal cell death. For example, its resemblance to an ion channel subunit suggests a possible mechanism for this functional role [38, 39]. Assembly of a channel in the membrane might be a swift means of triggering either a particular signalling event or may be the mechanism of cell death itself. The secretory form of PrP, in contrast, would serve a radically different function, not only because its folding and physical properties are totally different from that of the transmembrane form, but also because phosphatidylinositol anchor cleavage will release it from the cell, perhaps unmasking yet another unknown physiologic function in communication with other cells.

An interesting analogy can be seen in the control of B lymphocyte differentiation. An immature B lymphocyte bears surface IgM because the mu heavy chain is expressed as a transmembrane protein. Upon activation of surface IgM (by its cognate antigen), differentiation to a mature plasma cell proceeds with concomitant expression of mu heavy chain as a secretory form, as a result of alternate RNA splicing. Thus the change in topology of this gene product is the key to converting a transmembrane receptor into a secretory effector. In the case of PrP, regulation of secretory and transmembrane expression takes place by another mechanism other than RNA splicing (i.e. receptor alterations at the ER membrane, see above). Moreover, initial expression of PrP is in the secretory form with the transmembrane form being the induced phenotype culminating in cell death.

In the disease scrapie, control over this remarkable form of regulation is lost through the fortuitous introduction of a modified form of exogenous PrP. The modification which distinguishes normal from "infectious" PrP could be fairly trivial, perhaps aggregation , altered conformation, or some other association which allows a few molecules of the heterologous PrP to evade immune surveillance mechanisms and achieve access to neuronal cell surfaces. The key feature of scrapie pathogenesis would be that, once triggered, an irreversible terminal event of differentiation, neuronal cell death, occurs.

If the three initial assumptions prove correct, why is this formulation a more fruitful view of scrapie and related disorders? Let us consider an analogy to other endocrine systems. Suppose insulin were placed under positive feedback control resulting in a disease of "infectious hypoglycemia". Insulin injection would trigger an increase rather than a decrease in endogenous insulin production (i.e. positive rather than negative feedback) which would result in both hypoglycemia and a higher "titer" of the infectious agent, i.e. insulin itself, which could be demonstrated by injection into another individual. Formulation of the problem as one of aberrant gene expression rather than of infectious hypoglycemia would likely lead to an understanding of its pathogenesis. The problem with this analogy of course is that the insulin gene is not under positive feedback control and is involved in maintaining glucose homeostasis rather than in killing the cell of synthesis. This is precisely why recognized prion diseases may be so unusual: they involve a protein with unprecedented forms of regulation involving the transcriptional and co-translational levels and because they are designed to control a remarkable developmental sequence of events rather than to simply maintain homeostasis. If this general principle is correct however, there may be a plethora of as yet unrecognized degenerative or developmental disorders in which subtle or profound aberrations in control at the level of expression or topology in any of a large family of such genes have profound effects on protein phenotype.

The topogenesis of PrP suggests a model for developmental regulation of protein localization at the level of translocation and stop transfer in the ER. Another implication of a receptor-mediated hypothesis for stop transfer and transmembrane protein biogenesis is that alteration of topogenic sequences through evolutionary time might dissociate stop transfer from transmembrane integration and thereby allow specialized problems of biogenesis to be overcome. Apolipoprotein B (apo B) appears to be a candidate for such a process.

BIOGENESIS OF APOLIPOPROTEIN B

Apo B is a huge amphipathic secretory polypeptide which serves to solubilize cholesterol and triglyceride allowing their efficient transport and metabolism. Paradoxically, apo B is known to be insoluble in the absence of lipid and yet achieves the bulk of its lipid at a site distal to that of protein synthesis in the rough ER [40]. This paradox might be explained by a variation on the theme of translocation and transmembrane integration. Suppose that the newly-synthesized apo B chain were to periodically stop in the ER membrane, only to subsequently restart its translocation rather than being integrated into the bilayer. Such transient stop events would provide an opportunity (during the short-lived transmembrane state) for association of the chain with a minimum complement of lipid necessary for the chain to remain soluble during transit from site of synthesis to site of lipid loading. Even though apo B is an extremely hydrophobic polypeptide, it lack regions of more than 13 contiguous hydrophobic amino acid residues, and is therefore unlikely to integrate into the membrane following a stop transfer event.

Technical obstacles made this hypothesis difficult to test. First of all, the size of full-length apo B (500,000 daltons) precludes efficient full-length translation in existing cell-free systems. Secondly, efficient translocation has been established with microsomal membranes from pancreas which does not engage in lipoprotein assembly, but not from liver or intestine, the tissues which synthesize apo B. We bypassed the first of these problems by noting that mutants encoding amino-terminal fragments of apo B considerably smaller than the full-length species were also packaged as lipoprotein particles and secreted [41]. This suggested that the key issues could be addressed by expression of managable amino-terminal fragments of apo B. The second problem also seemed moot since non-liver or intestine-derived mammalian cell lines transfected with apo B are capable of lipoprotein particle assembly and secretion [42]. This suggested that any apo B specific variations in biogenesis are the result of recruitment or use of a subset of components found in all cells rather than the presence of specialized biosynthetic machinery unique to liver or intestine.

We expressed the amino terminal 70 kd of apo B (apo B-15) in the WG cell-free translation system [43]. In the presence of dog pancreas microsomal membranes the chain was glycosylated, suggesting translocation of at least some domains. Upon digestion with proteases a heterogeneous topology was observed: some chains were fully protected from proteases, which others were converted into smaller-sized fragments. All of the fragments were reactive to peptide-specific antisera to the authentic amino terminus of apo B. This finding was consistent with a model in which heterogeneous transmembrane orientation observed was a result of progressively longer amino terminal lengths of apo B being translocated across the ER membrane.

This topologically heterogeneous set of apo B-15 chains was subjected to carbonate extraction at pH 11.5 and found to be completely extractable from the membrane, in contrast to the behavior of a known intregral transmembrane protein included in the extraction as a control. This result suggested that all members of the heterogeneous family of apo B-15 transmembrane chains were either within an aqueous channel or associated with the membrane in some fashion distinct from that of a typical integral membrane protein.

Finally, digestion with proteases was carried out under "pulse-chase" conditions to determine if there was a temporal relationship in generation of the family of transmembrane proteolytic fragments. That is, synthesis was initiated in the presence of ^{35}S cystiene and, after a period of incubation (the pulse time), the reaction was supplemented with cold cystiene in 10^3-fold excess and synthesis allowed to proceed for the time necessary to complete the initiated chains, before treatment with RNAse A to terminate further translation. At this point an aliquot was taken to ice for digestion of proteases and subsequent aliquots taken at later time points for the same purpose (chase points). Analysis by SDS-PAGE revealed that the heterogeneous family of transmembrane apo B-15 chains observed on steady state labelling could be resolved into a precursor-product relatonship in which the cohort of newly completed apo B-15 chains progressed through a series of stages characterized by larger transmembrane (protease-protected) products, culminating in full-length chains. Moreover, apyrase (an ATP degrading enzyme), was observed to block this apparent post-translational lengthening of the protected domains.

Thus, apo B-15 displays two extraordinary features in its biogenesis: first, a progressive family of transmembrane intermediates *post-translationally* converted into a seemingly fully translocated species; second, a distinctive association of the transmembrane intermediates with the ER membrane (see figure 4). Taken together, the data suggest that apo B biogenesis may indeed involve dissociation of the receptor-mediated features of stop transfer from events leading to transmembrane integration . Why should apo B display a variation on the general mechanism of protein translocation? This unusual mode of biogenesis combines features typical of a secreted protein (which ultimately, it is) with that of a transmembrane polypeptide (which it is transiently). Such a variation may be necessitated by the extreme hydrophobicity or other unusual amphipathic physical properties of apo B together with the paradox of assembly described earlier. The precise reason for the series of transmembrane pause events remains unclear. One tempting hypothesis is that these events allow partial dissembly of the aqueous channel and association of a small complement of lipid rendering the chain soluble in the ER lumen pending accumulation of the bulk of lipid in a distal compartment. Studies are in progress to extend the analysis to larger lengths of apo B, to correlate these findings in cell-free systems with those observed in living cells, and to identify the machinery and sequence determinants by which these unusual events are triggered.

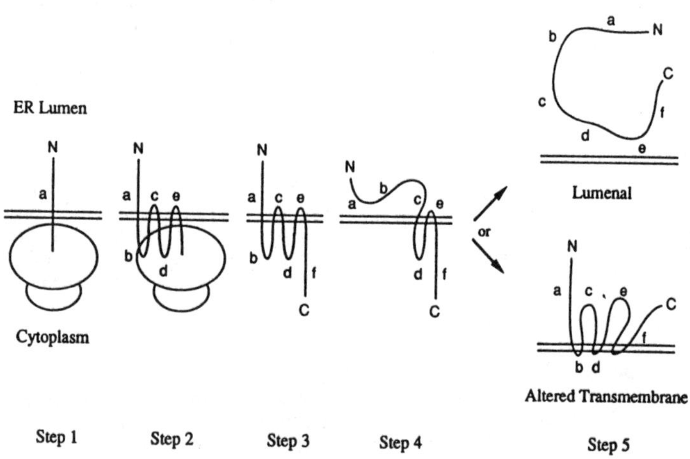

Figure 4.

Regardless of the precise molecular details, the existence of such a specialized variation on translocation for apo B has some intriging implications. First of all, the corollary of "Murphy's Law" (anything that can go wrong, will go wrong) applied to pathogenesis suggests that genetic as well as degenerative lesions in this translocational process may occur in humans. In either scenario, a consequence may be improper lipid packaging and ultimately, aberrant lipoprotein particles. In view of studies suggesting [44] that a large fraction of patients with hypercholesterolemia have a defect in their LDL and since apo B is the sole polypeptide component of apo B, aberrations in this pathway may be a cause of some cases of hypercholesterolemia by giving rise to altered VLDL and hence abnormal LDL. Secondly, knowledge of the details of this pathway may provide an additional approach to therapy of hypercholesterolemia through the use of drugs which specifically inhibit these steps.

BALANCE AND PROSPECTS

We have seen that a universal mechanism of eukaryotic secretory and transmembrane protein biogenesis can have organ-specific variations. In one case, a special cytoplasmic factor distinct from the core machinery for chain translocation seems to be involved (RRL cytosolic factor and PrP). In another case the conserved universal machinery is engaged by a protein (apo B) to carry out an unusual, if not unique, mechanism. These findings suggest that the ER is more than a barrier to be overcome in protein export, playing in some cases a regulatory role in gene expression (e.g. alternate fates of PrP) and in other cases as a specialized assembly line for biogenesis of proteins with unusual properties. It seems likely that many other examples of proteins using these two mechanisms will be found, as well as entirely different variations on the mechanisms of protein biogenesis.

REFERENCES

1. G. Blobel, Proc. Natl. Acad. Sci. USA 77 ,1496-1500 (1980).
2. V. Siegel and P. Walter, Cell 52, 39-49 (1988).
3. R. Gilmore, P. Walter and G. Blobel, J. Cell Biol. 95, 470-477 (1982).
4. D.I. Meyer, E. Krause and B. Dobberstein, Nature 297, 647-650 (1982).
5. T. Connolly and R. Gilmore, Cell 57, 599-610 (1989).
6. M. Weidmann, T. Kurzchalia, E. Hartmann, and T.A. Rapoport, Nature 328, 830-833 (1987).
7. C. V. Nicchitta and G. Blobel, Cell 60, 259-269 (1990).
8. J. P. Vogel, L. M. Misra and M. D. Rose, J. Cell Biol. 110, 1885-1 1897 (1990).
9. N. K. Mize, D. W. Andrews and V. R. Lingappa, Cell 47, 711-719 (1986).
10. R. Gilmore and G. Blobel, Cell 46, 497-505 (1985).
11. M. E. E. Watson, Nuc. Acids Res. 12, 5145-5164 (1984).
12. G. Von Heijne, J. Mol. Biol. 184, 99-105 (1985).
13. C. A. Kaiser, D. Preuss, P. Grisafi and D. Botstein, Science 235, 312-316 (1987).
14. D. Andrews, E. Perara, C. Lesser and V. R. Lingappa, J. Biol. Chem. 263, 15791-15798 (1988).
15. T. Maniatis, S. Boodbourn, and J.A. Fischer, Science 236, 1237-1242 (1987).
16. M.W. Hentze, S. Wright Caughman, T.A. Rouault, J.G. Barriocanal, A. Dancis, J. P. Harford, and R. D. Klausner, Science 238, 1570-1573 (1987).
17. J. Bonifacino, S. A. McCarthy, J.E. McGuire, T. Nakayama, D.S. Singer, R. D. Klausner and A. Singer, Nature 344, 247-252 (1990).

18. B. E. Roberts and B.M. Patterson Proc. Natl. Acad. Sci. USA 70, 2330-2334 (1973).
19. C.W. Anderson, J. W. Straus, and B. S. Dudock, Meth. Enz. 101, 635-644 (1983).
20. H. R. B. Pelham and R. J. Jackson, Eur J. Biochem 67, 247-256 (1976).
21. W. C. Merrick, Meth. Enz. 101, 606-615 (1983).
22. D. Melton, Nuc. Acids Res. 12, 7035-7056 (1984).
23. D. Anderson and G. Blobel, Meth Enz. 96, 367-375, (1983).
24. G. Blobel and B. Dobberstein, J. Cell Biol. 67, 835-851 (1975).
25. G. Blobel and B. Dobberstein, J. Cell Biol. 67, 852-867 (1975).
26. F.N. Katz, J.E. Rothman, V. R. Lingappa, G. Blobel, and H. F. Lodish, Proc Natl. Acad. Sci. USA 74, 3278-3282 (1977).
27. Y. Fujiki, A. L. Hubbard, S. Fowler, and P.B. Lazarow, J. Cell Biol. 93, 97-102 (1982).
28. R. E. Rothman, D. W. Andrews, C. Calayag and V. R. Lingappa, J. Biol. Chem. 263, 10470-10480 (1988).
29. M. McKinley, B. Hay, V. R. Lingappa and S. B. Prusiner, Dev. Biol. 121, 105-110 (1987).
30. B. Hay, I. Lieberburg, R. Barry, S. B. Prusiner and V. R. Lingappa, Mol. Cell. Biol. 7, 914-919 (1987).
31. B. Hay, S. B. Prusiner and V. R. Lingappa, Biochem. 26, 8110-8115 (1987).
32. C. S. Yost, C. D. Lopez, S. B. Prusiner, R. M. Myers and V. R. Lingappa, Nature 343, 669-672 (1990).
33. C. D. Lopez, C. S. Yost, S. B. Prusiner, R. M. Myers and V. R. Lingappa, Science 248, 226-229 (1990).
34. R.I. Carp, P.A. Merz, R.J. Kascsak, G.S. Merz and H.M. Wisniewski, J. Gen. Virol 66, 1357-1368 (1985).
35. S. B. Prusiner, New Eng. J. Med. 317, 1571-1581 (1987).
36. W. M. Cowan, J. Fawcett, D. O'Leary and B. Stanfield, Science 225, 1258-1265 (1984).
37. H. A. Kretzschmar, L. E. Stowring, D. Westaway, W. H. Stubblebine, S.B. Prusiner and S. J. DeArmond DNA 5, 315-324 (1986).
38. J. F. Bazan, R. J. Fletterick, M. P. McKinley, and S. B. Prusiner, Prot. Eng. 1, 125-135 (1987).
39. C.J. Brandl and C.M. Deber, Proc. Natl. Acad. Sci. USA 83, 917-923 (1986).
40. C.A. Alexander, R. L. Hamilton and R. J. Havel J. Cell Biol. 69, 241-263 (1976).
41. S.G. Young, Bertics, L. K. Curtiss, J. L. Witztum, J. Clin. Invest. 79, 1831-1841 (1987).
42. B. Blackhart, Z. Yao and B.J. McCarthy, personal communication.
43. S. Chuck, Z. Yao, B. Blackhart, B.J. McCarthy and V. R. Lingappa, Nature in press.
44. G. L. Vega and S. M. Grundy, J. Clin. Invest. 78, 1410-1414 (1986).
45. V. R. Lingappa, J. Clin. Invest 83, 739-751 (1989).
46. P. Novick, S. Ferro, and R. Schekman Cell 25, 461-469 (1981)
47. H. Ruohola, K.A. Kabcenell and S. Ferro-Novick J. Cell Biol. 107, 1465-1476 (1987).
48. G. Carlson, D.T. Kingsbury, P. Goodman, S. Coleman, S.T. Marshall, S.J. DeArmond, D. Westaway, and S.B. Prusiner Cell 46, 503-511 (1986)
49. M. G. Low, Biochem. J. 244, 1-13 (1987).
50. N. Stahl, D.R. Borchelt, K. Hsiao, and S. B. Prusiner Cell 51, 229-240 (1987).
51. S. Kornfeld, J. Clin. Invest. 77, 1-6 (1986).
52. D. Westaway, P.A. Goodman, C.A. Mirenda, M.P. McKinley, G.A. Carlson, and S. B. Prusiner, Cell 51, 651-662 (1987).

Regulation of VLDL Assembly and Secretion

Roger A. Davis

University of Colorado Health Sciences Center, Denver, Colorado

ABSTRACT

The secretion of VLDL varies in response to metabolic state. The availability of apo B, the major protein component of nascent VLDL, determines the capacity of the liver cell to secrete triglyceride. While the secretion rate of apo B varies greatly, the mRNA abundance does not, suggesting that post-transcriptional mechanisms regulate its secretion. In contrast, the editing of apo B mRNA, a process that determines the ratio of apo B48:apo B100 of apo B secreted by rat liver, does change in parallel with the secretion of VLDL, suggesting coordinate regulation. We examined the mechanisms through which VLDL secretion is regulated post-transcriptionally. Hepatic rough microsomes were incubated with trypsin. While about half of both molecular weight forms of apo B were degraded, albumin was not. Similar experiments using smooth ER and Golgi fractions showed that apo B in these fractions was not accessible to trypsin. Furthermore, the microsomes remained intact and oriented right side out as demonstrated by a 90% latency for the dephosphorylation of mannose-6-phosphate. Additional data show that the trypsin accessible pool of apo B could not be chased into the trypsin insensitive pool, suggesting that there are two distinct pools of apo B in the endoplasmic reticulum that are not inter-convertible. Using a different experimental approach to examine the possible cytoplasmic distribution of apo B, monoclonal antibodies prepared against apo B were covalently linked to magnetic beads. When incubated with microsomes, the magnetic beads could specifically isolate microsomes, whereas magnetic beads containing control IgG and IgG against albumin could not.

The combined data suggest that apo B is inefficiently translocated across the endoplasmic reticulum, forming two functionally distinct pools. The translocated, trypsin insensitive pool is assembled into VLDL and is secreted. The nontranslocated, trypsin accessible pool does not enter the lumen and is degraded. Regulated translocation of apo B may be the post-translational mechanism responsible for controlling VLDL assembly and secretion.

INTRODUCTION

Very low density lipoproteins (VLDL) are the major lipid secretory product of the liver. They serve as a vehicle with which to transport triglycerides from the liver to extrahepatic cells where they are utilized for energy and anabolic purposes. In addition, most, if not all, higher density plasma lipoproteins are derived from VLDL. Thus, the rate of VLDL secretion will play an important role in determining plasma lipoprotein levels.

Apolipoprotein B (apo B) is an usually large amphipathic protein that is essential for the assembly of VLDL. There are two molecular weight forms of apo B: the large form (apo B100) is over 512 Kd, whereas the small form (apo B48) is derived from the amino-terminal 48% of apo B100. Both forms are

Published 1990 by Elsevier Science Publishing Co., Inc.
Molecular Biology of Atherosclerosis
A.D. Attie, Editor

derived from a single gene and mRNA via a unique editing of the mRNA. At nucleotide 6666, a C can be edited to a U, forming a UAA termination codon resulting in a truncated form of apo B [1-3]. Rat liver secretes both molecular weight forms, which can be varied in response to metabolic state [4-6]. Feeding rat sucrose-rich diets increases the activity of many lipogenic enzymes, increases the synthesis of all lipids secreted as VLDL, increases the secretion of all VLDL components and increases the ratio of apo B48:apo B100 of the secreted apo B [4]. Conversely, fasting rats for three days causes a coordinate decrease in the activity of lipogenic enzymes, decreases the synthesis of all lipids secreted as VLDL and decreases the ratio of apo B48:apo B100 of the secreted apo B [5,6]. These data suggest that there is a coordinate regulation of lipogenic enzymes, VLDL assembly, and apo B secretion.

Editing of apo B is sensitive to metabolic state [7]. Thus, fasted rat liver has a marked reduction in apo B mRNA editing and a selective decrease in the secretion of apo B48 (no change in the secretion of apo B100) [7]. While regulated editing can explain the change in edited apo B mRNA, since the total amount of apo B mRNA does not change, a post-transcriptional mechanism is likely responsible for the decreased secretion of total (apo B100 plus apo B48) by the fasted rat liver [7].

Previous studies show that movement out of the rough endoplasmic reticulum is the rate limiting step governing apo B secretion [8]. Additional data show that only a fraction of _de novo_ synthesized apo B is secreted, the remainder is degraded [8]. Degradation appears to occur in a compartment proximal to the Golgi [9].

The goal of these studies was to better characterize the interaction of apo B with the endoplasmic reticulum and to determine its topography.

RESULTS

Rat livers were homogenized and separated into individual membrane fraction by sucrose density ultracentrifugation, as described in detail [8]. Equal quantities of rough, smooth and Golgi were subjected to trypsin at a concentration previously found to degrade all of the proteins in the presence of detergents to disrupt the membranes. After incubation at room temperature for 30 minutes, excess soybean trypsin inhibitor was added (to inhibit further degradation by trypsin) and the microsomes were re-isolated by centrifugation and subjected to Western blot analyses using antibodies against apo B or albumin. The results showed that in the rough microsomes (but not the smooth ER or Golgi) about 50% of both molecular weight forms of apo B were degraded by trypsin, whereas albumin was not. Furthermore, adding deoxycholate to the microsomes prior to the reaction caused a complete degradation of both albumin and apo B, these data show that there was sufficient trypsin present. These data suggest that a portion of apo B is exposed on the cytoplasmic surface of the endoplasmic reticulum.

To rule out the possibility that the microsomes were orientated the wrong way or that they were permeable to the trypsin, we assayed the ability of glucose-6-phosphatase to dephosphorylate mannose-6-phosphate. Glucose-6-phosphate is an integral protein of the endoplasmic reticulum that has its active site located in the lumen. Its natural substrate (glucose-6-phosphate) gains access to the active site because it is translocated into the lumen by a specific transporter. While glucose-6-phosphatase can dephosphorylate mannose-6-phosphate, under normal conditions this reaction is prevented because the glucose-6-phosphate transporter cannot transport mannose-6-phosphate. Thus, the inability to dephosphorylate mannose-6-phosphate is an accurate determinant for demonstrating the orientation of the microsomes and the degree to which they have remained intact. Measurement of the dephosphorylation of mannose-6-phosphate showed that there was almost no activity and that none of the treatments significantly affected this. Furthermore, adding deoxycholate to the microsomes prior to the assay show a marked 10-fold elevation of the ability to dephosphorylate mannose-6-phosphate, showing the enzyme was active. None of the treatments affect any of these parameters. The combined data show that the accessibility of apo B to the degradation by trypsin is not caused by either leaky membranes or improperly oriented microsomes.

We next determined if the trypsin accessible pool of apo B was a transient form that eventually becomes trypsin insensitive. Cultured rat hepatocytes were pulse labeled with ^{35}S-methionine and then chased with a 1000-fold excess of unlabeled methionine, as described in detail [8]. A total microsomal fraction was obtained at each time point and subjected to trypsin. The results show that the portion of apo B that was accessible to trypsin increased, but did not decrease during the time of the chase. These data suggest that the trypsin accessible form of apo B is not a transient form.

We sought another independent method to determine whether there is a portion of apo B in the endoplasmic reticulum that is exposed on the cytoplasmic surface. Monoclonal antibodies raised against rat apo B [9] were covalently coupled to magnetic beads. These were then incubated with microsomes and then isolated by a magnet. The activity of glucose-6-phosphatase was used to determine the recovery of microsomes. Beads containing the antibodies against apo B specifically isolated microsomes, whereas beads linked to either control IgG (from non-inoculated mouse serum) and IgG against rat serum albumin show non-specific affinity for microsomes. These data suggest that epitopes to rat apo B exist on the cytoplasmic surface of the endoplasmic reticulum.

DISCUSSION

The combined data suggest that there are two functionally distinct pools of apo B in the endoplasmic reticulum: a translocated intralumen form that is not accessible to trypsin and enters the VLDL assembly/secretion pathway, and a non-translocated form exposed on the cytoplasmic surface and is degraded by trypsin.

Our results are consistent with the concept that membrane integration obfuscates translocation. As a result of inefficient translocation, there are two functionally distinct pools of apo B in the ER. One pool is located in the lumen as demonstrated by protection from exogenous trypsin. This pool of apo B participates in the assembly of VLDL. The other pool is not translocated into the lumen; it is integrated into the cytoplasmic surface of the ER as shown by the ability of exogenous trypsin to degrade it. The pool of non-translocated apo B does not enter the Golgi, is shunted from the secretory pathway and does not participate in the assembly of VLDL. Non-translocated apo B probably accounts for the apo B that is synthesized but is not secreted by cultured rat hepatocytes [8].

These conclusions are supported by four different experimental protocols: 1) selective degradation by trypsin of endogenous apo B in rough microsomes as shown by Western blotting using specific polyclonal and monoclonal antibodies against apo B, 2) demonstration that the apo B that is accessible to trypsin is derived from the membrane associated pool of apo B, 3) demonstration that the _de novo_ synthesized [^{35}S]-labeled apo B degraded by trypsin does not enter the trypsin insensitive pool, and 4) demonstration that apo B epitopes recognized by monoclonal antibodies are present on the surface of microsomes and are effective antigens to immuno-isolate hepatic microsomes.

Apo B could be translocated arrested by a stop-transfer sequence, resulting in its integration into the ER as a trans-membrane protein. While several different algorithm analyses of the amino acid sequence of apo B predict that no hydrophobic domains in apo B are sufficiently long to act as alpha-helical trans-membrane spanning domains, it is possible that other motifs (e.g., beta-sheets) may span the membrane bilayer. Our data do not address this issue of whether or not apo B is a trans-membrane protein in the ER. The trypsin-sensitive non-translocated pool of apo B could be all cytoplasmic or the major part of a protein that is trans-membrane. The manner in which apo B is integrated into the ER membrane may be similar to the way porin is integrated into the outer membrane of E. coli. Porin does not contain any trans-membrane spanning domains, but does contain hydrophobic beta-sheets. Like porin, apo B contains several hydrophobic beta-sheet structures situated throughout the molecule. Apo B associates with lipoproteins mainly via these hydrophobic beta-sheets. It is reasonable to expect that similar structures are responsible for the association of apo B with the ER membrane.

Diversion of apo B from the VLDL assembly pathway may provide an explanation for the observation that only a fraction of apo B that is synthesized is secreted; the remainder is degraded intracellularly. The recent finding that proteolytic fragments of apo B exist in the rough and smooth microsomal fractions, but not in Golgi fractions, led to the hypothesis that the degradation of apo B occurs in the ER [9].

While all of the trypsin degraded apo B was membrane associated, clearly not all of the membrane-associated apo B was degraded by trypsin. This suggests that apo B is also integrated into the lumenal side of the ER membrane, which is probably the initial step in the assembly of VLDL. Physiologic variation in the translocation of apo B may provide a unique mechanism accounting for the post-translational regulation of VLDL assembly.

REFERENCES

1. Chen, S.-H., Habib, G., Yang, C.-Y., Gu, Z.-W., Lee, B.R., Wang, S.A., Silberman, S.R., Cai, S.-J., Deslypere, J.P., Rosseneu, M., Gotto, A.M., Jr., Li, W.-H., and Chan, L., Apolipoprotein B-48 is the product of a messenger RNA with an organ-specific in-frame stop codon. Science 238, 363-366 (1987)
2. Hospattankar, A.V., Higuchi, K., Law, S.W., Meglin, N., Cartwright, J., and Brewer, H.B., Jr., Identification of a novel in-frame translational stop codon in human intestine apoB mRNA. Biochem. Biophys. Res. Commun. 148, 279-285 (1988)
3. Powell, L.M., Wallis, S.C., Pease, R.J., Edwards, Y.H., Knott, T.J., and Scott. J., A novel form of tissue-specific RNA processing produces apolipoprotein-B48 in intestine. Cell 50, 831-840 (1987)
4. Boogaerts, J.R., Malone-McNeal, M., Archambault-Schexnayder, J., and Davis, R.A., Dietary carbohydrate induces lipogenesis and very-low-density lipoprotein synthesis. Am. J. Physiol. 246, E77-E83 (1984)
5. Davis, R.A., Boogaerts, J.R., Borchardt, R.A., Malone-McNeal, M., and Archambault-Schexnayder, J., Intrahepatic assembly of very low density lipoproteins. Varied synthetic response of individual apolipoproteins to fasting. J. Biol. Chem. 260, 14137-14144 (1985)
6. Davis, R.A., Dluz, S.M., Leighton, J.K. and Brengaze, V.A., Increased translatable mRNA and decreased lipogenesis are responsible for the augmented secretion of lipid-deficient apolipoprotein E by hepatocytes from fasted rats. J. Biol. Chem. 264, 8970-8977 (1989)
7. Leighton, J.K., Joyner, J., Deines, M.D., Zamarripa, J. and Davis, R.A. (In Press) J. Lipid Res.
8. Borchardt, R.A., and Davis, R.A., J. Biol. Chem. 262, 16394-16402 (1987)
9. Davis, R.A., Prewett, A.B., Chan, D.C.F., Thompson, J.J., Borchardt, R.A., and Gallaher, W.R., J. Lipid Res. 30, 1185-1196 (1989)

An "LPL-Receptor" on Adipocytes Regulates LPL Degradation

André Bensadoun,[1] Laura A. Cisar,[2] Arlene J. Hoogewerf, Mary Cupp, and Jeffrey Weinfeld[3]

Cornell University, Division of Nutritional Sciences and the Division of Biological Sciences, Ithaca, New York

INTRODUCTION

Lipoprotein lipase (LPL; EC 3.1.1.34) is a ubiquitous enzyme synthesized in most extrahepatic tissues. The enzyme is synthesized in parenchymal cells, and by unknown mechanisms, the enzyme is transported to the luminal surface of capillary endothelium where it interacts with heparan sulfate proteoglycans [1,2]. Hydrolysis of plasma VLDL and chylomicron triglycerides to free fatty acids by the action of LPL is the only mechanism whereby plasma triglyceride fatty acids are transferred to tissues. Inhibition of LPL by specific antibodies results in a quantitative inhibition of triglyceride hydrolysis in chylomicrons and VLDL [3]. Robinson and associates [4] have clearly shown that LPL activity in a given tissue parallels the influx of triglyceride fatty acids into the tissue. During the past five years considerable progress was achieved in our understanding of the regulation of LPL. As the enzyme from several sources was purified, tools necessary for molecular studies of the regulation of the enzyme, namely, antibodies, immunoprecipitation techniques and cDNA's became available. In isolated rat adipocytes [5] Ong, et al. demonstrated that insulin increases the synthetic rate of the enzyme and this was paralleled by an increase in LPL mRNA. However, in studies with 3T3-L1 adipocytes Semenkovich, et al. [6] concluded that regulation by insulin occurred mainly at the post-transcriptional and post-translational levels. Similarly Doolittle, et al. [7] reports that regulation of LPL in response to fasting and feeding occurs mainly at the post-translational level. A post-translational mechanism which could be significant *in vivo* is modulation of the degradation rate of the enzyme with little or no change in its synthetic rate. Three laboratories [8,9,10] have shown, independently, that in isolated cultured adipocytes 70 to 80 percent of the newly synthesized enzyme is degraded before appearing in the extracellular fluid. This report summarizes recent experiments conducted with avian cultured adipocytes on the regulation of secretion and degradation of LPL.

Avian preadipocytes can be prepared from chicken adipose tissue by digestion with collagenase followed by low speed centrifugation [8]. A somatovascular fraction containing preadipocytes pellets whereas mature adipocytes float. The somatovascular fraction is then seeded in plastic dishes and differentiated over a two week period in the presence of a cell culture medium (RPMI 1640) enriched with insulin, glucose and dexamethasone. This system is very convenient to measure enzyme synthesis, secretion and degradation rates.

---

[1]To whom correspondence should be addressed.

[2]Present address UMDNS School of Osteo. Medicine, Department of Physiology, 675 Hoes Lane, Piscataway, NJ 08854

[3]Present address: University of Arizona, Department of Entomology, Forbes Hall, Tucson, AZ 85721

© 1990 by Elsevier Science Publishing Co., Inc.
Molecular Biology of Atherosclerosis
A.D. Attie, Editor

To calculate these parameters a pulse chase protocol is utilized. Dishes of cells are pulsed with L[^{35}S]-methionine for 60 min and then chased over a 60 min period [8]. Enzyme mass and radioactivity is then measured in the intracellular pool, the cell surface, and the medium at various times during the chase. Fig. 1 presents the results of such an experiment, which was conducted in the presence of either control medium or medium supplemented with 10 U/ml heparin. Heparin was employed to perturb enzyme turnover, since this agent was known to enhance LPL secretion in cultured adipocytes [11,12].

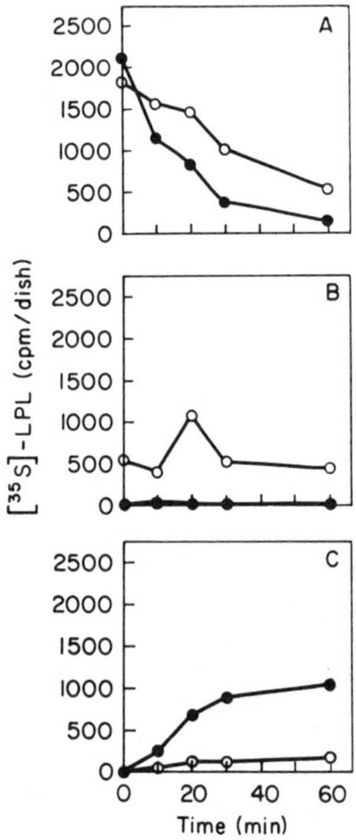

FIG. 1. Secretion of labeled lipoprotein lipase (LPL) during a 60-min chase in the presence of control medium (open circles) or medium containing 10 units/ml heparin (closed circles). Adipocytes were radiolabeled with L-[^{35}S]methionine (100 μCi/dish, 5 μM L-methionine) for 60 min at 37°C and then chased for the indicated time in label-free medium containing 105 μM L-methionine. Radiolabeled lipoprotein lipase was isolated by immunoadsorption followed by electrophoresis and fluorography. A cell extract; B, heparin releasable surface associated; and C, medium ^{35}S-labeled lipoprotein lipase.

Heparin treatment results in a more rapid loss of enzyme from the cellular compartment. By 60 min, in control cells, 76% of the radiolabeled LPL had been secreted or degraded. This was increased to 92% in the presence of heparin. Plotting the same data as semi-logarithmic plots indicates that the labeled LPL is lost from the intracellular pool by a first order process. There is no suggestion of concentration of newly synthesized enzyme in storage vesicles. In the presence of heparin there was very little detectable enzyme at the cell surface, whereas in control cells, a relatively constant level of labeled enzyme was measured. After 60 min of chase, radiolabeled LPL in the medium was 5-fold higher in heparin-treated cells than in control cells. The synthesis rates were calculated as the product of the intracellular pool size and the first order rate constant of disappearance of labeled LPL from the intracellular compartment. Secretion rates were directly measured by ELISA in medium samples. The degradation rates were then obtained by difference. These calculations yielded the following mean values for 3 experiments:

TABLE I. Turn-over of LPL in Culture Adipocytes in the Presence and Absence of Heparin

Treatment	Synthesis	Secretion	Degradation
		ng/h/60 mm dish	
Control	8.1	1.9	6.2
Heparin (10 U/ml)	9.1	7.2	1.9

Adapted from Cupp, et al. (1987) J. Biol. Chem. 262: 6383-6388.

The degradation rate can also be calculated directly from the same data (13). The degradation rate constant can be calculated as follows:

$$K = \frac{A_o - A_{60}}{\int_o^{60} Cdt}$$

A_0 and A_{60} are the total LPL radioactivity in the intracellular, cell surface and medium pools at t = 0 and at t = 60 min. C is the function describing the intracellular LPL radioactivity as a function of time. The derivation assumes: a three pool model consisting of intracellular, cell surface and medium compartments; first order processes and degradation in the intracellular pool; the degradation rates can then be calculated by multiplying the rate constant by the intracellular LPL pool size. Similarly, the secretion rate can also be measured independently as:

$$S = \frac{M_{60}}{\int_o^{60} ydt}$$

where M_{60} is the radioactive LPL accumulating at t = 60 in the medium and y is a function describing the specific activity of the immediate precursor pool. In control cells the cell surface compartment is the immediate precursor pool. In heparin treated cells, the intracellular LPL specific activity can be employed. The methodology described above could be employed for the study of any secreted cellular protein studied in cell culture.

The striking result in the above turn-over experiment is that in control cells, 77% of the synthesized enzyme is degraded, whereas in heparin-treated cells this is reduced to 21%. On the basis of the above data we proposed [14] the following hypothesis: In control cells LPL is transported to the cell surface where it binds to cell surface heparan sulfate. The enzyme is then either released to the medium or internalized as a heparan sulfate-enzyme complex. The internalized enzyme would then be degraded or recycled to the cell surface. When heparin is present in the medium it would compete with cell surface heparan sulfate for the binding of LPL and effectively prevent internalization and degradation. Consistent with the above hypothesis one would expect a decrease in compartment sizes of intracellular and cell surface associated LPL. Indeed for the experiments discussed above the mean intracellular and surface associated LPL were:

TABLE II. Intracellular and Cell Surface Associated LPL in Control and Heparin Treated Adipocytes

	Intracellular	Cell Surface
	ng/60 mm dish	
Control	6.9	3.0
Heparin (10 U/ml)	4.3	0.3

Adapted from Cupp, et al. (1987) J. Biol. Chem. 262: 6383-6388.

Of relevance to the above model, Conrad and his group [15,16] have shown recently that hepatocytes continuously secrete heparan sulfate proteoglycans into the culture medium and the cell surface matrix and internalize them from both compartments. In addition, the same group has shown that bacterial phosphatidylinositol-specific phospholipase C stimulates the release of heparan sulfate proteoglycans into the medium [16]. The cleaved heparan sulfate proteoglycan would then bind to a postulated inositol phosphate receptor. In the same report [16] it was shown that the fraction of cell matrix HSPG which was released by 5 mM myo-inositol hexaphosphate increased from 29 to 73% as medium insulin was increased from 0 to 20 μg/ml. These results were consistent with a report that insulin activates a cell surface phospholipase C [17]. With increased medium insulin, phospholipase C was presumably activated and a greater proportion of HSPG molecules were released and bound to myo-inositol-phosphate receptors than in control cells.In chicken adipocytes we have shown that phosphatidylinositol-specific phospholipase C stimulates the release of heparan sulfate into the medium (Hoogewerf and Bensadoun, unpublished data). Chajek-Shaul, et al. [18] recently demonstrated that the same bacterial phospholipase C stimulates LPL release into the medium of cultured rat heart cells. Incorporating all of the elements discussed above, we propose the following model for the regulation of secretion of LPL in adipocytes.

To test the model we have evaluated several segments of the intracellular and extracellular transport of LPL. Equilibrium-binding experiments with ^{125}I-labeled avian LPL demonstrate the presence of a class of high affinity binding sites on adipocytes [14]. The association constant was calculated to be 0.6 x $10^8 M^{-1}$. If cells are pretreated with heparinase or heparitinase, the binding activity is essentially equal to the non-specific binding measured in the absence of enzymatic treatment. This is direct evidence that the lipase is binding to heparan sulfate (HS) chains probably associated with heparan sulfate proteoglycans (HSPG). At 37°C, cell surface associated labeled enzyme is internalized, a fraction of the internalized enzyme is recycled to the cell surface or medium and the balance is degraded [14]. The degradation presumably occurs in the lysosomes, since the lysosomotropic agent chloroquine inhibits degradation. If the above model is correct, one would expect that agents which affect the integrity of heparan sulfate would result in decreased LPL degradation and enhanced secretion. Indeed, treatment of adipocytes with heparinase or heparitinase results in an increase enzyme secretion rate. Similarly, in pulse chase experiments it was shown that treating cells with a mixture of heparinase and heparitinase resulted in a quantitative inhibition of degradation 30 min after endoglycosidase treatment [14]. An inositol monophosphate receptor may be involved in the internalization of the HSPG-LPL complex. Addition of myoinositol-2-monophosphate to the medium results in a dose dependent increase in enzyme secretion. In addition, enzyme degradation is greatly inhibited (L. Cisar and Bensadoun, unpublished data). The internalization of the HSPG-LPL complex may perhaps occur only after the HSPG phosphatidyl inositol anchor is cleaved, and after interaction with the putative inositol monophosphate receptor.

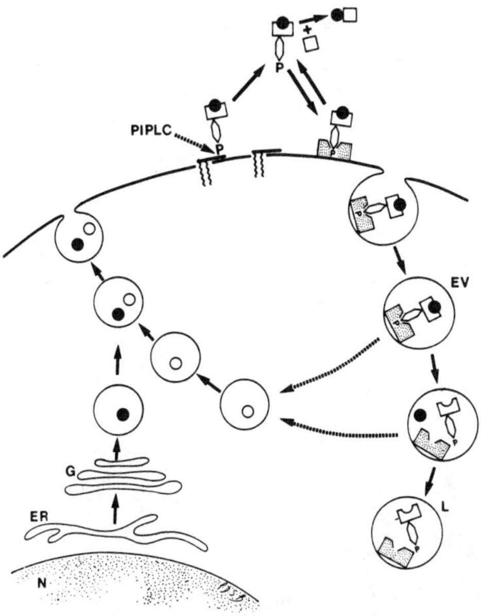

FIG. 2. Proposed pathway of lipoprotein lipase. •, denotes newly synthesized LPL; o, recycled LPL; ⊏⊐, molecules with high affinity for LPL, such as heparin or lipoproteins. The newly synthesized LPL is shown bound to a HSPG anchored via a phosphatidyl-inositol moiety. After release from the cell surface the HSPG would be recognized by an inositol phosphate receptor, shown as the stippled form on the cell surface, endocytic vesicle (EV), and lysosome (L).

To further characterize the interaction of LPL with cell surface HSPG, the HSPG fractions with high affinity for LPL were purified. Adipocyte cell extracts metabolically labeled with $[^{35}S]SO_4$ and Trans $[^{35}S]$ label^{TM} were passed through an affinity column containing LPL covalently coupled to Affigel-10. The column was then developed with a salt gradient. A fraction containing 13% of the initial starting material was eluted. This fraction was shown to bind quantitatively when recycled over the column. The fraction was further purified by gel filtration and ion-exchange chromatography. Two major fractions were separated by gel filtration. A high molecular weight fraction with an average M_r of 250,000 eluted first. This fraction was identified as HSPG by its sensitivity to a mixture of heparinase and heparitinase and the appearance of a major core protein with an approximate M_r of 90,000. A lower molecular weight fraction (average M_r 31,000) was eluted next and is also sensitive to mixtures of heparinase and heparitinase, but yielded no core proteins when preparations were digested. The low molecular weight fraction may be mainly intracellular HS chains, intermediates in either the biosynthesis or degradation of HSPG. It is unlikely that the HSPG's which bind to LPL-Affigel-10 column are specific HSPG species binding only LPL. It is more probable that, like in the case of antithrombin III [19], LPL binds to specific heparan sulfate sequences. It is therefore inappropriate to refer to the LPL binding activity on the surface of adipocytes as a specific receptor molecule.

The model described above may be a significant mechanism whereby the secretion of LPL and other molecules with affinity for the cell surface HSPG may be regulated. Different events could perturb the steady state of LPL degradation and secretion. A sudden change in extracellular concentration of molecules with high affinity for LPL, like lipoproteins, free fatty acids [20] or endogenous heparin from mast cells would be expected to decrease enzyme internalization and enhance desorption of lipase from the adipocyte surface. Alternatively, endogenous endoglycosidases may degrade HS chains and limit the number of specific LPL binding domains. Oldberg, et al. [21] have purified from human platelets an endoglycosidase which specifically cleaves heparin and heparan sulfate, but does not digest glycosidic bonds in other mucopolysaccharides. Rosenberg and associates [22] have suggested that this lysosomal endoglycosidase present at low levels *in vivo* may play a role in modulating the HSPG pool sizes in the environment of vascular smooth muscle cells. All of the above mechanisms would result in a rapid modulation of enzyme efflux with no change in synthesis rate. Quantitatively, inhibition of LPL degradation could result in a maximum 4 to 5-fold increase in LPL secretion. This magnitude of stimulation of enzyme activity could account for the fold increases observed *in vivo* when comparing enzyme secretion by adipocytes prepared from control and insulin injected rats [23].

The previous model is compatible with a simple mechanism whereby LPL could be transported from subendothelial cells to the luminal surface of the endothelium. LPL in buffers is notoriously unstable, especially at 37°C. It has been documented that heparin stabilizes enzyme activity [24,25]. Similarly HSPG may maintain the catalytic activity of the enzyme and prevent its inactivation by irreversible aggregation [26]. LPL would be secreted by adipocytes as soluble LPL-HSPG complexes. Because of the high binding capacity of the endothelial surface for LPL [27], a concentration gradient of LPL-HSPG between the extracellular fluid in the proximity of the adipocyte and the endothelium would be created. This concentration gradient would provide the driving force for the transport process.

ACKNOWLEDGEMENTS

We thank Jean Hsu and Kristan Melford for expert technical assistance and Connie Soper for preparation of the manuscript. This work was supported by N.I.H. grant HL-14990.

REFERENCES

1. Cheng, C.-F., Oosta, G.M., Bensadoun, A. and Rosenberg, R.D., J. Biol. Chem. 256: 12893-12898 (1981).
2. Shimada, K., Gill, P.J., Silbert, J.E., Doublas, W.H.J. and Fanburg, B.L., J. Clin. Invest. 68: 995-1012 (1981).
3. Kompiang, I.P., Bensadoun, A. and Yang, M.W., J. Lipid Res. 17: 498-505 (1976).
4. Speake, B.K., Parkin, S.M. and Robinson, D.S., Biochem. Soc. Trans. 13: 29-31 (1985a).
5. Ong, J.M., Kirchgessner, T.G., Schotz, M.C. and Kern, P.A., J. Biol. Chem. 263: 12933-12938 (1988).
6. Semenkovich, C.F., Wims, M., Noe, L., Etienne, J. and Chan, L., J. Biol. Chem. 264: 9030-9038 (1989).
7. Doolittle, M.H., Ben-Zeev, O., Elovson, J., Martin, M. and Kirchgessner, T.G., J. Biol. Chem. 265: 4570-4577 (1990).
8. Cupp, M., Bensadoun, A. and Melford, M., J. Biol. Chem. 262: 6383-6388 (1987).
9. Semb, H. and Olivecrona, T., Biochim. Biophys. Acta 921: 104-115 (1987).
10. Vannier, C. and Ailhaud, G., J. Biol. Chem. 264: 13206-13216 (1989).

11. Glick, J.H. and Rothblat, G.H., Biochim. Biophys. Acta 618: 163-172 (1980).
12. Vannier, C. and Ailhaud, G., Biochim. Biophys. Acta 875: 324-333 (1986).
13. Cisar, L.A., Melford, K.H., Sensel, M. and Bensadoun, A., Biochim. Biophys. Acta 1004: 196-204 (1989).
14. Cisar, L.A., Hoogewerf, A.J., Cupp, M., Rapport, C.A. and Bensadoun, A., J. Biol. Chem. 264: 1767-1774 (1989).
15. Bienkowski, M.J. and Conrad, H.E., J. Biol. Chem. 259: 12989-12996 (1984).
16. Ishihara, M., Fedarko, N.S. and Conrad, H.E., J. Biol. Chem. 261: 13575-15580 (1986) .
17. Saltiel, A.R. and Cuatrecasas, P., Proc. Natl. Acad. Sci. USA 83: 5793-5797 (1986).
18. Chajek-Shaul, T., Halimi, O., Ben-Naim, M., Stein, O. and Stein, Y., Biochim. Biophys. Acta 1014: 178-183 (1989) .
19. Choay, J., Lormeau, J.C., Petitoce, M., Sinay, P. and Fareed, J., Ann. N.Y. Acad. Sci. 370: 644-649 (1981).
20. Saxena, V., Witte, L.D. and Goldberg, I.J., J. Biol. Chem. 264: 4349-4355 (1989) .
21. Oldberg, A., Heldin, C.H., Wasteson, A., Busch, C. and Höök, M., Biochemistry 19: 5755-5762 (1980).
22. Oosta, G.M., Favreau, L.V., Beeler, D.L. and Rosenberg, R.D., J. Biol. Chem. 257: 11249-11255 (1982).
23. Garfinkel, A.S., Nilsson-Ehle, P. and Schotz, M.C., Biochim. Biophys. Acta 424: 264-273 (1976).
24. Iverius, P-H., Lindahl, V., Egelrud, T. and Olivecrona, T., J. Biol. Chem. 247: 6610-6616 (1972).
25. Bengtsson, G. and Olivecrona, T., Biochem. J. 226: 409-413 (1985).
26. Osborne, J.C., Jr., Bengtsson-Olivecrona, G., Lee, N.S. and Olivecrona, T., Biochemistry 24: 5606-5611 (1985).
27. Cheng, C.-F., Oosta, G.M., Bensadoun, A. and Rosenberg, R.D., J. Biol. Chem. 256: 12893-12898 (1981).

The Editing of Apolipoprotein-B mRNA

Donna M. Driscoll

Southwest Foundation for Biomedical Research, San Antonio, Texas

ABSTRACT

A novel form of RNA editing generates two forms of apolipoprotein-B (apo-B) from a single gene. The apo-B gene and hepatic apo-B mRNA contain C at nucleotide 6666 whereas intestinal mRNA contains U at this position. This converts codon 2153 from glutamine (CAA) to an in-frame stop codon (UAA) resulting in the production of a shorter apo-B protein by the intestine. We have previously developed an *in vitro* system for the editing of apo-B mRNA using synthetic RNA substrates and cell-free extracts from a rat hepatoma cell line. Editing of apo-B mRNA was detected by a sensitive primer extension assay. To identify a tissue source of the editing activity for biochemical purification, extracts were prepared from enterocytes isolated from baboon small intestine. These extracts edit apo-B RNA with very high efficiency. Approximately 20% of the input RNA is edited *in vitro*. The editing activity is sensitive to proteinase K treatment but not to micrococcal nuclease which suggests that a protein component but not an RNA component is required. Partial purification of the editing protein(s) has been achieved by fractionation of the extracts by column chromatography. The possibility that this mechanism may also regulate the expression of genes other than apo-B is discussed.

INTRODUCTION

Molecular biologists have always thought that if they could determine the nucleotide sequence of a gene, they could predict the sequence of the mRNA and protein that the gene encodes. This principle has been questioned recently by the exciting and unexpected discovery of RNA editing. RNA editing can be defined as any mechanism that posttranscriptionally modifies an mRNA, altering its nucleotide sequence and consequently its coding capacity. The end result is that a new protein is synthesized from the edited mRNA which is different from the protein encoded in the genome. Not only is RNA editing a novel mechanism for regulating gene expression but this process also raises questions regarding the central dogma of molecular biology. RNA editing has been found in a number of organisms including trypanosomes, viruses, and plants. This paper focuses on the only example of RNA editing in a mammalian system, the editing of apolipoprotein-B (apo-B) mRNA. Apo-B mRNA is modified in the intestine by a mechanism which converts a cytosine (C) to a uracil (U) resulting in the tissue-specific

© 1990 by Elsevier Science Publishing Co., Inc.
Molecular Biology of Atherosclerosis
A.D. Attie, Editor

expression of two apo-B proteins from a single gene. These two proteins have functionally different roles in the assembly and metabolism of plasma lipoproteins.

Apo-B is Important in Lipid Metabolism

Apo-B plays a key role in the assembly, transport, and metabolism of plasma lipoproteins [1]. In humans there are two forms of apo-B which circulate in the plasma. Apo-B100, a 512 kD protein is required for the assembly and secretion of VLDL from the liver [1]. In the plasma, VLDL is converted to LDL which contains apo-B100 as its principal protein component. Apo-B100 is the ligand that binds to the LDL receptor delivering cholesterol to cells by receptor-mediated endocytosis [2]. There is strong epidemiologic and genetic evidence showing a positive correlation between plasma LDL levels and coronary heart disease [3]. Apo-B48, a 242 kD protein, is synthesized by the intestine and represents the amino-terminal half of apo-B100 [1,4]. As a structural component of chylomicrons, apo-B48 is important in the absorption and transport of dietary lipid [1].

Although it is well established that apo-B100 and apo-B48 differ in size, site of synthesis and function in lipid metabolism, it is not known why the intestine synthesizes a truncated form of apo-B. One possible explanation may have to do with the LDL-receptor binding domain which has been localized to the carboxy-terminal half of apo-B100. Apo-B48 lacks this domain and consequently the intestinal lipoproteins that contain apo-B48 and dietary fat cannot be cleared by the LDL receptor [5]. It has been proposed that apo-B48 may be produced by the intestine to target dietary lipid to the liver where it is cleared by a lipoprotein receptor different from the LDL receptor [6]. However, there may be additional explanations since apo-B48 is missing over 50% of the apo-B100 sequence. For example, sequences in the carboxy-terminal half of apo-B100 may be required for the assembly of VLDL in the liver but not for the assembly of triglyceride-rich chylomicrons in the intestine.

Apo-B48 is Produced by an RNA-editing Mechansim

Because apo-B100 and apo-B48 are physiologically important, there has been considerable interest in investigating the biosynthesis of these two proteins. Epitope mapping studies as well as peptide mapping experiments indicated that apo-B48 represented the amino-terminal half of apo-B100 [4,7]. Given that apo-B100 and apo-B48 are encoded by the same gene [8], there were two likely mechanisms which could account for the synthesis of apo-B48. The primary apo-B mRNA transcript could be spliced differently in the intestine compared to the liver. Alternatively, posttranslational cleavage of the primary apo-B translation product could occur in the intestine. To everyone's surprise, neither of these proposed mechanisms was correct. Because apo-B is a notoriously insoluble and difficult protein to work with, it was not until the apo-B gene and corresponding cDNAs were cloned and sequenced that the mechanism was elucidated.

Apo-B48 is produced by an unusual RNA editing mechanism which posttranscriptionally modifies apo-B mRNA in the intestine. Using DNA sequencing techniques, several laboratories have shown that both the apo-B gene and hepatic mRNA contain C at nucleotide 6666 whereas intestinal mRNA contains U at this position [9-11]. This nucleotide change converts codon 2153 from glutamine (CAA) to a premature in-frame stop codon (UAA) resulting in the synthesis of apo-B48 by the intestine. The insertion of a stop codon into the coding sequence of an mRNA is an unprecedented mechanism for regulating gene expression. The C to U change in apo-B mRNA is a posttranscriptional event but very little is currently known about the mechanism of this reaction.

Primer Extension Assay for Apo-B mRNA

We are interested in investigating the editing of apo-B mRNA at the molecular level. As a first step, we have developed a sensitive primer extension assay which distinguishes between the apo-B100 and apo-B48 mRNAs [12]. A ^{32}P-labeled primer is annealed to apo-B mRNA downstream of the editing site at nucleotide 6666. The primer is extended with reverse transcriptase in the presence of dideoxy GTP which is a chain terminator. Because of the nucleotide change at the editing site, apo-B100 and apo-B48 mRNAs generate extension products of different sizes which can be analyzed by electrophoresis [12]. Primer annealed to apo-B100 mRNA is extended to the C at nucleotide 6666, generating a product of 42 nucleotides. Primer annealed to apo-B48 mRNA is extended to the next upstream C, generating a product of 52 nucleotides. This assay is sensitive and can detect apo-B48 mRNA when it represents less than 1% of the total apo-B mRNA [12].

In Vitro Editing of Apo-B mRNA

To identify the cellular factors and RNA sequences required for the editing of apo-B mRNA, we have recently established an *in vitro* system for the editing of apo-B mRNA [12]. A synthetic apo-B100 RNA of 480 nucleotides was incubated *in vitro* with cell-free extracts prepared from the McArdle 7777 cell line [12]. These cells are derived from a rat hepatoma and synthesize both apo-B100 and apo-B48 mRNAs [12,13]. RNA editing was detected by the primer extension assay. Approximately 3% of the apo-B100 RNA was edited *in vitro* [12]. This low efficiency may reflect low levels of editing activity in McArdle 7777 cells since only 15% of their endogenous apo-B mRNA is edited *in vivo* [12,13]. The results of the primer extension assay were confirmed by cloning and sequencing the products of an editing reaction. The C at nucleotide 6666 was the only nucleotide in the synthetic RNA that was modified during the reaction [12]. The *in vitro* editing activity was specific for RNA, not DNA, and was not detected in extracts from Hep3B cells which synthesize only apo-B100 or in extracts from HeLa cells which do not synthesize apo-B [12]. These studies definitively establish that apo-B mRNA undergoes a posttranscriptional editing reaction and provide the basis for investigating this mechanism at the biochemical level.

Intestinal Cell Extracts Edit In Vitro

One of our goals is to purify the protein or protein complex which edits apo-B mRNA. McArdle 7777 cells are not a good source of extracts for this purpose since these cells contain low levels of editing activity and are difficult to grow in large quantities. To identify a large tissue source for the biochemical purification of the editing protein, we investigated whether extracts prepared from baboon small intestine contain editing activity. Like the human and rabbit small intestine, the baboon small intestine edits over 95% of its apo-B mRNA [unpublished observations]. Intestinal epithelial cells were isolated from baboon small intestine using NaCitrate [14]. S100 extracts were prepared from these cells as described [15] with the modification that extensive precautions were taken against proteases and ribonucleases. These extracts contain cytoplasmic proteins and some nuclear proteins which have leaked out of the nucleus during cell fractionation. The extracts from baboon intestinal cells edit synthetic apo-B100 RNA *in vitro* with high efficiency. Approximately 20% of the apo-B RNA is edited by the intestinal cell extracts, compared to 3% by the McArdle 7777 cell extracts [unpublished observations]. The identification of a tissue source that provides a large amount of starting material with high levels of activity should facilitate the purification of the editing protein. In preliminary experiments we have successfully fractionated the intestinal extracts by ammonium sulfate precipitation, ion-exchange chromatography, and heparin-agarose chromatography. Compared to the crude extracts, the partially purified fractions are enriched approximately 20-fold for the editing activity.

Characterization of the Editing Mechanism In Vitro

The editing of apo-B mRNA involves the alteration of a single base in a 14,121 nucleotide mRNA and may be similar to the base modification reactions that occur during the biosynthesis of tRNAs [16]. The C to U change in apo-B mRNA may be mediated by a sequence-specific cytidine deaminase. Although cytidine deaminases play an important role in nucleotide metabolism in mammalian cells, none have been found to act at the polynucleotide level [17]. Editing may be performed by a transglycosylase that catalyzes a base replacement reaction exchanging C for U. Similar enzymes in rat liver catalyze the exchange of guanine for queuine [18] or adenine for hypoxanthine [19] in certain tRNAs. Alternatively, the edited nucleotide in apo-B48 mRNA may represent a modified base which is read as U by reverse transcriptase and the ribosome.

We have used the *in vitro* editing assay to investigate the mechanism of the editing reaction. The editing of apo-B mRNA does not appear to be an ATP-dependent process. The *in vitro* reaction is not stimulated by the addition of ribonucleotide triphosphates and creatine phosphate [12] and is not inhibited by the addition of nonhydrolyzable ATP analogs or by treatment of the extracts with ATPase [unpublished observations]. The editing mechanism requires a protein moiety and does not require an RNA component. Treatment of the extracts with proteinase K abolishes the editing activity [12] whereas micrococcal nuclease treatment has no effect [unpublished observations]. We have also tested several known inhibitors of the mammalian enzyme cytidine deaminase for their effect on the *in vitro* editing reaction. The addition of uridine, dihydrouridine, or tetrahydrouridine (a particularly potent inhibitor) does not inhibit the activity of the partially purified editing protein [unpublished observations]. Whether the editing of apo-B mRNA involves base-exchange, deamination, or a more complex mechanism still remains to be determined.

Editing of Apo-B mRNA May be a Nuclear Event

Before transport to the cytoplasm, most newly transcribed mRNAs undergo a number of modification reactions including capping, splicing, and polyadenylation. Two lines of evidence indirectly suggest that the editing of apo-B mRNA may also occur in the nucleus. The rat liver is unusual in that it produces apo-B48 by the same RNA editing mechanism as the intestine [12, 13]. We have used subcellular fractionation techniques to isolate nuclei from rat liver by ultracentrifugation through 2 M sucrose. The nuclei isolated by this method are intact and free of cytoplasmic debris [unpublished observations]. Total RNA isolated from the purified nuclei was then analyzed by the primer extension assay for apo-B mRNA. Apo-B48 mRNA represented approximately 10% of the apo-B mRNA in the nucleus which suggests that editing can be a nuclear event [unpublished observations]. Editing may be a late event in the processing of apo-B mRNA. This may explain the low level of edited apo-B mRNA found in the nucleus compared to the newly transcribed apo-B100 mRNA.

The second line of evidence comes from studies by Bostrom et al. [20]. When apo-B100 cDNAs were transfected into $CaCO_2$ cells, two different apo-B mRNAs were expressed. One mRNA is the expected size and represents primarily unedited apo-B mRNA. The other mRNA, which has undergone editing, is shorter due to the use of a cryptic polyadenylation site [20]. These results suggest that editing may occur before polyadenylation, a known nuclear event.

Sequence Requirements for Editing In Vitro

How the mechanism that edits apo-B mRNA achieves its high degree of specificity is not known. Editing involves a single nucleotide change in a 14,121 nucleotide mRNA which suggests that the editing protein recognizes a specific sequence in apo-B mRNA. To identify sequences in apo-B mRNA required for editing, a series of apo-B deletion mutants spanning nucleotide 6666 were constructed [12]. All constructs were derived from exon 26 and contained only coding sequences. Synthetic RNAs transcribed from these plasmids were used as substrates in the *in vitro* editing reaction. RNAs containing 2385, 483, or 55 nucleotides of human apo-B mRNA sequence were all edited *in vitro*. However, an RNA containing a 26 nucleotide sequence that is highly conserved across species was not edited [12]. The 55 nucleotide RNA which is edited *in vitro* contains only coding sequences and lacks the sequences for splicing and polyadenylation. At least *in vitro*, editing is not obligatorily coupled to transcription, accurate splicing, or polyadenylation or translation.

Sequence Requirements for Editing in Transfected Cells

Similar apo-B deletion mutants were also transfected into McArdle 7777 cells. All four RNAs, including the RNA containing the 26 nucleotide sequence, were edited [13]. This result differs from our *in vitro* study discussed above and the transfection studies by Bostrom et *al.* in which a chimeric RNA containing 63 nucleotides of apo-B mRNA sequence was not edited [20]. In all three studies, the apo-B sequences were flanked by additional sequences that may have influenced editing. Our transfection studies used an apo-B minigene that contained sequences from the editing site as well as sequences from other regions of the apo-B cDNA [13]. The synthetic apo-B RNAs assayed in the *in vitro* editing reaction contained additional sequences from the polylinker of the vector [12]. In the study by Bostrom et al. [20], the apo-B sequences in the chimeric gene were flanked by sequences from apo-E cDNA.

Clearly the sequence requirements for editing need to be further defined by mutational analysis of apo-B mRNA. The 26 nucleotide region edited in transfected cells is highly conserved across species and contains a high proportion (approximately 74%) of A + U residues [13]. This region also has the potential to form a stem loop structure containing a 7 nucleotide loop. It will be interesting to determine whether the editing mechanism recognizes a primary sequence or secondary structure or both in apo-B mRNA.

Hormonal and Developmental Regulation of the Editing Activity

In humans and rabbits, apo-B mRNA is edited in the intestine but not in the liver [9-11]. The rat liver is unusual in that it produces both apo-B100 and apo-B48 although the physiologic reason for this is not known. Studies by Davidson et al. [4] have shown that the editing mechanism may be hormonally regulated in the rat liver. The percentage of apo-B48 mRNA in the rat liver increases from 60% to almost 100% with the administration of thyroid hormone [21]. It remains to be investigated whether thyroid hormone increases editing activity since the stability of the apo-B100 and apo-B48 mRNAs may be differentially affected by thyroid hormone. Since treatment with thyroid hormone also increases cortisone and growth hormone levels, the changes in apo-B48 mRNA may be an indirect rather than direct effect of thyroid hormone. In fact, a recent report suggests that growth hormone may have different effects on the synthesis of apo-B100 and apo-B48 in the rat liver [22]. The results of these studies provide the basis for experiments designed to manipulate the editing of apo-B mRNA both *in vivo* and *in vitro*.

The editing mechanism may also be developmentally regulated. The adult human intestine synthesizes and secretes apo-B48. However, studies using tissue slices have shown that the human fetal intestine synthesizes only apo-B100 early in gestation [23]. After 16 weeks of gestation, the intestine produces both forms of apo-B whereas only apo-B48 is synthesized after 21 weeks [23]. These studies have measured newly synthesized apo-B protein but the results suggest that this switch from apo-B100 to apo-B48 during development may be mediated at the level of RNA editing. The developing fetal intestine should be a good model for investigating the regulation of the activity that edits apo-B mRNA.

Does the Apo-B mRNA Editing Activity Regulate the Expression of Other Genes?

The fact that RNA editing occurs in several organisms suggests that this process may be a more common mechanism for regulating gene expression than has been appreciated. It seems unlikely that in mammals RNA editing is restricted to the intestine and it is possible that the editing activity that edits apo-B mRNA also edits other mRNAs. Although the editing activity is not detected in HeLa cells [12,13], studies by Bostrom et al. suggest that this activity is expressed in other cell types. When plasmids containing apo-B100 cDNAs were transfected into mammalian cell lines, apo-B mRNA was edited in A431 cells derived from a human epidermoid carcinoma and MG63 cells derived from a human osteosarcoma [K. Bostrom, personal communication]. In transgenic mice carrying the human apo-B gene, the human apo-B mRNA was edited in several tissues in addition to the liver and intestine [24]. These studies raise the possibility that the mechanism that edits apo-B mRNA may be expressed in other tissues, possibly to regulate the expression of genes other than apo-B.

To investigate whether the editing protein is present in lower eukaryotes, a plasmid containing human apo-B100 cDNA was transfected into yeast in an experiment done in collaboration with Dr. Steve Sturley. Human apo-B100 mRNA was not edited when expressed in yeast cells [unpublished observations]. This is not a surprising finding given that the editing protein may have arisen late in evolution. Although the editing activity may be expressed in a number of mammalian tissues, a very recent study has shown that the chicken intestine does not synthesize apo-B48 [25]. This suggests that the editing mechanism may have evolved after the divergence of birds and mammals.

Other Examples of RNA Editing

RNA editing has been found in a number of other organisms, including trypanosomes, viruses, and plants. These examples are quite different from the editing of apo-B mRNA and involve very unusual mechanisms for regulating gene expression at the posttranscriptional level.

RNA editing was first discovered in 1986 in the trypanosome when the mitochondrial genome was sequenced [reviewed in 26,27]. It was found that the genome contained only defective or incomplete genes whereas the mitochondrial mRNAs were perfectly normal. It was later shown that these defective genes are transcribed and that the primary mRNA transcripts are edited by the insertion or deletion of uridines at specific sites. This editing creates new amino acid sequences, uncovers cryptic reading frames, and generates the AUG initiation codons that are lacking in many of the mitochondrial genes [26,27]. Editing can be quite extensive and in some cases up to several hundred uridines can be added. Recent studies have suggested that this editing reaction may be a templated process involving short antisense mRNAs. The discovery of these "guide mRNAs" may explain how this editing process achieves its high degree of specificity [28].

In the paramyxoviruses such as SV5 and measles viruses, about half of the P protein mRNAs have the same nucleotide sequence as the P protein gene. However, the other P protein mRNAs contain an additional one or two guanosine (G) residues in the carboxy-terminus of the mRNA. This insertion uncovers a cryptic reading frame and leads to the production of two proteins from the same mRNA [29,30]. These two proteins have the same amino-terminus but different carboxy-termini. This process may be a co-transcriptional rather than posttranscriptional event since the insertion of the extra G's may occur when the RNA polymerase stutters during transcription [29,30].

The most recent example of RNA editing has been found in plant mitochondria. An RNA editing mechanism converts C to U at several positions in a number of plant mitochondrial mRNAs, resulting in amino acid changes and the conservation of protein sequences [31-33]. The edited sites in the mitochondrial mRNAs do not share any sequence homology or secondary structure with each other or with the edited site in apo-B mRNA although these sites are all edited by C to U conversions. However, it is possible that these sequences all have a common secondary or tertiary structure that we have not been able to identify by computer analysis. In collaboration with Dr. Patrick Covello, we have investigated whether the plant mitochondrial mRNAs and apo-B mRNA are edited by the same mechanism. The mitochondrial mRNA coding for cytochrome oxidase subunit II (COXII) is edited in wheat at multiple sites by C to U conversions. A synthetic mRNA corresponding to unedited COXII sequence was not edited in our in vitro assay by the intestinal cell extracts which edit apo-B mRNA with high efficiency. These results suggest that the mammalian editing protein does not recognize the editing sites in the plant mitochondrial mRNAs.

SUMMARY

The discovery of RNA editing has been one of the most exciting and unexpected findings in molecular biology. Apo-B is an attractive system for studies on RNA editing because an in vitro system for the editing reaction has been established and a minimum sequence in apo-B mRNA that is required for editing has been identified. The development of a functional assay for editing will enable us to purify the editing activity and to subsequently isolate cDNA clones that can be used to analyze the structure and function of the editing protein. Using cDNA clones, we will also be able to study how the expression of the editing protein is regulated both during development and in response to hormones.

One important area of research concerns the role of apo-B48 in lipoprotein biosynthesis and metabolism. By using gene targeting strategies, we may be able to create transgenic mice that no longer edit apo-B mRNA or that edit apo-B mRNA both in the intestine and liver. The results of these studies may give some insight into why the intestine produces apo-B48.

Finally, one of the most intriguing questions is whether this editing activity also regulates the expression of other genes. Our hypothesis is that these other mRNAs, which may undergo editing will share sequence or secondary structure homology with apo-B mRNA. By identifying the sequences in apo-B mRNA that are recognized by the editing protein, we may be able to use this information to identify other mRNAs which may be edited by this same mechanism.

REFERENCES

1. J.P. Kane, Ann. Rev. Physiol. 45, 637-650 (1983).
2. M.S. Brown and J.L. Goldstein, Science 232, 34-37 (1986).
3. R.J. Havel, J.L. Goldstein, and M.S. Brown in: Metabolic Control and Disease, P.K. Bondy and L.E. Rosenberg, eds. (Saunders, Philadelphia, PA 1980) pp. 672-712.
4. Y.L. Marcel, T.L. Innerarity, C. Spillman, R.W. Mahley, A.A. Protter, and R.W. Milne, Arteriosclerosis 7, 166-175 (1987).
5. T.J. Knott, R.J. Pease, L.M. Powell, S.C. Wallis, S.C. Rall, T.L. Innerarity, B. Blackhart, W.H. Taylor, Y. Marcel, R. Milne, D. Johnson, M. Fuller, A.J. Lusis, B.J. McCarthy, R.W. Mahley, B. Levy-Wilson, and J. Scott, Nature 323, 734-738 (1986).
6. M.S. Brown and J.L. Goldstein, Nature 330, 113-114, (1987).
8. S.G. Young, S.J. Bertics, T.M. Scott, B.W. Dubois, L.K. Curtiss, and J.L. Witzum, J. Biol. Chem. 261, 2995-2998 (1986).
9. L.M. Powell, S.C. Wallis, R.J. Pease, Y.H. Edwards, T.J. Knott, and J. Scott, Cell 50, 831-840 (1987).
10. S.-H. Chen, G. Habib, C.-Y. Yang, Z.-W. Zu, B.R. Lee, S.-A. Weng, S.R. Silberman, S.-J. Cai, J.P. Desylpere, M. Rosseneu, A.M. Gotto, Jr., W.-H. Li, and L. Chan, Science 328, 363-366 (1987).
11. A.V. Hospattankar, K. Higuchi, S.W. Law, N.M. Meglin, and H.B. Brewer Jr., Biochem. Biophys. Res. Comm. 148, 279-285 (1987).
12. D.M. Driscoll, J.K. Wynne, S.C. Wallis, and J. Scott, Cell 58, 519-525 (1989).
13. M.S. Davies, S.C. Wallis, D.M. Driscoll, J.K. Wynne, G.W. Williams, L.M. Powell, and J. Scott, J. Biol. Chem. 264, 13395-13398 (1989).
14. M.W. Weiser, J. Biol. Chem. 248, 2536-2541 (1973).
15. T.D. Dignam, R.M. Lebovitz, and R.G. Roeder, Nucl. Acids Res. 11, 1475-1489 (1983).
16. G.R. Bjork, J.U. Ericson, C.E.D. Gustafsson, T.G. Hagervall, Y.H. Jonsson, and P.M. Wikstrom, Ann. Rev. Biochem. 56, 263-287, (1987).
17. P. Nygaard, Adv. Exp. Med. Biol. 195B, 415-420 (1986).
18. N. Shindo-Okada, N. Okada, T. Ohgi, T. Goto, and S. Nishimura, Biochemistry 19, 395-400 (1980).
19. M.S. Elliott and R.W. Trewyn, J. Biol. Chem. 259, 2407-2410 (1984).
20. K. Bostrom, S.J. Lauer, K.S. Poksay, Z. Garcia, J.M. Taylor, and T.L. Innerarity, J. Biol. Chem. 264, 15701-15708 (1989).
21. N.O. Davidson, L.M. Powell, S.C. Wallis, and J. Scott, J. Biol. Chem. 263, 13482-13485 (1988).
22. J. Oscarsson, A. Sjoberg, S. Eden, G. Bondgers, and S.-O. Olofsson, Arteriosclerosis 9, 716a (1989).
23. R.M. Glickman, M. Rogers, and J.N. Glickman, Proc. Natl. Acad. Sci. USA 83, 5296-5300 (1986).
24. J. Scott, S.C. Wallis, M.S. Davies, J.K. Wynne, L.M. Powell, and D.M. Driscoll, Gut, suppl. 30, 35-43 (1989).
25. P. Tarugi, L. Albertazzi, S. Nicolini, and S. Calandra, J. Lipid Res. 31, 417-427 (1990).
26. R. Benne, Biochim. Biophys. Acta. 1007, 131-139 (1989).
27. L. Simpson and J. Shaw, Cell 57, 355-366 (1989).
28. B. Blum, N. Bakalara, and L. Simpson, Cell 60, 189-198 (1990).
29. S.M. Thomas, R.A. Lamb, and R.G. Paterson, Cell 54, 891-902 (1988).
30. R. Catteneo, K. Kaelin, K. Baczko, and M.A. Billeter, Cell 56, 759-764 (1989).
31. J.M. Gualberto, L. Lamattina, G. Bonnard, J.-H. Weil, and J.-M. Grienenberger, Nature 341, 660-662 (1989).
32. P.S. Covello and M.W. Gray, Nature 341: 662-666 (1989).
33. W. Schuster, B. Wissinger, M. Unseld, and A. Brennicke, EMBO J. 9, 263-269 (1990).

Regulation of c-*myc* mRNA Stability in Cells and Cell-Free Extracts

Jeff Ross, Phil Bernstein, and Gary Brewer*

*McArdle Laboratory for Cancer Research and Department of Pathology, University of Wisconsin-Madison, Madison, Wisconsin; *Present address: Bowman Gray School of Medicine, Department of Microbiology and Immunology, Winston-Salem, North Carolina*

ABSTRACT

The levels of many mRNAs are determined more by their stability than by their synthetic rate. We have developed an *in vitro* mRNA decay system to analyze how mRNA stability is regulated. This system seems to mirror mRNA decay rates in intact cells, since mRNAs that are unstable in cells are also unstable *in vitro*.

c-*myc* mRNA levels increase when cells are exposed to inhibitors of translation. In exponentially growing human erythroleukemia cells exposed for two hours to cycloheximide, a four-fold increase in c-*myc* mRNA occurs as a result of prolongation of its half-life from 40 to 160 minutes. c-*myc* mRNA is approximately four-fold more stable *in vitro* in reactions containing extracts from cycloheximide-treated cells than in extracts from untreated cells. Mixing experiments reveal that untreated cells contain a cytosolic destabilizer activity which is itself unstable in cycloheximide-treated cells. Therefore, the increase in c-*myc* mRNA half-life in cycloheximide-treated cells might result from destruction or inactivation of the destabilizer. Several properties of the destabilizer suggest that it consists of RNA or ribonucleoprotein. These data indicate that the stability of some mRNAs is regulated by cytosolic factors that are not associated with polysomes.

INTRODUCTION

Messenger RNA levels can be regulated by changing not only gene transcription rates but also mRNA turnover rates, and the half-lives of some mRNAs can vary by an order of magnitude or more [reviewed in references 55, 56, 63]. For example, mRNAs like c-*myc*, whose products probably influence cell replication, are usually relatively unstable, with half-lives of an hour or less [2, 13]. Therefore, modest changes in their turnover rates affect their steady-state levels over a short time, ensuring that the amount of each mRNA is maintained within a limited range. Such precise regulation appears necessary, because inappropriate expression of these mRNAs and their protein products interferes with cell replication and differentiation [1, 7, 12, 30, 31, 39, 47]. The stability of many mRNAs seem to be regulated [3, 13, 15, 16, 19, 20, 35, 36, 41, 62, 65, 7-73, 80].

For this reason, it is important to identify stability-regulating factors. To this end, we and others [46, 48, 57, 58, 67, 68] have developed *in vitro* mRNA decay systems, with the following important properties: i) These systems apparently mimic the authentic degradation pathways of at least some mRNAs. For example, c-*myc* mRNA is degraded *in vitro* by a pathway involving poly(A) removal followed by degradation of the mRNA body [6], and some polyadenylated mRNAs seem to be degraded by a similar pathway in cells [20, 69, 70, 74]. ii) Structural mutations that affect mRNA stability in cells have similar effects *in vitro* [17, 26, 46, 48, 51, 53]. iii) Most importantly, the *in vitro* systems seem to be useful

Published 1990 by Elsevier Science Publishing Co., Inc.
Molecular Biology of Atherosclerosis
A.D. Attie, Editor

for investigating how mRNA stability might be regulated. For example, histone mRNA is destabilized *in vitro* when histone proteins and a post-ribosomal supernatant fraction (S130) are added to reactions containing polysomes [49]. The effect is highly specific for histones and histone mRNA and requires the S130. This autoregulatory pathway might also function to control histone production during the S and M phases of the cell cycle [36].

The experiments described here were designed to identify cytoplasmic components that regulate the stability of proto-oncogene mRNAs such as c-*myc* and c-*myb*. We chose to focus on c-*myc* mRNA for three reasons. i) It is as unstable *in vitro* as in whole cells [6, 13, 72; this paper]. ii) Portions of the c-*myc* mRNA decay pathway *in vitro* parallel those observed in cells [6, 69, 70]. iii) In some cells, c-*myc* mRNA is stabilized when translation is inhibited, and its decay rate varies during the early stages of the mitogen-induced transition from G_0 to G_1 phase [13, 27, 32, 72]. Therefore, regulatory factors probably modulate its stability [see also 44], and we reasoned that such factors might be functional *in vitro*.

MATERIALS AND METHODS

Cell culture and preparation of polysomes and S130. The culturing of human erythroleukemia cells, K562 [14, 33], and the isolation of their polysomes and post-polysomal supernatant (S130) were as previously described [57]. For some experiments, S130 was concentrated approximately four-fold at 4°C in a Centricon-10 tube (Amicon Corp.).

***In vitro* mRNA decay reactions**. In all experiments reported here, we analyzed the *in vitro* degradation of polysome-associated mRNAs. Reaction mixtures (25 µl) included 0.7 A260 units of polysomes (from ~4 x 10^6 cells) and, where noted, variable amounts of S130 [58]. RNase protection mapping, using RNases P1 and T1, and blotting of c-*myc* mRNA were carried out as described [6]. The c-*myc* probes were derived from a cDNA clone, pM1-11, kindly provided by Grace Ju and colleagues [42]. To detect c-*myb* mRNA, a ^{32}P-labeled v-*myb* probe (from G. Holland and R. Risser, Univ. of Wisconsin) was hybridized to the blot for 18 hr at 60°C as per Church and Gilbert [10].

Biochemical characterization of the destabilizer activity. For proteinase K treatment, 100 µl aliquots of S130 (500 µg of protein) were incubated at 30°C for 30 min under the following conditions: proteinase K at 1 mg/ml, proteinase K at 1 mg/ml + 1 mM phenylmethylsulfonylflouride (PMSF), 1 mM PMSF, or 1% ethanol. (PMSF was dissolved in 100% ethanol and diluted 1:100 into the protease reactions.) For micrococcal nuclease treatment, S130 (100 µg of protein) was mixed with $CaCl_2$ and micrococcal nuclease to 1 mM and 1000 units/ml, respectively. The reaction mixtures were then incubated at 30°C for 10 min, EGTA was added to a final concentration of 2 mM, thereby blocking further nuclease action, and the treated S130 was left on ice for 10 min.

RESULTS

Destabilization of c-*myc* and c-*myb* mRNAs by a cytosolic activity(ies)

The rapid fluctuations in c-*myc* and c-*myb* gene expression that accompany changes in cell proliferation or protein synthesis might result, in part, because the stabilities of their mRNAs are modulated [27, 32, 72]. Preliminary experiments using actinomycin D revealed that the half-lives of c-*myc* mRNA were 20 and 170 min in untreated and cycloheximide (CHX)-treated cells, respectively (data not shown). Polysomes were then prepared from untreated cells and from cells exposed to CHX for two hours. The *in vitro* decay of polysome-associated c-*myc* mRNA first determined in reactions containing polysomes (no S130). c-*myc* mRNA was degraded at similar rates with polysomes from control or CHX-treated cells (data not shown). Therefore, the *in vitro* activity of the polysome-associated mRNase(s) that degrades c-*myc* mRNA was unaffected by CHX treatment.

To determine if non-polysomal cytosolic factors affected c-*myc* mRNA turnover *in vitro*, polysome-containing reactions were supplemented with S130 from control or CHX-treated cells. The S130 fraction is known to contain components that influence histone mRNA turnover [49] and was thus a logical source to search for other regulatory factors. Two major observations were made. First, c-*myc* mRNA was degraded at least 8-fold faster with S130 from untreated cells than with BSA (Fig. 1, compare lanes 6-10 with 11-14). Second, the S130 from CHX-treated cells (CHX S130) did not affect c-*myc* mRNA decay (compare lanes 6-10 with 15-19); the mRNA was degraded at comparable rates in reactions with BSA, CHX S130, or no additions (Fig. 1 and unpublished observations). This experiment, coupled with those presented below, suggested that exponentially growing cells con

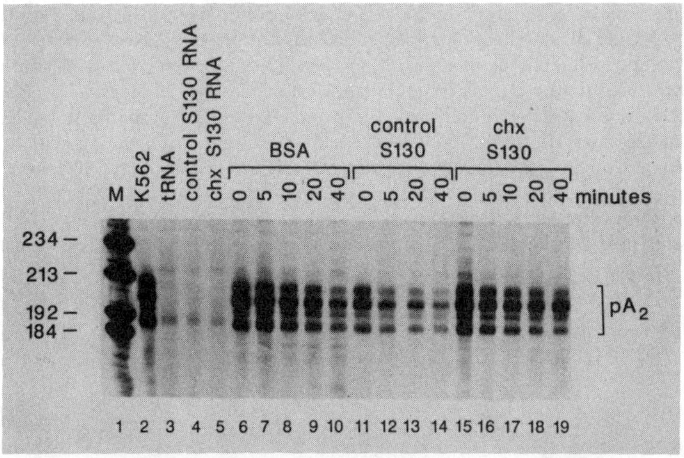

Fig. 1. Effects of K562 cell S130s on the *in vitro* degradation of c-*myc* mRNA.

Standard *in vitro* decay reactions containing equivalent amounts of polysomes from exponentially growing cells were supplemented with 100 µg of either BSA, S130 protein from exponentially growing cells (control S130), or S130 protein from cells harvested after a 2 hr exposure to CHX at 100 µg/ml (CHX S130). After incubation *in vitro* for the indicated times, RNA was extracted, and 30 µg from each reaction was analyzed by the RNase P1 plus T1 protection assay, as per Fig. 1. The gel was exposed for 2 days with an intensifying screen.

Lane 1: marker; HaeIII-digested pBR322 DNA, as per Fig. 1. Lane 2: 30 µg of total RNA from K562 cells. Lane 3: 30 µg of *E. coli* tRNA. Lane 4: RNA extracted from 100 µg of control S130. Lane 5: RNA extracted from 100 µg of CHX S130. Lanes 6-10: RNAs from reactions supplemented with BSA. Lanes 11-14: RNAs from reactions supplemented with control S130. Lanes 15-19: RNAs from reactions supplemented with CHX S130.

tain a cytosolic factor or factors, referred to here as a destabilizer activity, that accelerates c-*myc* mRNA decay. Since the destabilizer activity was diminished or eliminated when cells were exposed to CHX for two hours, continuous protein synthesis is probably required to maintain it at a detectable level.

Several controls supported these conclusions. i) c-*myc* mRNA was degraded at the same rate in reactions supplemented with control S130 or control S130 and CHX at 100 µg/ml (unpublished observatons). Therefore, residual inhibitor could not account for the low destabilizer activity of the CHX S130. This experiment also suggests that the destabilizer functions independently of translational elongation, because the added cycloheximide should inhibit residual *in vitro* protein synthesis. ii) None of the S130 preparations contained detectable c-*myc* mRNA (see Fig. 2); the mRNA analyzed in these experiments was derived from the polysome fraction. iii) Control S130 did not change the stability of delta or gamma globin (see below) or H4 histone [49] mRNAs. Therefore, the destabilizer is not a general ribonuclease activity.

c-*myb* mRNA is at least as unstable as c-*myc* mRNA in cells [72] and was also destabilized in reactions with control S130 (data not shown). We do not know if both mRNAs are affected by the same factor(s).

Mixing experiments with S130s from control and cycloheximide-treated cells

To confirm that S130 from untreated cells contained a destabilizer, the decay of c-*myc* mRNA was compared in reactions with 100 μg of control S130 protein, CHX S130 protein, or a mixture containing 100 μg of each (total of 200 μg). If CHX inactivated a destabilizer, the mixture should display decay kinetics similar to control S130 alone. c-*myc* mRNA was degraded at approximately equivalent rates in reactions supplemented with control S130 alone or with the mixture (Fig. 2, compare lanes 8-11 or 12-15 with lanes 4-7). However, it was degraded approximately 6-fold faster with the mixture, as compared with CHX S130 alone (compare lanes 12-15 with 16-19). These data indicate that growing cells contain a destabilizer that requires continuous protein synthesis to maintain high levels of activity.

Partial characterization of the destabilizer

The destabilizer was heat-labile *in vitro*, most of its activity being lost by preincubation

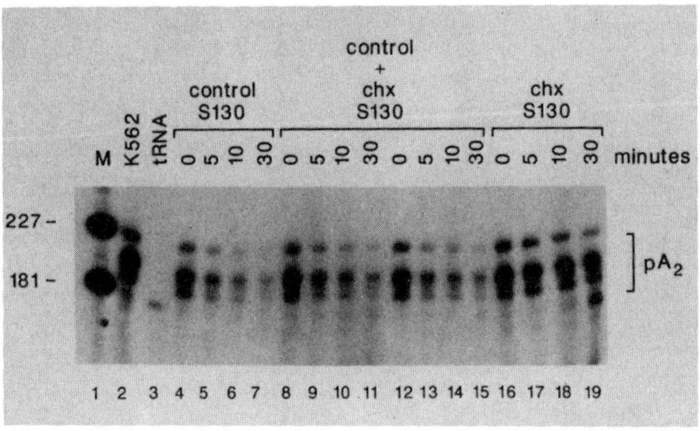

Fig. 2. Effect of mixing control and CHX S130s on c-*myc* mRNA decay: evidence for a destabilizer in the control S130.

Standard *in vitro* decay reactions containing polysomes from untreated cells were supplemented with 100 μg of control S130 (from exponentially growing cells), 100 μg of control S130 plus 100 μg of S130 from CHX-treated cells (CHX S130), or 100 μg of CHX S130. 15 μg of RNA from each reaction was analyzed by RNase P1 plus T1 mapping. The gel was exposed for 7 hr with an intensifying screen.

Lane 1: marker; pBR322 ^{32}P-labeled DNA cleaved with HaeII; sizes in nucleotides are noted on the left. Lane 2: 15 μg of total RNA from K562 cells. Lane 3: 15 μg of *E. coli* tRNA. Lanes 4-7: control S130. Lanes 8-15: two separate decay reactions containing the 1:1 mix of control and CHX S130s. Lanes 16-19: CHX S130.

at 45°C for 15 min (data not shown). Surprisingly, it was not inactivated by preincubation with proteinase K (Fig. 3), in spite of the fact that most of the S130 proteins that were visible in a stained gel were degraded by this treatment (Fig. 3B, lane 5). Experiments are in progress to determine if the destabilizer lacks protein components or if it contains proteinase-resistant protein(s), as described for the scrapie prion protein and for other proteins (reviewed in reference 38).

To determine if a nucleic acid component was associated with the destabilizer, S130 was preincubated with calcium and micrococcal nuclease at 30°C for 10 min. Further nuclease action was blocked by adding excess EGTA, and destabilizer activity was assayed. Nuclease pretreatment inactivated the destabilizer, because c-*myc* mRNA was degraded at comparable rates with nuclease-treated S130 or BSA (Fig. 4A and B, compare lanes 2, 3, and 5). Calcium-responsive factors in the S130 might also influence mRNA stability (compare lanes 3, 4, and 5), consistent with the fact that calcium fluxes affect mRNA abundance in cells [43, 54]. Several controls revealed that the micrococcal nuclease was cleaving RNA but not protein (data not shown). Taken together, the data indicate that micrococcal nuclease inactivated the destabilizer by destroying an essential nucleic acid component.

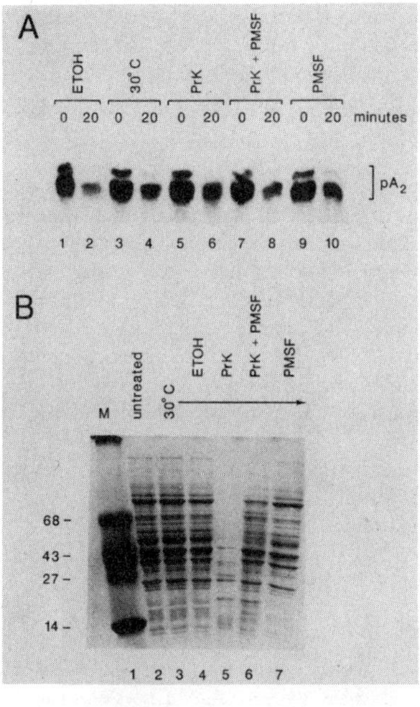

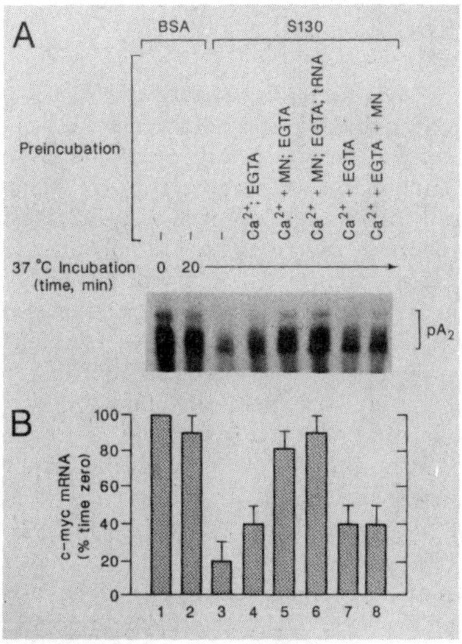

Fig. 3 (left side). Resistance of S130 destabilizer activity to digestion by proteinase K.

Panel A - mRNA decay reactions: 100 µl aliquots of concentrated S130 from exponentially growing cells were preincubated at 30°C for 30 min as indicated. These S130s were then chilled in ice water for 5 min, and 100 µg of protein from each was added to mRNA decay reactions, which were incubated at 37°C for either zero min (lanes 1, 3, 5, 7, 9) or 20 min (lanes 2, 4, 6, 8, 10). c-*myc* mRNA was analyzed by RNase P1 plus T1 mapping, and the mini-gel was autoradiographed for 14 hr with an intensifying screen.

Lanes 1 and 2: 1% ethanol. Lanes 3 and 4: no additives. Lanes 5 and 6: proteinase K, 1 mg/ml. Lanes 7 and 8: proteinase K, 1 mg/ml, plus 1mM PMSF. Lanes 9 and 10: 1 mM PMSF.

Panel B - effect of proteinase K on S130 proteins: Aliquots of the preincubated S130s from panel A were electrophoresed in a 10% SDS-polyacrylamide mini-gel and stained by Coomassie blue. Lane 1 contains pre-stained markers (BRL); sizes in kDa are indicated on the left. Lanes 2-7: S130s preincubated as noted in panel A.

Fig. 4 (right side). Sensitivity of S130 destabilizer activity to digestion by micrococcal nuclease.

Panel A - mRNA decay reactions with preincubated S130s: Aliquots of S130 from exponentially growing cells were preincubated at 30°C for 10 min as indicated (Materials and Methods). The plus (+) signs indicate that the reagents were added together in the indicated order. Semicolons (;) indicate sequential additions. Thus, for lane 4, Ca^{2+} was added, the reactions were preincubated, and then EGTA was added; for lane 8, Ca^{2+}, EGTA, and micrococcal nuclease were added together in that order. Following preincubation, each reaction mixture was chilled in ice water for 10 min, and 100 µg of the indicated protein was added to *in vitro* decay reactions. Following incubation at 37°C for either zero min (lane 1) or 20 min (lanes 2-8), RNA was extracted and analyzed by RNase P1 plus T1 mapping assay; the mini-gel was exposed for 14 hr with an intensifying screen.

Panel B - quantitation of the effect of micrococcal nuclease on the S130 destabilizer: Autoradiograms from the experiment shown in panel A and from three similar experiments were scanned, to estimate the relative decay of c-*myc* mRNA. Results are plotted as the percentage of undegraded mRNA after a 20 min incubation, as compared with time zero. The line above each bar denotes the standard deviation.

DISCUSSION

These data indicate that a 130,000 x g cytoplasmic supernatant fraction (S130) from exponentially growing cells contains a labile activity(ies) that destabilizes polysome-associated c-*myc* (and perhaps c-*myb*) mRNA *in vitro*. The significance of this observation is highlighted by the apparent correlation between destabilizer activity *in vitro* and c-*myc* mRNA turnover in intact cells. Furthermore, the steady-state levels of c-*myc* and c-*myb* mRNAs are two- to four-fold higher in CHX-treated cells, which are deficient in the activity, than in untreated cells, which contain the activity [13, 72]. The S130 is not an indiscriminate ribonuclease, and its expression probably requires continuous protein synthesis to replace what is lost, by whatever mechanism, during its normal turnover. Its half-life might be significantly less than two hours.

Preliminary characterization suggests that the destabilizer contains nucleic acid, presumably RNA, and is resistant to proteinase K. However, protein-free nucleic acid isolated from control S130 by phenol extraction lacks destabilizer activity (data not shown), suggesting that the destabilizer is a ribonucleoprotein. If so, it would be important to know if it has enzymatic activity, as reported for other RNPs [4, 18, 21, 25, 28, 76], and if its putative RNA component is complementary to any portion of the mRNA(s) it destabilizes [11]. Until we characterize it further, we cannot explain the apparent paradox that the activity diminishes in CHX-treated cells but is not inactivated (*in vitro*) by proteinase K. We also do not know if the same factor(s) affects both c-*myc* and c-*myb* mRNAs. However, the v-*myc* and v-*myb* proteins share several properties, and the c-*myc* and c-*myb* genes are regulated in a similar fashion in response to cell growth factors [22, 34, 66, 72].

The destabilizer presumably interacts with mRNAs that share some common sequences and/or secondary structure features. We favor the notion that it recognizes a specific conformational feature of certain mRNAs and increases their susceptibility to nuclease attack by modifying that conformation. For example, the 3' region of c-*myc* mRNA contains several interspersed AU islands, with sections of 8 to 25 nucleotides consisting exclusively of A and U 8, [64]. These islands are interspersed have the capacity to generate alternative stem-loop structures; one AU island can base pair with two or more other such islands. Perhaps the destabilizer binds to one or more AU-rich stem-loops, unwinds them, and thereby permits new ones to form. As a result, the conformation of the mRNA is changed, rendering the mRNA more susceptible to nuclease digestion. Conformational switching of this sort accounts for some instances of transcriptional attenuation and mRNA stabilization in prokaryotes reviewed in references [61, 78].

The following observations suggest that mRNA stability regulatory factors play an important role in the expression of many genes. i) Various hormones trigger dramatic (10-

fold or more), reversible changes in the turnover of specific mRNAs, and at least some of these changes might be influenced by stabilizer or destabilizer factors (reviewed in reference 24 and 63). ii) Translation inhibitors induce the accumulation of various mRNAs, a phenomenon frequently referred to as superinduction (3, 13, 20, 35, 41, 71-73, 80). Superinduction might, in some instances, involve the inactivation of destabilizer activities. iii) Cytoplasmic components autoregulate the stability of histone and tubulin mRNAs by a mechanism that involves an interaction between the mRNA and the protein it encodes [9, 36, 45, 49, 79]. iv) Recently, Schuler and Cole [62] found that the stability of GM-CSF mRNA is regulated in *trans* in monocytic tumor cells. Their results provide strong evidence that mRNA stabilizers and/or destabilizers modulate mRNA levels in intact cells.

The existence of mRNA stability factors also supports the idea that mRNA turnover rates are frequently determined by multiple interactions. In the simplest case, an mRNA whose stability was regulated might be affected by two sorts of interactions: i) Some sequences would determine the intrinsic or unregulated half-life, independent of regulatory factors reviewed in [55, 56, 63]. These sequences might influence the susceptibility of the mRNA to ribonucleases. ii) Some sequences would interact with regulatory factors that modify the intrinsic half-life. Mutational analyses, coupled with *in vitro* assays of regulatory components, should distinguish whether the sequences that determine intrinsic half-life differ from those that respond to regulatory factors [26, 64, 74].

We suggest that the regulation of mRNA stability provides two major advantages for the cell. First, it permits the cell to respond rapidly to changes in its environment; changing the rate of gene transcription and of mRNA turnover would permit a faster response than simply changing one or the other, particularly for mRNAs that are intrinsically unstable (see below). Second, subsets of gene products could be coordinately regulated in various ways. For example, by mixing and matching at the mRNA decay level, specific mRNAs, encoded by genes whose transcription had been induced in response to unrelated stimuli and by unrelated factors, could be controlled coordinately by a single cytoplasmic regulator. The rationale for stabilizing certain mRNAs in response to stresses like translation inhibition seems straightforward; the cell might need the stabilized mRNAs for essential proteins, once the translation block is relieved. The more interesting question seems to be why destabilizers (and stabilizers?) would be used to regulate mRNAs like histone, c-*myc*, and c-*myb* that are already relatively unstable. Perhaps their protein products need to be maintained within specified levels, above or below which they interfere with essential cell functions [12, 29, 39, 77]. This idea is consistent with the rapid turnover rates of c-*myc* and c-*myb* proteins (reviewed in reference 34) and with the fact that additional control mechanisms are exploited to regulate the expression of their genes [5].

ACKNOWLEDGEMENTS

We are grateful to Grace Ju for the c-*myc* cDNA plasmid pM1-11 [42], Bill Dove, Peggy Farnham, Phil Hart, Alan Kinniburgh, Stuart Peltz, and Bill Sugden for reading the manuscript and helpful comments, and Carol Dizack and Terry Stewart for artwork and photography. This work was supported by Public Health Service grants CA23076 and CA07175 from the National Institutes of Health. G. B. was supported by Public Health Service grant CA09230 from the National Institutes of Health.

REFERENCES

1. Adams, J. M., A. W. Harris, C. A. Pinkert, L. M. Corcoran, W. S. Alexander, S. Cory, R. D. Palmiter, and R. L. Brinster. 1985. Nature 318, 533-538.
2. Almendral, J. M., D. Sommer, H. MacDonald-Bravo, J. Burckhardt, J. Perera, and R. Bravo. 1988. Mol. Cell. Biol. 8, 2140-2148.
3. Altus, M.S., D. Pearson, A. Horiuchi, and Y. Nagamine. 1987. Biochem. J. 242, 387-392.

4. Arrigo, A. P., K. Tanaka, A. L. Goldberg, and W. J. Welch. 1988. Nature 331, 192-194.
5. Bentley, D. L., and M. Groudine. 1986. Nature 321, 702-706.
6. Brewer, G., and J. Ross. 1988. Mol. Cell Biol. 8, 1697-1708.
7. Campisi, J., H. E. Gray, A. B. Pardee, M. Dean, and G. E. Sonenshein. 1984. Cell 36, 241-247.
8. Caput, D., B. Beutler, K. Hartog, R. Thayer, S. Brown-Shimer, and A. Cerami. 1986. Proc. Natl. Acad. Sci., USA 83, 1670-1674.
9. Caron, J. M., A. L. Jones, L. B. Rall, and M. W. Kirschner. 1985. Nature 317, 648-651.
10. Church, G., and W. Gilbert. 1984. Proc. Natl. Acad. Sci. USA 81, 1991-1995.
11. Clemens, M. J. 1987. Cell 49, 157-158.
12. Coppola, J. A., and M. D. Cole. 1986. Nature 320, 760-763.
13. Dani, C., J. M. Blanchard, M. Piechaczyk, S. El Sabouty, L. Marty, and P. Jeanteur. 1984. Proc. Natl. Acad. Sci. USA 81, 7046-7050.
14. Dean, A., T. J. Ley, R. K. Humphries, M. Fordis, and A. N. Schechter. 1983. Proc Natl. Acad. Sci. USA 80, 5515-5519.
15. Dony, C., M. Kessel, and P. Gruss. 1985. Nature 316, 636-639.
16. Edgar, B.A., M.P. Weir, G. Schubiger, and T. Kornberg. 1986. Cell 47, 747-754.
17. Eick, D., M. Piechaczyk, B. Henglein, J.-M. Blanchard, B. Traub, E. Kofler, S. Wiest, G. M. Lenoir, and G. W. Bornkamm. 1985. EMBO J. 4, 3717-3725.
18. Falkenburg, P. E., C. Haass, P. M. Kloetzel, B. Niedel, F. Kopp, L. Kuehn, and B. Dahlmann. 1988. Nature 331, 190-192.
19. Fey, G.H., and G.M. Fuller. 1987. Mol. Biol. Med. 4, 323-338.
20. Fort, P., J. Rech, A. Vie, M. Piechaczyk, A. Bonnieu, P. Jeanteur, and J-M. Blanchard. 1987. Nucl. Acids Res. 15, 5657-5667.
21. Gardiner, K., and N. R. Pace. 1980. J. Biol. Chem. 255, 7507-7509.
22. Gazin, C., S. D. de Dinechin, A. Hampe, J-M. Masson, P. Martin, D. Stehelin, and F. Galibert. 1984. EMBO J. 3, 383-387.
23. Gilmartin, G.M., M.A. McDevitt, and J.R. Nevins. 1988. Genes and Dev. 2, 578-587.
24. Gordon, D. A., G. S. Shelness, M. Nicosia, and D. L. Williams. 1988. J. Biol. Chem. 263, 2625-2631.
25. Greider, C. W., and E. H. Blackburn. 1987. Cell 51, 887-898.
26. Jones, T. R., and M. D. Cole. 1987. Mol. Cell. Biol. 7, 4513-4521.
27. Kindy, M. S., and G. E. Sonenshein. 1986. J. Biol. Chem. 261, 12,865-12,868.
28. Kole, R., and S. Altman. 1981. Cell 20, 1902-1906.
29. Lachman, H. M., G. Cheng, and A. I. Skoultchi. 1986. Proc. Natl. Acad. Sci. USA 83, 6480-6484.
30. Leder, A., P. K. Pattengale, A. Kuo, T. A. Stewart, and P. Leder. 1986. Cell 45, 485-495.
31. Lee, W. M., M. Schwab, D. Westaway, and H. E. Varmus. 1985 Mol. Cell. Biol. 5, 3345-3356.
32. Levine, R. A., J. E. McCormack, A. Buckler, and G. E. Sonenshein. 1986. Mol. Cell. Biol. 6, 4112-4116.
33. Lozzio, C. B., and B. B. Lozzio. 1975. Blood 45, 321-334.
34. Luscher, B., and R. N. Eisenman. 1988. Mol. Cell. Biol. 8, 2505-2512.
35. Majesky, M. W., E. P. Benditt, and S. M. Schartz. 1988. Proc. Natl. Acad. Sci. USA 85, 1524-1528.
36. Marzluff, W. F., and N. B. Pandey. 1988. Trends Biochem. Sci. 13, 49-52.
37. McDevitt, M. A., G. M. Gilmartin, W. H. Reeves, and J. R. Nevins. 1988. Genes and Dev. 2, 588-597.
38. McKinley, M.P., D. C. Bolton, and S. B. Prusiner. 1983. Cell 35, 57-62.
39. Meeks-Wagner, D., and L. H. Hartwell. 1986. Cell 44, 43-52.
40. Melton, D. A., P. A. Krieg, M. R. Rebagliati, T. Maniatis, K. Zinn, and M. R. Green. 1984. Nucl. Acids Res. 12, 7035-7056.
41. Mitchell, R. L., L. Zokas, R. D. Schreiber, and I. M. Verma. 1985. Cell 40, 209-217.
42. Miyamoto, C., R. Chizzonite, R. Crowl, K. Rupprecht, R. Kramer, M. Schaber, G. Kumar, M. Poonian, and G. Ju. 1985. Proc Natl. Acad. Sci. USA 82, 7232-7236.
43. Morgan, J. I. and T. Curran. 1986. Nature 322, 552-555.
44. Nepveu, A., K. B. Marcu, A. I. Skoultchi, and H. M. Lachman. 1987. Genes and Dev. 1, 938-945.
45. Pachter, J. S., T. J. Yen, and D. W. Cleveland. 1987. Cell 51, 283-292.
46. Pei, R., and K. Calame. 1988. Mol. Cell. Biol. 8, 2860-2868.
47. Pellegrini, S., and C. Basilico. 1986. J. Cell. Physiol. 126, 107-114.
48. Peltz, S. W., G. Brewer, G. Kobs, and J. Ross. 1987. J. Biol. Chem. 262, 9382-9388.
49. Peltz, S. W., and J. Ross. 1987. Mol. Cell. Biol. 7, 4345-4356.
50. Perry, R. P. 1976. Ann. Rev. Biochem. 45, 605-629.
51. Piechaczyk, M., J-Q. Yang, J-M. Blanchard, P. Jeanteur, and K. B. Marcu. 1985. Cell 42, 598-597.
52. Puckett, L., S. Chambers, and J. E. Darnell. 1975. Proc. Natl. Acad. Sci. USA 72, 389-393.
53. Rabbitts, P. H., A. Forster, M. A. Stinson, and T. H. Rabbitts. 1985. EMBO J. 4, 3727-3733.
54. Radzioch, D., B. Bottazzi, and L. Varesio. 1987. Mol. Cell. Biol. 7, 595-599.
55. Raghow, R. 1987. Trends Biochem. Sci. 12, 358-360.
56. Ross, J. 1988. Mol. Biol. Med. 5, 1-14.

57. Ross, J., and G. Kobs. 1986. J. Mol. Biol. 188, 579-593.
58. Ross, J., G. Kobs, G. Brewer, and S. W. Peltz. 1987. J. Biol. Chem. 262, 9374-9381.
59. Ross, J., S. W. Peltz, G. Kobs, and G. Brewer. 1986. Mol. Cell. Biol. 6, 4362-4371.
60. Ross, J., and A. Pizarro. 1983. J. Mol. Biol. 167, 607-617.
61. Sandler, P., and B. Weisblum. 1988. J. Mol. Biol. 203, 905-915.
62. Schuler, G. D., and M. D. Cole. 1988. Cell 55, 1115-1122.
63. Shapiro, D. J., J. E. Blume, and D. A. Nielsen. 1987. BioEssays 6, 221-226.
64. Shaw, G., and R. Kamen. 1986. Cell 46, 659-667.
65. Simcox, A.A., C.M. Cheney, E.P. Hoffman, and A. Shearn. 1985. Mol. Cell. Biol. 5, 3397-3402.
66. Slamon, D. J., T. C. Boone, D. C. Murdock, D. E. Keith, M. F. Press, R. A. Larson, and L. M. Souza. 1986. Science 233, 347-351.
67. Stolle, C. A., and E. J. Benz, Jr. 1988. Gene 62, 65-74.
68. Sunitha, I., and L. I. Slobin. 1987. Biochem. Biophys. Res. Communs. 144, 560-568.
69. Swartwout, S. G., and A. J. Kinniburgh. 1989. Mol. Cell. Biol. 9, 288-295.
70. Swartwout, S. G., H. Preisler, W. Guan, W., and A. J. Kinniburgh. 1987. Mol. Cell. Biol. 7, 2052-2058.
71. Theodorakis, N.G., and R.I. Morimoto. 1987. Mol. Cell. Biol. 7, 4357-4368.
72. Thompson, C. B., P. B. Challoner, P. E. Neiman, and M. Groudine. 1986. Nature 319, 374-380.
73. Thorens, B., J.J. Mermod, and P. Vassalli. 1987. Cell 48, 671-679.
74. Wilson, T., and R. Treisman. 1988. Nature 336, 396-399.
75. Wilson, J. T., L. B. Wilson, J. K. deRiel, L. Villa-Komaroff, A. Efstratiadis, B. G. Forget, and S. M. Weissman. 1978. Nucleic Acids Res. 5, 563-581.
76. Wong, T. W., and D. A. Clayton. 1986. Cell 45, 817-825.
77. Wurm, F. M., K. A. Gwinn, and R. E. Kingston. 1986. Proc. Natl. Acad. Sci. USA 83, 5414-5418.
78. Yanofsky, C. 1988. J. Biol. Chem. 263, 609-612.
79. Yen, T. J., D. A. Gay, J. S. Pachter, and D. W. Cleveland. 1988. Mol. Cell. Biol. 8, 1224-1235.
80. Young, H.A., L. Varesi, and P. Hwu. 1986. Mol. Cell. Biol. 6, 2253-2256.

Regulated Degradation of Apolipoprotein II mRNA

Roberta Binder, Sheng-Ping L. Hwang, Ratneswaran Ratnasabapathy, Moisés Eisenberg, and David L. Williams

Department of Pharmacological Sciences, Health Sciences Center, State University of New York at Stony Brook, Stony Brook, New York

ABSTRACT

In addition to regulating gene expression at the transcriptional level, estrogen also alters the stability of induced mRNAs. In chick liver, the degradation rates of two induced mRNAs, apolipoprotein (apo) II and vitellogenin (VTG) II, are altered depending on the duration of prior estrogen treatment. During the two days required to attain the new steady state, the turnover rates for these messages were identical in the presence of estrogen and upon hormone withdrawal ($t_{½}$ = 13 hours). However, these messages turned over rapidly when hormone was withdrawn following a prolonged estrogen treatment (at least five days; $t_{½}$ = 1.5 hours). In order to understand how specific messages can be targeted for degradation, we have examined several aspects of apoII mRNA. The results of these studies demonstrate that apoII mRNA displays endonucleolytic degradation intermediates which result from cleavages that occur at 5′-AAU-3′/5′-UAA-3′ elements in single-stranded loop domains of the 3′-untranslated region (UTR). These cleavages occur in two larger domains of secondary structure which have been shown to bind specifically and independently to two different cytosolic proteins. The localization of endonucleolytic cleavages within binding domains for specific proteins suggests that these proteins may recognize the structural domains and play some role in the degradation of apoII mRNA or in the regulation of this process.

INTRODUCTION

In an increasing number of studies it is clear that mRNA stability plays an important role in gene regulation (1). However, little is known about the mechanisms responsible for regulating turnover of a specific mRNA. Regulation of mRNA stability has been studied in a class of genes that responds to estrogenic steroids by changing both mRNA transcription and decay rates. Estrogen was shown to induce the accumulation of ovalbumin, conalbumin, ovomucoid, and lysozyme mRNAs in chick oviduct (2), VTG II and apoII mRNAs in chick liver (3), and VTG mRNA in Xenopus liver (4). It has been proposed that these messages are also stabilized by estrogen because they are rapidly degraded upon hormone withdrawal (5,6). We have previously shown that the rapid degradation of chick liver apoII and VTG II mRNAs upon hormone withdrawal ($t_{½}$ = 1.5 hours) requires a period of estrogen induction of at least five days (7). If estrogen is withdrawn within the first few days of induction, both messages display the same half-life, 13 hours, as in the presence of estrogen. These results suggest that estrogen induces an activity that selectively destabilizes apoII and VTG II mRNAs upon hormone withdrawal. We have proposed that the mechanism of the hormone induced alteration in message stability may involve the interaction of cellular factors with specific sequence or structural elements of apoII and VTG II mRNAs.

ApoII mRNA has been characterized further in order to gain an understanding as to how its stability can be regulated. We present evidence that hepatocytes contain low levels of apoII mRNA degradation intermediates that arise endonucleolytically within 5′-AAU-3′/5′-

© 1990 by Elsevier Science Publishing Co., Inc.
Molecular Biology of Atherosclerosis
A.D. Attie, Editor

UAA-3′ elements in single-stranded loop domains of the 3′-UTR. Cytosolic proteins bind specifically to different regions of apoII mRNA, some of which are the target sites for the endonucleolytic cleavages. These proteins may be a part of the machinery that regulates the level of apoII mRNA by directly or indirectly modulating cleavage activity in the 3′-UTR.

IDENTIFICATION OF SPECIFIC ENDONUCLEOLYTIC DEGRADATION INTERMEDIATES IN THE 3′-UTR OF APOII mRNA

Previous studies using Northern analysis were unable to detect apoII mRNA degradation intermediates, suggesting that levels of intermediates may be low and/or unstable (7). When RNA was analyzed using more sensitive approaches, degradation intermediates were detected (8). In order to enrich for degradation intermediates, S1 nuclease mapping was carried out on the poly(A)$^-$ fraction, which should contain no full-length, polyadenylated apoII mRNA. These RNA samples were isolated from livers homogenized in guanidine isothiocyanate (GTC). This is a rigorous method that should yield RNA which reflects the *in vivo* state of apoII mRNA. To eliminate the possibility that the degradation intermediates occurred during the isolation of RNA, an *in vitro* synthesized ^{32}P-labeled, capped and polyadenylated apoII mRNA was added to the initial GTC homogenate and taken through all subsequent RNA isolation steps, including oligo(dT)-cellulose chromatography. This labeled apoII transcript displayed no appreciable degradation at any step (8). The S1 mapping probe was a 3′ end-labeled HinfI restriction fragment which extended from nucleotide 329 in the coding region to beyond the site of polyadenylation. The S1 mapping probe detected apoII mRNAs that were truncated at discrete locations within the 3′-UTR at sites 3′ to and including nucleotide 471. Fig. 1 is a representative S1 mapping experiment in which truncated apoII mRNAs were found to be enriched in the poly(A)$^-$ fractions from liver RNA samples pooled from either 24 hour estrogen-treated chickens (lane 5) or 24 hour estrogen-treated chickens that were withdrawn from hormone for 2 hours (lane 7). After correcting for the amount of sample analyzed and normalizing to the same amount of apoII mRNA, truncated apoII mRNAs were 2.8-fold more abundant in RNA from hormone-withdrawn animals. Similar truncated apoII molecules were detected with chickens treated with estrogen for 2 weeks, without or with subsequent hormone withdrawal (data not shown).

To demonstrate that these truncated apoII mRNAs were the result of an endonuclease, we assayed for the 3′ side of the degradation intermediates by primer extension of an oligonucleotide that hybridizes to the 3′ most end of the message, adjacent to the poly(A) tail (8). As shown in Fig. 2 (lanes 2-4), primer extension yielded cDNAs terminated at positions which corresponded to most sites of truncation as determined by S1 nuclease mapping. These cleavage sites were distinguished from reverse transcriptase pause sites by their greater abundance in animals withdrawn from hormone (lanes 2-4 as compared with lane 1). Pause sites were equally abundant in all samples and verified as pause sites because they also appear in reverse transcription of an unlabeled, *in vitro* synthesized apoII transcript (data not shown). The presence of the 3′ mRNA fragments indicates that most truncated apoII mRNAs resulted from endonucleolytic cleavage in the 3′-UTR.

When the sequence context of the cleavage sites mapped by primer extension and S1 nuclease protection are examined, the sites fall into three categories (Fig. 3). Class I and class II sites (or clusters of sites) are prominent cleavages identified by both S1 mapping and primer extension analyses. An exception is the site at nucleotides 636-637 which is too close to the oligonucleotide primer to be seen by primer extension. Class I sites occur within or adjacent to the trinucleotides 5′-AAU-3′ or 5′-UAA-3′. Class II sites occur at the dinucleotide 5′-UA-3′. Class III sites were detected only by S1 mapping, suggesting that these sites did not result from endonucleolytic cleavage but may have resulted from 3′→5′ exonuclease trimming, perhaps from endonucleolytic cleavages at sites further to the 3′ side.

Fig. 4 shows that the cleavage sites are primarily located within single-stranded loop regions in a secondary structure model of the 3′-UTR. This model is based on data from various chemical and enzymatic structural probes of the naked mRNA (9). Taken together, these data suggest that degradation of apoII mRNA is targeted to AU-rich, single-stranded regions. In addition, the consensus sequence 5′-AAU-3′/5′-UAA-3′ may also serve as a target site for cleavage. In order to determine whether the cleavage regions are accessible in the

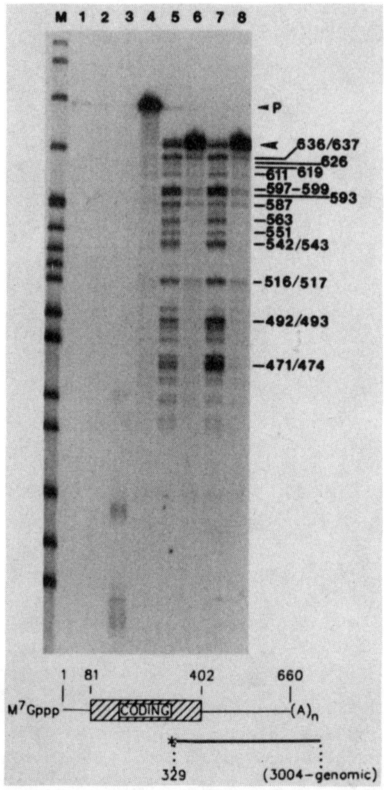

FIG. 1. S1 nuclease mapping detection of specific apoII degradation intermediates. Liver RNA (10 μg) pooled from three chickens treated with estrogen for 24 h was separated into poly(A)$^-$ (lane 5) and poly(A)$^+$ (lane 6) fractions, and 10 μg of liver RNA pooled from two chickens treated with estrogen for 24 h and withdrawn for 2 h was separated into the poly(A)$^-$ (lane 7) and poly(A)$^+$ (lane 8) fractions. These samples were annealed with 5000 cpm of the 3′ end-labeled 417 nucleotide S1 probe described below and in the text. Unprotected probe was digested with 2000 units/ml of S1 nuclease. Samples (600 cpm) from each of these reactions were loaded in lanes 5-8. Lane M, pBR322/Msp I markers; lane 1, unincubated probe; lane 2, probe incubated with yeast RNA; lane 3, probe incubated with annealing buffer; lane 4, probe incubated with poly(A)$^+$ RNA but undigested. Undigested probe (P), S1-resistant products reflecting full length (large arrowhead) and cleaved apoII molecules are indicated along the right side of the gel (reproduced with permission, from ref. 8).

native polyribosomal mRNP, chemical and nuclease modification studies were carried out in liver homogenates under conditions which do not result in nonspecific degradation of apoII mRNA (8). The results of these studies, summarized in Fig. 4, demonstrate that the regions containing cleavage sites were also accessible to modification in polyribosomes, suggesting that they would also be accessible to the degradation machinery *in vivo*.

BINDING OF DISTINCT CYTOSOLIC FACTORS TO TWO INDEPENDENT DOMAINS WITHIN THE 3′-UTR

Although a variety of mRNA binding proteins have been identified (10, 11), only the CAP binding protein and the poly(A) binding protein have been well characterized in terms

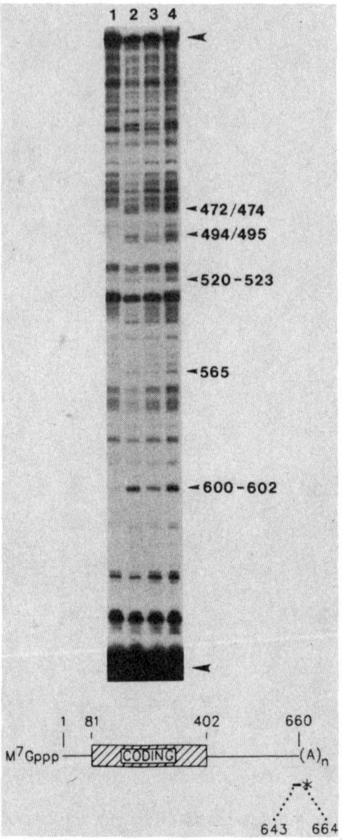

FIG. 2. Primer extension analysis confirms the presence of the 3′ side of apoII mRNA cleavage products. Equal amounts of apoII mRNA from guanidine isothiocyanate-extracted liver RNA made from a 24 h estrogen-induced chicken (lane 1) or from three 24 h estrogen-induced and 2 h withdrawn chickens (lanes 2-4) were primer extended using 30,000 cpm of the 5′ end-labeled primer described below the gel. Full length message (large arrowhead) and coordinates for cleavage sites are indicated along the right side of the gel (reproduced with permission, from ref. 8).

of their function and binding domains (12-17). Other mRNP proteins may be involved in directing aspects of mRNA metabolism such as message subcellular localization, translatability, and stability. For this reason, we sought to identify liver cytosolic factors that bound to the apoII 3′-UTR in a specific fashion. Using gel shift and label transfer assays, cytosolic factors were identified which bound preferentially to the 3′-UTR as compared to the coding region (18). These experiments were performed using [α- ^{32}P]UTP uniformly labeled, *in vitro* synthesized apoII mRNA, either as the full length, capped, and polyadenylated transcript, or as smaller fragments of the RNA. The smaller RNAs were generated from the full length RNA using a combination of oligonucleotide-directed RNase H cleavage to define the 5′ ends and either restriction enzyme digestion of the transcription vector or oligonucleotide-directed RNase H cleavage to define the 3′ ends (18). Liver cytosol consisted of a 100,000 x g supernatant prepared from two to three day estrogen-treated roosters (18).

Initial gel shift assays showed that the upstream domain of the 3′-UTR (nucleotides 400-547) incubated with cytosolic extracts exhibited reduced mobility on a native polyacrylamide gel (Fig. 5A, lanes 1 and 2). Addition of excess unlabeled upstream domain was able to compete with ^{32}P-labeled upstream domain for protein binding, eliminating the shift in mobility (Fig. 5A, lanes 3 and 4). However, neither excess downstream domain of the 3′-UTR (nucleotides 568-643) (lanes 5 and 6) nor excess coding region (nucleotides 90-380) (lanes 7 and 8) were able to compete for binding with the upstream domain. These results suggest that the factors which bind to the 400-547 fragment are specific for some sequence or structural element in this fragment. Binding of this fragment can also be competed by the full-length RNA (Fig. 5B, lanes 3 and 4), suggesting that the same specific sequence/structure elements responsible for binding of the 400-547 fragment are also active in the full length RNA.

In order to visualize the proteins which bind to different regions of apoII mRNA [α-^{32}P]UTP uniformly labeled full length apoII mRNA or mRNA fragments were UV cross linked to the cytosolic proteins. Samples were then treated with RNase A in order to remove non-cross linked RNA and analyzed by SDS-10% polyacrylamide gel electrophoresis. Fig. 6 shows that when full length RNA is incubated with cytosol a variety of proteins are labeled (lane 2). When only the 3′-UTR (nucleotides 400-643) is cross linked to cytosolic proteins, fewer

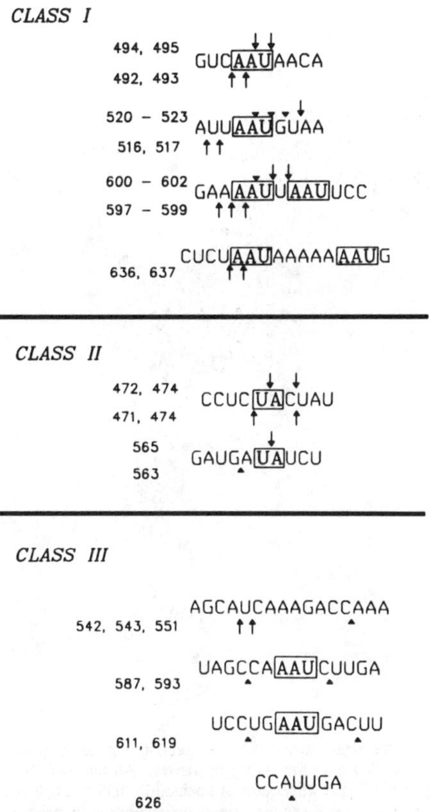

FIG. 3. Summary of cleavage sites in the 3′-UTR. Sites mapped by primer extension are indicated along the top of the sequences, and sites mapped by S1 nuclease protection are indicated along the bottom of the sequences by arrows (stronger cleavages) and arrowheads (weaker cleavages). Class I sites occur at and adjacent to 5′-AAU-3′ (boxed) and 5′-UAA-3′ trinucleotides. Class II sites occur at and adjacent to 5′-UA-3′ dinucleotides (boxed). Class III sites were detected only by S1 mapping (reproduced with permission, from ref. 8).

proteins are labeled, and these proteins appear to be a subset of those labeled by the full length RNA (lane 3). Within the 3′-UTR, the upstream domain (nucleotides 400-547) (lane 4) labeled a different set of proteins than the downstream domain (nucleotides 568-643) (lane 5). Each fragment labeled a subset of the proteins which were labeled by the entire 3′-UTR. The upstream domain labeled predominantly a 34 kd protein and the downstream domain labeled predominantly a 60 kd protein.

Competition experiments showed that the pattern of protein labeling for the individual domains of the 3′-UTR is specific. Excess unlabeled competitor of each domain could efficiently compete for its own protein labeling but had no effect on protein labeling of the other fragment. In addition, the coding region was unable to compete for protein labeling by either fragment (18).

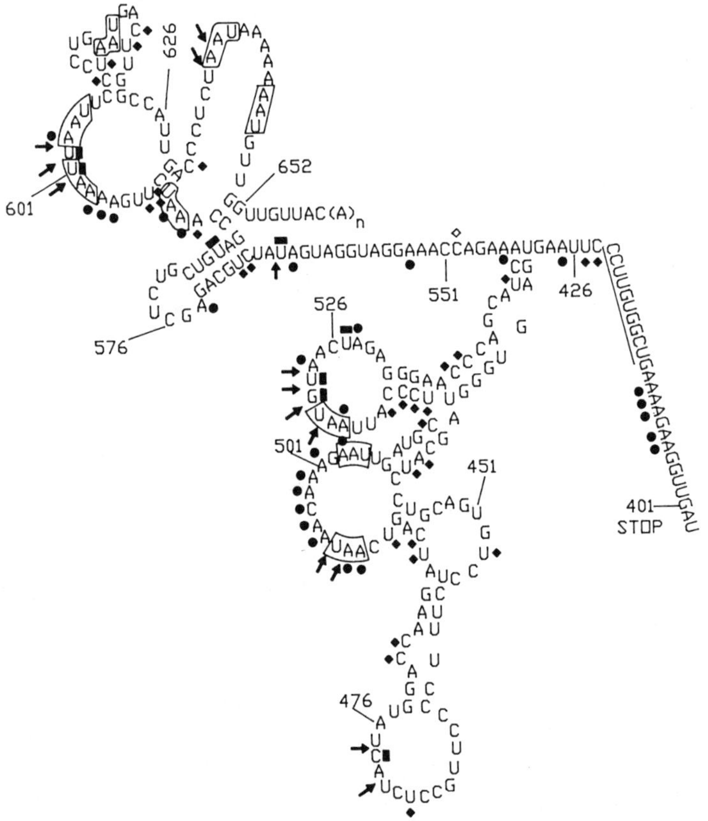

FIG. 4. Comparison of in vivo cleavage sites with sites accessible to exogenous modifications in apoII polyribosomal mRNP. The in vivo cleavages are shown by arrows. All but two sites are taken from primer extension mapping as summarized in Fig. 2. The sites at nucleotides 636 and 637 could only be mapped by S1 nuclease protection; this region is too close to the primer for resolution by primer extension. Sites in the mRNP which are sensitive to cobra venom RNase are indicated by diamonds. Sites in the mRNP which are sensitive to dimethylsulfate modification are indicated by circles. All of these sites are also mapped in the naked RNA with the exception of the cobra venom RNase site at nucleotide 550, which is only seen in the mRNP (open diamond). Sites that are targets of endogenous endonucleolytic cleavage in liver homogenates are indicated by rectangles. The underlined region, spanning nucleotides 414-423, is base paired to the coding region in a larger model from which the region shown here was taken (reproduced with permission, from ref. 8).

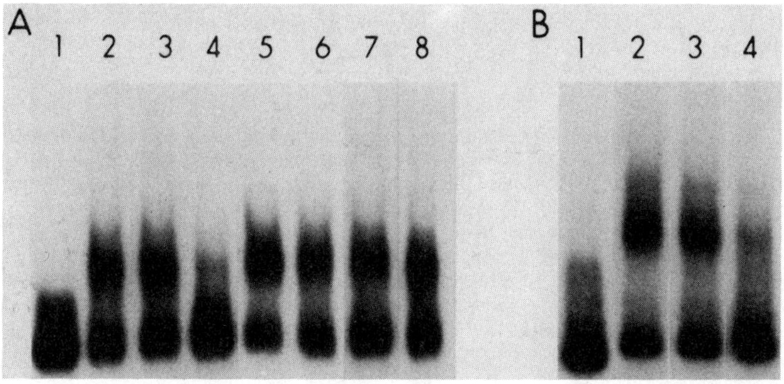

FIG. 5. Gel shift assays demonstrate that nucleotides 400-547 of the 3´-UTR bind cytosolic proteins in a specific fashion. (Panel A) An apoII mRNA fragment from nucleotides 400-547, labeled with [α-^{32}P]UTP, was incubated without (lane 1) or with (lanes 2-8) 20 μg of cytoplasmic extract. Competitor fragments were added prior to addition of extract. Lane 2, no competitor; lane 3 and 4, 5 fold and 50 fold molar excess of the nucleotides 400-547 fragment as competitor, respectively; lanes 5 and 6, 5 fold and 50 fold molar excess of nucleotides 568-643 fragment as competitor; lanes 7 and 8, 5 fold and 50 fold molar excess of nucleotides 90-380 fragment as competitor. (Panel B) The nucleotides 400-547 fragment was incubated without (lane 1) or with (lanes 2-4) 20 μg of cytoplasmic extract. Lane 2, no competitor; lanes 3 and 4, 5 fold and 50 fold molar excess of full-length apoII mRNA as competitor (reproduced with permission, from ref. 18).

The upstream and downstream binding domains of the 3´-UTR correspond to two larger regions of secondary structure on the structure model of apoII mRNA. These are shown as shaded regions in Fig. 7. It is tempting to speculate that the structures represent two different mRNP complexes. Both regions contain the target sites for apoII mRNA degradation (arrowheads).

CONCLUSIONS

There are limited examples where regulation of eukaryotic message stability can be associated with specific protein binding or appearance of degradation intermediates (19-22). It may be functionally significant that in apoII mRNA, domains of complex secondary structure serve as unique recognition sites for binding of specific proteins. Because these regions also contain the target sites for endonucleolytic cleavage, the proteins may play a role in the degradation of apoII mRNA. While we have no direct evidence to conclude that the cleavages are a result of the physiological mRNA turnover mechanism, the sequence and structural properties for these sites, together with their localization to the two protein binding domains is suggestive of functional significance.

The best example of post-transcriptional regulation via a specific RNA-protein interaction is the iron regulation of ferritin and transferrin receptor expression (23). Both messages contain a similar stem-loop that binds a 90 kd cytoplasmic protein. One copy of the stem-loop is located in the 5´-UTR of ferritin mRNA and five copies of the stem-loop are located in the 3´-UTR of transferrin receptor mRNA. The stem-loop-protein interaction has different functions in the two messages. In the absence of iron, the cytoplasmic protein binds to the stem-loop(s) and either represses translation of ferritin mRNA or stabilizes the transferrin receptor mRNA. However, in the case of transferrin receptor, the stem loop that binds the protein is not the same RNA element that imparts instability when the protein is removed. The investigators proposed that when the protein is not bound a rapid-turnover determinant is exposed, perhaps because the message forms an alternate conformation (24). A similar complex model may have to be invoked in order to understand how estrogen modifies apoII mRNP components in order to alter stability of the message.

The protein binding and degradation intermediate data suggests various models to explain regulation of apoII mRNA stability. The endonuclease activity does not seem to be a new turnover mechanism induced together with the rapid decay mode because the same cleavages occur after one day or 14 days of estrogen treatment and are not altered upon hormone withdrawal. Endonuclease activity appears to require an AU-rich or 5´-AAU-3´/5´-UAA-3´ sequence context located within single stranded domains that are in accessible regions of the apoII polysomal mRNP. Neither an AU rich element alone nor a single stranded element alone is sufficient to serve as a target site. Induction of the rapid decay mode may involve increased targeting of apoII mRNA to this preexisting degradation pathway. The 34 kd and 60 kd proteins may play a role in regulating accessibility to the degradation pathway.

One possible model to explain induction of the rapid decay mode is presented in Fig. 8. The model shows the 34 kd and 60 kd proteins binding to their respective recognition sites. When the proteins are bound to the 3´-UTR they simultaneously direct an endonuclease to the 3´-UTR and block the nuclease from clipping the RNA (panel A, left). As ribosomes move through the coding region, the interaction between the coding region and the 3´-UTR is melted

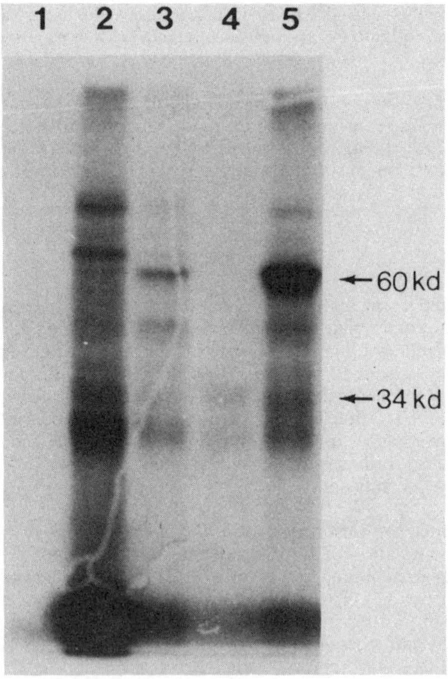

FIG. 6. Domains of the 3´-UTR are UV-cross linked to unique cytosolic proteins. Full length apoII mRNA and mRNA fragments labeled with [α-^{32}P]UTP were incubated without (lane 1) or with (lanes 2-5) 40 μg of cytoplasmic extract and UV-irradiated as described (18). After treatment with RNase A, samples were run on an SDS-10% polyacrylamide gel and subjected to autoradiography. Lane 1, full-length apoII mRNA not incubated with extract; lane 2, full-length apoII mRNA; lane 3, 3´-UTR fragment, nucleotides 400-643; lane 4, 3´-UTR upstream fragment, nucleotides 400-547; lane 5, 3´-UTR downstream fragment, nucleotides 568-643 (reproduced with permission, from ref. 18).

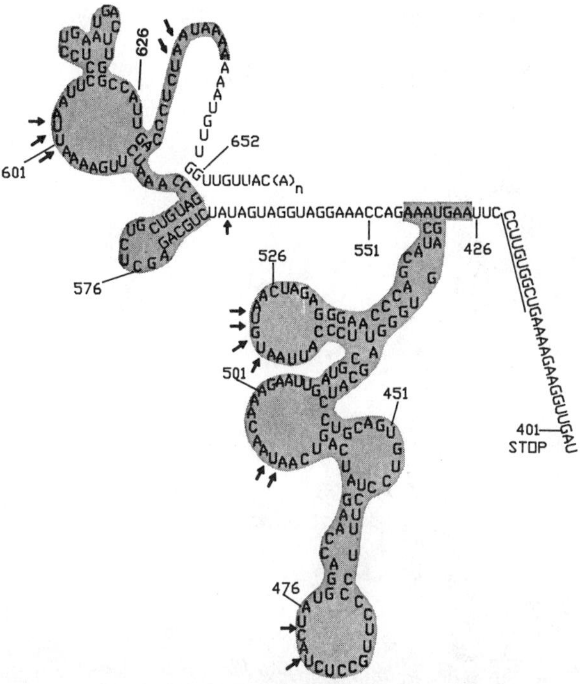

FIG. 7. Protein binding domains and degradation target sites in the 3´-UTR of apoII mRNA. The arrows show the endonuclease cleavage sites as sites as shown in Fig. 4. The shaded areas represent the upstream and downstream protein binding domains discussed in the text (reproduced with permission, from ref. 18).

out and the mRNP proteins now have a reduced affinity for the resulting alternate secondary structure that is formed (panel A, right). The nuclease may now recognize the alternate structure and cleave the RNA. We previously reported that apoII mRNA can form alternate secondary structures: 82% of the messages form a stable interaction between the 3´-UTR and a portion of the coding region, while the remainder of the messages do not form this interaction (9). These two structures may reflect the state of protein synthesis, similar to what is shown in the model. Alternatively, the mRNP proteins may remain bound, while ribosome translocation alters the secondary structure sufficiently to present a new target for the nuclease (not shown in this model). In the model, five days of estrogen treatment is sufficient to induce a cytoplasmic estrogen-binding protein (panel B). Upon hormone withdrawal, the hormone-free form of this protein binds to the nuclease and increases its activity (panel C, right). Induction of such a protein could account for the switch to the rapid decay mode upon hormone withdrawal. While there are reports of cytoplasmic estrogen-binding proteins, no functions have yet to be associated with them (25, 26). In the model presented here estrogen augments the activity of a preexisting and perhaps a general mRNA degradation pathway by inducing a factor that activates the ribonuclease. Such a mechanism has a biologically relevant role for rapidly shutting off egg yolk protein synthesis upon cessation of a laying cycle.

In summary, specific sequence/structure elements in apoII mRNA may serve as target sites for the cellular degradative machinery. The mRNA binding proteins may direct a

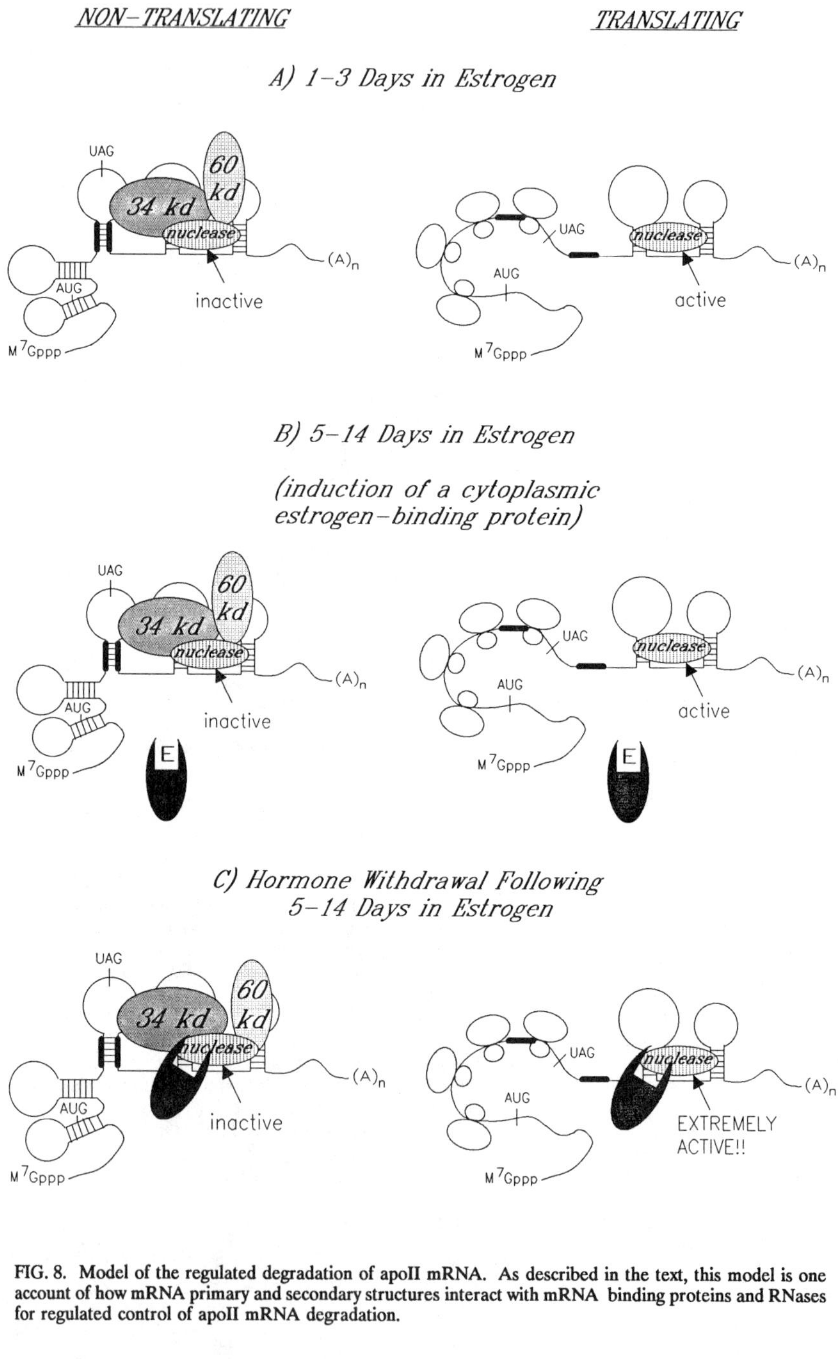

FIG. 8. Model of the regulated degradation of apoII mRNA. As described in the text, this model is one account of how mRNA primary and secondary structures interact with mRNA binding proteins and RNases for regulated control of apoII mRNA degradation.

nuclease(s) to the target sites. Alternatively, these proteins may protect the target sites from cleavage by limiting access to the target sites or by stabilizing an inaccessible secondary structure. Identification of the apoII sequences which regulate stability and bind proteins along with the identification of these proteins are in progress.

ACKNOWLEDGEMENTS

We would like to thank Mary Reyland and Martha Sensel for critical reading of the manuscript.

REFERENCES

1. G. Brawerman, Cell 48, 5-6 (1987).
2. N.E. Hynes, B. Groner, A.E. Sippel, S. Jeep, T. Wurtz, M.C. Nguyen-Huu, K. Giesecke, and G. Shütz, Biochem. 18, 616-624 (1979).
3. R. Wiskocil, P. Bensky, W. Dower, R.F. Goldberger, J.I. Gordon, and R.G. Deeley, Proc. Natl. Acad. Sci. USA 77, 4474-4478 (1980).
4. D.J. Shapiro and H.J. Baker, J. Biol. Chem. 252, 5244-5250 (1977).
5. M.L. Brock and D.J. Shapiro, Cell 34, 207-214 (1983).
6. D.J. Shapiro, J.E. Blume, and D.A. Nielsen, BioEssays 6, 221-226 (1987).
7. D.A. Gordon, G.S. Shelness, M. Nicosia, and D.L. Williams, J. Biol. Chem. 263, 2625-2631 (1988).
8. R. Binder, S-P.L. Hwang, R. Ratnasabapathy, and D.L. Williams, J. Biol. Chem. 264, 16910-16918 (1989).
9. S-P.L. Hwang, M. Eisenberg, R. Binder, G.S. Shelness, and D.L. Williams, J. Biol. Chem. 264, 8410-8418 (1989).
10. J.R. Greenberg, Nucleic Acids Res. 8, 5685-5701 (1980).
11. J.R. Greenberg and E. Carrol, Mol. Cell. Biol. 5, 342-351 (1985).
12. J. Pelletier and N. Sonenberg, Mol. Cell. Biol. 5, 3222-3230 (1985).
13. J.R. Greenberg and V.E. Burn, Nucleic Acids Res. 16, 3437-3454 (1988).
14. G. Blobel, Proc. Natl. Acad. Sci. USA 70, 924-928 (1973).
15. S.W. Kwan and G. Brawerman, Proc. Natl. Acad. Sci. USA 69, 3247-3250 (1972).
16. A. Jacobsen and M. Favreau, Nucleic Acids Res. 11, 6353-6368 (1983).
17. A.B. Sachs and R.W. Davis, Cell 58, 857-867 (1989).
18. R. Ratnasabapathy, S-P.L. Hwang, and D.L. Williams, J. Biol. Chem., in press (1990).
19. J. Ross, S.W. Peltz, G. Kobs, and G. Brewer, Mol. Cell. Biol. 6, 4362-4371 (1986).
20. J. Ross and G. Kobs, J. Mol. Biol. 188, 579-593 (1986).
21. D.M. Koeller, J.L. Casey, M.W. Hentze, E.M. Gerhardt, L-N.L. Chan, R.D. Klausner, and J.B. Harford, Proc. Natl. Acad. Sci. USA 86, 3574-3578 (1989).
22. E.W. Müllner, B. Neupert, and L.C. Kühn, Cell 58, 373-382 (1989).
23. R.D. Klausner and J.B. Harford, Science 246, 870-872 (1989).
24. J.L. Casey, D.M. Koeller, V.C. Ramin, R.D. Klausner, and J.B. Harford, EMBO J. 8, 3693-3699 (1989).
25. H. Eriksson, S. Upchurch, J.W. Hardin, E.J. Peck, Jr., and J.H. Clark, Biochem. Biophys. Res. Commum. 81, 1-7 (1978).
26. M.A. Hayward and D.J. Shapiro, Develop. Biol. 88, 333-340 (1981).

ANIMAL MODELS

Size and Composition of High Density Lipoproteins Is Determined by a Polymorphism Affecting Apolipoprotein A-II Translational Efficiency

R.C. LeBoeuf, M.H. Doolittle,* C. Warden,† L. Bee,† and A.J. Lusis†

*Department of Medicine, University of Washington, Seattle, Washington; *Wadsworth VA Medical Center, Los Angeles, California; †Department of Medicine, Department of Microbiology and Molecular Biology Institute, University of California, Los Angeles, California*

ABSTRACT

High density lipoproteins (HDL) are heterogeneous particles consisting of about equal amounts of lipid and protein that are thought to mediate the transport of cholesterol from peripheral tissues to liver. We show that a previously identified polymorphism affecting HDL electrophoretic mobility in mice is due to a monogenic variation controlling HDL size and apolipoprotein composition. Thus, the HDL particles of various inbred strains of mice exhibit a striking difference in the ratio of the two major apolipoproteins of HDL, apoA-I and apoA-II. The HDL size polymorphism and an apoA-II plasma concentration variation cosegregate with the apoA-II structural gene on mouse chromosome 1 among sets of Recombinant Inbred strains. This indicates that a mutation of the apoA-II gene locus is responsible. Studies of rates of apoA-II and A-I synthesis, turnover, cDNA in vitro translation and mRNA quantity suggest that a mutation at the apoA-II gene controls apoA-II translational efficiency. We conclude that the assembly of apoA-II into HDL does not have a set stoichiometry but is controlled by the production of apoA-II. As apoA-II levels increase, the HDL particles become larger and acquire more lipid, but apoA-I content per particle remains unchanged.

INTRODUCTION

The regulation of high density lipoprotein (HDL) concentration and chemical features is a multigenic process involving several tissues and metabolic systems. The major HDL proteins, apolipoprotein (apo) A-I and A-II, are synthesized in liver and intestine and assembled, with lipid, either at these tissues or in the plasma compartment. HDL are modified and remodeled in plasma by several enzymes, and we perceive them in our sampling of blood, as a collection of particles, heterogeneous in size and chemical composition. This report discusses the role of apoA-II in determining HDL size and composition.

RECOMBINANT INBRED STRAINS

A major tool used here involves the analysis of Recombinant Inbred (RI) strains. RI strains are commercially available mouse strains constructed by inbreeding F_2 progeny derived from two different pre-existing progenitor strains (1-3). Several RI strains can be derived independently, each strain forming a stable segregant population consisting of a unique mixture of alleles derived from the two parental strains. Genes are made homozygous by rigorous brother-sister mating. A key feature of RI strain analysis is that if the RI strains exhibit phenotypes resembling one or the other parent, the phenotype is likely to be controlled by a single gene. This is because each RI strain has a 50:50 chance of inheriting an allele from one or the other parent. If RI strains exhibit non-parental phenotypes (greater, lower, or intermediate values), the trait is multigenic in inheritance. An added advantage of using RI strains is that data for the segregation of genetic markers is cumulative and each RI strain needs to be typed for a

© 1990 by Elsevier Science Publishing Co., Inc.
Molecular Biology of Atherosclerosis
A.D. Attie, Editor

marker only once. Thus, it is possible to map genes responsible for single gene phenotypes by identifying cosegregation between new phenotypes and previously typed gene markers among the RI strains. RI strains used in this report, seven strains of CXB (BALB/c X C57BL/6) and twelve strains of BXH (C57BL/6 X C3H), have been typed for dozens of markers making them useful RI sets for the mapping of new genes.

A POLYMORPHIM AFFECTING HDL SIZE AND APOLIPOPROTEIN COMPOSITION

We have previously reported that HDL size varies among inbred strains of mice (4). There are two common phenotypes, as evidenced by HDL electrophoretic mobility in nondenaturing polyacrylamide gradient gels (5). HDL mobilities observed for inbred strains C57BL/6, BALB/c, and C3H exemplify the two common phenotypes: a rapid migration phenotype of strain C57BL/6 (average particle diameter of 8.5 nm), and a slow migration phenotype of BALB/c and C3H (average particle diameter of 10.5 nm).

This size polymorphism appears to be controlled by one major gene with Mendelian inheritance. HDL size phenotypes for the RI strains resemble one parent or the other in about a 1:1 ratio for the CXB and BXH sets of RI strains (6). F_1 animals exhibit intermediate phenotypes indicating codominant inheritance of this gene. The HDL size phenotype cosegregates with the structural gene for apoA-II, which is located on mouse chromosome 1 (4). On the other hand, the phenotype strain distribution pattern is discordant with the segregation pattern of the apoA-I gene on mouse chromosome 9. These results suggest that the HDL phenotype is determined by a mutation of the apoA-II locus.

Although structural differences exist for apoA-II between mouse strains, the mutation accounting for differences in HDL size is more likely due to quantitative differences in apoA-II. The apoA-II concentration of C57BL/6 is half that seen for BALB/c and C3H (15 mg/dl and 32 mg/dl, respectively), as quantitated by immunoblot analysis. The apoA-II level variation cosegregates with the apoA-II structural gene and the HDL size variation among CXB and BXH RI strains (6).

Further confirmation of the association between apoA-II and HDL size was obtained from the examination of congenic strain B6.C-*H-25*^{c}, which carries the chromosome 1 minor histocompatibility allele, *H-25*^{c}, transferred from BALB/c onto the genetic background of C57BL/6 (7). The congenic strain resembles the BALB/c donor strain with respect to apoA-II concentration and HDL size, but is like the C57BL/6 background strain with respect to apoA-I. Thus, the genetic background, or C57BL/6 alleles of other proteins, do not influence HDL size.

The biochemical consequence of this apparent genetic relationship between HDL size and apoA-II was explored by examining the chemical composition of HDL from C57BL/6 and BALB/c (6). Although total percent composition for HDL was similar for the two strains (57% protein, 22% phospholipid, 19% cholesterol, and 1% triglyceride), the ratio of the two major apolipoproteins, A-I/A-II, was different (1.63 for C57BL/6 and 0.68 for BALB/c). The difference in apoA-II concentration between strains accounts for the molar ratio differences, since apoA-I concentrations were similar for BALB/c and C57BL/6 (110mg/dl) (8).

THE HDL POLYMORPHISM DUE TO A CIS-ACTING MUTATION AT THE APOA-II GENE

The apoA-II quantitative phenotype appears to be under cis regulation, as suggested by its expression in F_1 animals. Isoelectric focusing gel electrophoresis was initially used to identify apoA-II charge variations between inbred mouse strains (4). Basic (BALB/c and C3H) and acidic (C57BL/6) forms were identified. F_1 heterozygotes derived from crosses between C57BL/6 and BALB/c, and C57BL/6 and C3H exhibited both parental forms of the protein band. In addition, the two charge forms in F_1 animals showed the two-fold difference in concentration as seen in parental strains (e.g. acidic form was less abundant than basic form). This pattern of relative concentration in the F_1 is consistent with a <u>cis</u> mode of regulation of apoA-II concentration. If the mutation acted in trans, similar levels of the two charge forms would be expected.

GENETIC CONTROL OF APOA-II LEVELS DETERMINED BY APOA-II SYNTHETIC RATE

ApoA-II levels could be controlled in two ways. First, a polymorphism could affect transcription or translation, and thereby the absolute rates of apoA-II synthesis, or second, an apoA-II structural polymorphism could influence its turnover. The first possibility was tested by measuring (^{35}S)-methionine incorporation into newly synthesized apoA-II. In mouse, only the liver contains significant levels of apoA-II mRNA (6), so experiments were performed in liver tissue: isolated hepatocytes and perfused livers. The rate of hepatic incorporation was significantly less in C57BL/6 as compared to BALB/c mice, reflecting the differences seen in plasma apoA-II pool sizes (6).

To examine the molecular basis of the genetic variation in apoA-II synthetic rates, levels of hepatic apoA-II mRNA were examined in various strains of mice. Northern blots of RNA isolated from five animals of strains C57BL/6 and BALB/c were prepared, and mRNA specific for apoA-II was identified by hybridization with a cDNA probe for mouse apoA-II (6). Autoradiograms were densitometrically scanned, and the average quantity of apoA-II mRNA compared to alpha-tubulin (internal standard) determined. The apoA-II quantitative variation did not appear to be determined by levels of specific mRNA, which were similar for the two strains (6).

That the fractional catabolic rate (FCR) did not appear to control apoA-II plasma pool size was suggested from turnover studies. HDL from C57BL/6 and BALB/c were isolated, radioactively labeled using (^{125}I)-ICl, and reinjected via the tail vein into the homologous strain. ApoA-I and apoA-II turnovers were examined individually on SDS gels following immunoprecipitation in several turnover analyses, and significant differences in apoA-II FCR were not observed (6).

APOA-II PRODUCTION IS REGULATED AT THE LEVEL OF TRANSLATIONAL EFFICIENCY

Incorporation of (^{35}S)-methionine label into C57BL/6 apoA-II was nearly half that of incorporation into BALB/c apoA-II. Yet incorporation of label into apoA-I was similar in the two strains. The basis for the apoA-II difference appeared to be utilization of mRNA, based on results from cell free translations of total RNA isolated from BALB/c and C57BL/6. Under conditions in which the RNA added was rate limiting for the level of translation, the incorporation of label into immunoprecipitable apoA-II was significantly greater using RNA from strain BALB/c than strain C57BL/6, mirroring the difference in apoA-II synthesis observed upon labeling of isolated hepatocytes (6). In contrast, the rate of in vitro translation of apoA-I was similar between strains as was apoA-I labeling in hepatocytes. The difference in translational efficiency of apoA-II observed between strains must result from an inherent difference in the apoA-II mRNA, because it is not tissue dependent.

APOA-II STRUCTURAL GENE POLYMORPHISMS

The results presented above indicate that polymorphisms of the apoA-II gene affect translational efficiency, thereby resulting in differences in apoA-II concentrations and HDL size among inbred mouse strains. These polymorphisms must occur within the regions of the gene encoding apoA-II mRNA, since translational efficiency is affected in vitro as well as in vivo. To examine this variation, cDNA from several strains of mice exhibiting low and high apoA-II plasma concentrations were sequenced (6). A number of nucleotide substitutions occurring between strains were identified. Although some of these substitutions affect the amino acid sequence, a particularly interesting substitution was found about 50 nucleotides upstream from the authentic start site. An AUG sequence was present in apoA-II cDNA from C57BL/6 but not BALB/c. It is thought that initiation of translation is the most critical step in the regulation of protein synthesis (9), and it is possible that the slower rate of apoA-II synthesis in C57BL/6 is due to the delayed formation of the correct initiation complex as a result of the presence of the alternate AUG codon.

CONTRIBUTION OF APOA-II TO HDL SIZE AND COMPOSITION

Although it is clear that apoA-I is a necessary requirement for HDL biosynthesis, as indicated by the apoA-I/C-III deficiency syndrome (10-12), apoA-II shares with apoA-I the important function of controlling HDL structure and composition. Likely mechanisms for this involve the interaction of apoA-II with apoA-I. The higher apoA-II content of the larger HDL species suggests that these larger HDL must also contain more lipid than the smaller HDL, since lipid and protein percent composition were similar between strains. Studies with phosphatidylcholine (PC) liposomes have indicated that apoA-II interacts with apoA-I in such a way as to increase the ability of apoA-I to bind PC (13). In addition, overexpression of the human apoA-I gene in transgenic mice resulted in increasing numbers of small HDL_3-like particles (14). Thus, in the transgenic mouse, decreasing the apoA-II/A-I ratio by overproduction of apoA-I lead to decreased HDL size, in agreement with our results.

Studies in humans and experimental animals suggest that apoA-II influences the metabolism of HDL, leading to HDL remodeling in the circulation. For example, incorporation of increasing amounts of apoA-II and apoA-I containing liposomes stimulates lecithin:cholesterol acyltransferase activity (LCAT) (15). Similarly, immunoaffinity purification of HDL subpopulations indicated that there are significant differences in the distribution of LCAT and apoD on HDL particles containing both apoA-I and A-II in comparison to HDL containing only apoA-I (16,17). There are also substantial differences in the ability of the two types of HDL particles to support sterol efflux from cultured cells (18). In addition, hepatic lipase activity, a triglyceride- and phospholipase which is thought to be involved in the conversion of HDL_2 to HDL_3, is activated *in vitro* by apoA-II (19). These observations strongly suggest that variations in the content of apoA-II can profoundly affect the ability of HDL to serve as efficient substrates for the various lipid transfer and lipolytic enzymes.

Thus, it seems quite likely that similar polymorphisms of apoA-II may contribute to variation in HDL size in humans. However, in humans, polymorphisms of other genes, such as the cholesteryl ester transfer protein gene, inactive or nonexistent in rodents, can also contribute to variations in HDL size and composition.

Because of genetic heterogeneity and environmental influences, analysis of lipoprotein metabolism directly in humans is complex. In the mouse, on the other hand, it is possible to isolate and study individual genetic variations affecting lipoproteins. Studies of additional strains of mice may well reveal other genes influencing HDL composition.

REFERENCES

1. D.W. Bailey in: The Mouse in Biomedical Research, History, Genetics and Wild Mice, H.L. Foster, J.D. Small and J.G. Fox, eds. (Academic Press, New York 1981) Vol. 1, pp. 223-240.
2. B.A. Taylor in: Origins of Inbred Mice, H.C. Morse, III, ed. (Academic Press, New York 1978) pp.423-438.
3. A.J. Lusis and R.L. LeBoeuf in: Methods in Enzymology, J.P. Segrest and J.J. Albers, eds. (Academic Press, Inc. 1986) pp.877-894.
4. A.J. Lusis, B.A. Taylor, R.W. Wangenstein, and R.C. LeBoeuf, J. Biol. Chem. 248, 5071-5078 (1983).
5. A.V. Nichols, P.J. Blanche, and E.L. Gong in: CRC Handbook of Electrophoresis. Vol III. Lipoprotein Methodology and Human Studies, Lena A. Lewis, ed. (CRC Press, Ohio 1983) pp.29-47.

6. M.H. Doolittle, R.C. LeBoeuf, C. Warden, L. Bee, and A.J. Lusis, J. Biol. Chem. in press (1990).
7. D.W. Bailey, Immunogentics 2, 249-256 (1975).
8. R.C. LeBoeuf, M.H. Doolittle, A. Montcalm, D.C. Martin, K. Reue, and A.J. Lusis, J. Lipid Res. 31, 91-101 (1990).
9. K. Moldave, Annu. Rev. Biochem. 54, 1109-1149 (1985).
10. R.A. Norum, J.B. Laker, S. Goldstein, A. Angel, R.B. Goldberg, W.D. Block, D.K. Noffze, P.J. Dolphin, J. Edelglass, D.D. Bogorad, and P. Alanpovic, New Engl. J. Med. 306, 1513-1519 (1982).
11. S.K. Karathanasis, R.A. Norum, V.I. Zannis, and J.L. Breslow, Nature 301, 718-720 (1983).
12. S.K. Karathanasis, V.I. Zannis, and J.L. Breslow, Nature 305, 823-825 (1983).
13. J.D. Morrisett, R.L. Jackson, and A.M. Gotto, Jr., Biochim. Biophys. Acta 472, 93-133 (1977).
14. A. Walsh, Y. Ito, and J.L. Breslow, J. Biol. Chem. 264, 6488-6494 (1989).
15. C.H. Chen and J.J. Albers, Eur. J. Biochem 155, 589-594 (1986).
16. M.C. Cheung and J.J. Albers, J. Biol. Chem. 259, 12201-12209 (1984).
17. M.C. Cheung, A.C. Wolf, K.D. Lum, J.H. Tollefson, and J.J. Albers, J. Lipid Res. 27, 1135-1144 (1986).
18. C.J. Fielding and P.E. Fielding, Proc. Natl. Acad. Sci. USA 78, 3911-3914 (1981).
19. C.E. Jahn, J.C. Osborne, E.J. Schaeffer, and H.B. Brewer, Eur. J. Biochem. 131, 25-29 (1983).

Apolipoprotein-A1 Metabolism in WHAM Chickens

Sandra A. Schreyer, Ferry Poernama, and Alan D. Attie

Departments of Biochemistry and Comparative Biosciences, University of Wisconsin-Madison, Madison, Wisconsin

ABSTRACT

A mutant chicken strain identified by a white skin phenotype was shown to have a profound deficiency in both HDL cholesterol and apo-A1. HDL plasma turnover studies showed that while the mutant chicken clears HDL 40% faster than the control, this could not explain the differences in HDL plasma concentrations (14.0 mg/dl vs. 100.1 mg/dl). The predominant defect responsible for the HDL deficiency is lower HDL production; the mutants produce 0.83 mg/dl/hr of HDL compared to 7.54 mg/dl/hr for the control. Similar results were observed when autologous HDL that had been preincubated with ^{125}I-apo-A1 was used as the tracer. From these data we conclude that the principal defect in the mutant chickens is reduced production of apo-A1.

Because the mutation is sex-linked, we determined if the apo-AI gene is on the Z chromosome. Apo-AI was shown to be autosomal, indicating that the mutation defines a *trans*-acting factor encoded by the Z chromosome that influences apo-A1 expression.

The mutant chickens did not have a reduction in apo-A1 mRNA abundance, suggesting that the mutation does not affect transcription or mRNA turnover. Additionally, the apo-A1 mRNA from the mutant chicken was shown to be translationally competent in a rabbit reticulocyte lysate system. Finally, immunoblots performed on liver, intestine, and muscle extracts showed a profound difference in intracellular apo-AI concentration between control and mutant chickens. These results suggest that the defect responsible for the low plasma apo-AI phenotype is in either apo-AI translation or intracellular degradation of the apo-AI protein.

INTRODUCTION

The plasma concentration of high density lipoprotein (HDL) is inversely correlated with an increased risk of developing coronary heart disease (Castelli, 1986; Third et al., 1984). Apolipoprotein AI (apo-AI) is a principal protein component of HDL and this protein may play a key role in HDL metabolism.

We have recently described a mutant animal model that has a dramatic reduction in plasma HDL compared to its normal counterpart (Poernama et al.,

© 1990 by Elsevier Science Publishing Co., Inc.
Molecular Biology of Atherosclerosis
A.D. Attie, Editor

1990). The mutation in these chickens is linked to the Z chromosome (the sex chromosome of the chicken) (Bitgood, 1988). We have shown that this deficiency is due to a defect in apo-A1 expression and have named these chickens the Wisconsin Hypo-Alpha Mutants or WHAM chickens.

RESULTS

Lipoprotein analysis. The mutant chickens have white shanks and beaks in contrast to the yellow coloration of controls. The plasma from the mutant birds is relatively pale in appearance. Since the xanthophylls that are responsible for the skin color and the darker appearance of the plasma are transported on lipoproteins, it is plausible that the abnormal color could be due to a lipoprotein abnormality.

There was a striking seven-fold reduction in plasma cholesterol in the female mutant compared to the controls; male mutants had a five-fold reduction in cholesterol. When the individual lipoproteins were isolated, a 13-fold difference in HDL cholesterol was seen (controls, 82.5 mg/dl; mutants, 6.3 mg/dl). Additionally, a 50% reduction in cholesterol was observed in the low density lipoprotein (LDL) fraction.

Two-dimensional polyacrylamide gels showed no differences in apo-A1 isoforms between control and mutant chickens (data not shown). Apo-A1 plasma concentrations were measured by radioimmunnoassay (RIA) using antibodies generated against chicken apo-A1.

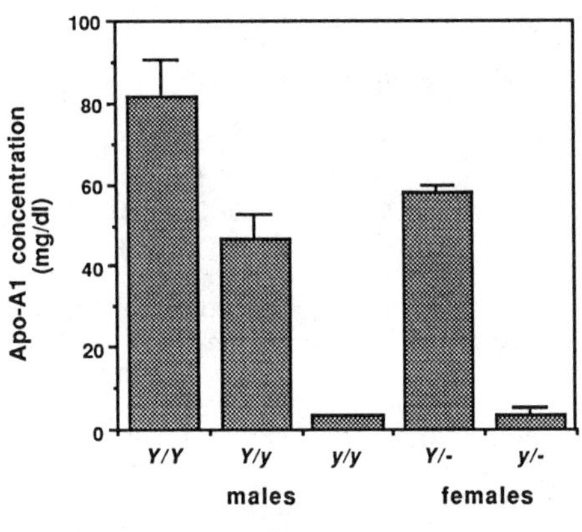

Figure 1. Plasma apo-A1 concentrations for mutant and control male and female chickens. (Reprinted with permission from: *Journal of Lipid Research* (1990) 31, 955-963.)

Figure 1 shows a 13-fold difference in plasma apo-A1 concentration between control and mutant male chickens with the heterozygotes having an intermediate value. Additionally, the control females have an apo-A1 concentration similar to the heterozygous males. These data suggest that the factor affecting apo-A1 expression is expressed in a gene dosage-dependent manner.

HDL turnover studies. HDL turnover studies were performed to determine if the defect is due to reduced synthesis or increased catabolism of the HDL particle in the mutants. Control and mutant HDL were isolated and labeled with ^{125}I or ^{131}I. The tracers were simultaneously injected into control and mutant female chickens and plasma samples collected over a fifty-hour time period.

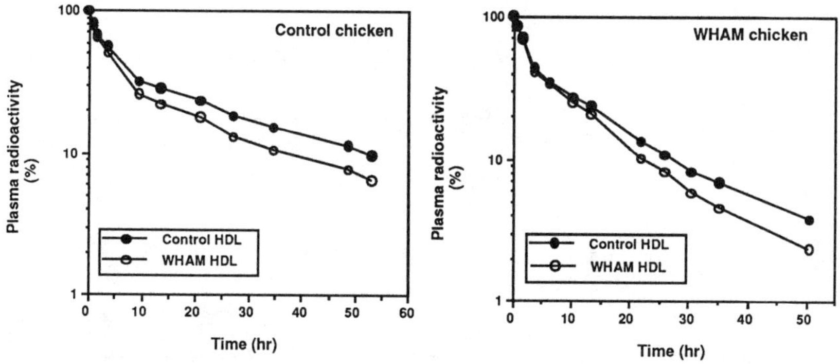

Figure 2. Plasma disappearance of radiolabeled control and mutant HDL. (Reprinted with permission from: *Journal of Lipid Research* (1990) 31, 955-963.)

Table I. HDL Fractional Catabolic Rate (pools/hr)

Chicken	Control HDL	Mutant HDL
Control	0.076	0.093
WHAM	0.106	0.127

The mutant chicken cleared both control and mutant HDL 40% faster than the control chickens (figure 3). In hypertriglyceridemic humans, an increase in HDL FCR is also observed (Brunzell *et al.*, 1983). Therefore, we were interested in ascertaining whether the mutant chickens were also hypertriglyceridemic. While total plasma triglycerides were near normal (28.9 mg/dl for control and 23.0 mg/dl for mutants), a 2.5-fold reduction of HDL triglyceride was seen in the mutants; control chickens had HDL triglycerides of 14.2 mg/dl plasma while the mutants had 5.6 mg/dl. Hence, the HDL deficiency cannot be a consequence of hypertriglyceridemia.

The mutant HDL is cleared by either chicken 20% faster than control HDL. To determine if the mutant HDL particle is abnormal, an HDL compositional analysis was performed.

Mutant HDL particles are reduced in cholesterol esters and enriched in triglycerides, relative to control HDL (table II). In humans, it has been suggested that triglyceride-rich HDL particles are cleared faster than triglyceride-poor particles (Fidge *et al.*, l980). Our results are consistent with this suggestion.

The differences in the HDL turnover, while significant, did not fully account for the gross deficiency of HDL in the mutants; there was a pronounced reduction in the HDL synthetic rate. The HDL synthetic rates were 7.54 mg/dl/hr for controls and 0.83 mg/dl/hr for the mutants. To directly measure apo-A1 turnover rates apo-A1 was purified, labeled with ^{125}I and incubated with either control or mutant HDL(Shepherd *et al.*, 1978). The HDL's were then injected into control and mutant chickens, respectively, and the plasma disappearance was followed. The particles were hypercatabolized in the mutant chickens and there was also an 80% reduction in the apo-A1 synthetic rate (Table III). Because the hypercatabolism also occurs when the triglyceride-enriched mutant HDL particles are injected into normal chickens, we propose that the primary defect is the diminished apo-A1 production rate. "Production" in this context refers to all events preceding the appearance of apo-A1 in the bloodstream.

Table II. HDL Lipid Composition

Chicken	Mass (%) Protein	Phospholipid	Cholesterol	Cholesterol ester	Triglycerides
Control	46.4	18.6	5.2	23.4	6.4
WHAM	37.6	23.6	2.6	12.8	23.4

TABLE III. Turnover of ^{125}I apo-A1-labeled HDL in male chickens

Chicken	FCR (pools/hr)	Apo-A1 Conc. (mg/dl)	Production Rate (mg/dl/hr)
Control	0.042	136.9	5.7
WHAM	0.105	10.6	1.11

Chromosomal location of the apo-A1 gene. Since the mutation in the WHAM chicken is Z-linked, we were interested in determining if apo-A1 is located on the Z chromosome. This would allow us to infer whether the apo-A1 deficiency is due to a mutation in the apo-A1 structural gene. A Southern blot of genomic DNA from New Hampshire and White Leghorn chickens revealed a *Sac*1 restriction fragment length polymorphism (RFLP) in the apo-A1 gene. When the two strains were crossed, both the male and female offspring were heterozygous for the RFLP. Therefore, apo-A1 is located on an autosome in chickens. Because the apo-A1 structural gene and the mutation responsible for the apo-A1 deficiency are not on the same chromosome, the mutation involves a factor that acts in *trans* on apo-A1 expression.

Apo-A1 expression. By Northern blot analysis there was no decrease in apo-A1 mRNA abundance in the mutant was observed, suggesting that there is no major defect in either RNA synthesis or turnover. RNA samples from control and mutant chicken livers were translated *in vitro* using the rabbit reticulocyte lysate system. No differences in the size or abundance of apo-A1 protein product between the controls and the mutants was observed, indicating that the apo-A1 mRNA from the mutant is translationally competent.

Mutant liver and intestinal samples showed a pronounced decrease in the amount of apo-A1 protein (figure 3). The reduction in apo-A1 protein suggests that the mutation involves a defect in either translation or a defect leading to degradation of newly-synthesized apo-A1.

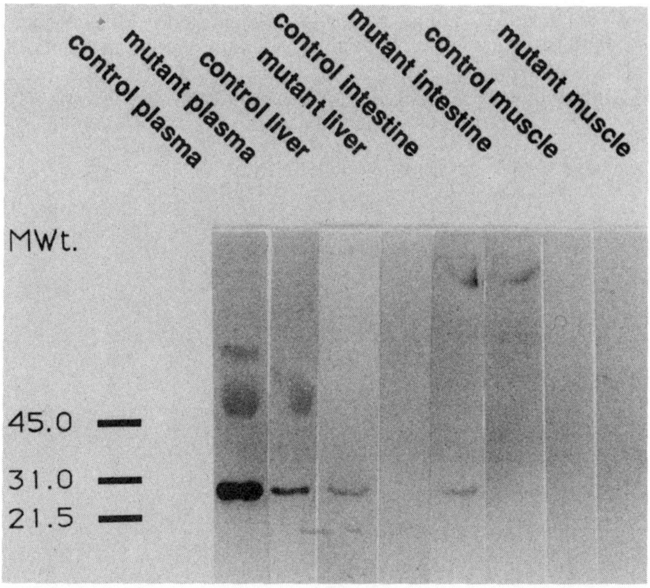

Figure 3. Immunoblot of control and mutant liver, intestine and muscle. Samples were homogenized in a buffer containing urea, SDS, and triton X-100 prior to electrophoresis. After transfer to nitrocellulose, the samples were probed with rabbit anti-chicken apo-A1 IgG.

CONCLUSIONS

The principal defect in the WHAM chicken is a major reduction in plasma HDL concentration due to reduced apo-A1 production. Apo-A1 mRNA from the mutants was similar in size and was not reduced in abundance, suggesting that the defect does not affect apo-A1 transcription. Intracellular apo-A1 protein was reduced in the mutant. We propose that either the apo-A1 mRNA is not being efficiently translated or that the protein is undergoing intracellular degradation rather than being secreted.

REFERENCES

Bitgood, J.J. (1988). Linear Relationship of the Loci for Barring, Dermal Melanin Inhibitor, and Recessive White Skin on the Chicken Z Chromosome. *Poultry Science* 67: 530-533.

Brunzell, J. D., Albers, J. J., Chait, A., Grundy, S. M., Groszek, E. and McDonald, G. B. (1983) Plasma lipoproteins in familial combined hyperlipidemia and monogenic familial hypertriglyceridemia. *J. Lipid Res.* 24: 147-155.

Castelli, W.P., Doyle, J.T., Gordon, T., Hames, G., Hjortland, M.C., Hulley, S.B., Kagan, A., and Zukel, W.J. (1986). Incidence of Coronary Heart Disease and Lipoprotein Cholesterol Levels. The Framingham Study. *JAMA* 256: 2835-2838.

Fidge, N., Nestel, P., Ishikawa, T., Reardon, M., and Billington, T. (I980). Turnover of Apoproteins A-I and A-II of High Density Lipoprotein and the Relationship to Other Lipoproteins in Normal and Hyperlipidemic Individuals. *Metabolism* 29: 643-653.

Poernama, F., Schreyer, S.A., Bitgood, J., Cook, M.E. and Attie, A.D. (I990). Spontaneous High Density Lipoprotein Deficiency Syndrome Associated with a Z-Linked Mutation in Chickens. *J. Lipid Res.* 31, 955-963.

Shepherd, J., Packard, C.J., Gotto, A.M. and Taunton, O.D. (l978).A comparison of two methods to investigate the metabolism of human apolipoproteins A-I and A-II. *J. Lipid Res.* l9:656-661.

Third, J.L.H.C., Montag, J., Freidel, J., Laskarzewski, P., and Glueck, C.J. (1984). Primary and Familial Hypoalphalipoproteinemia. *Metabolism* 33: l36-l46.

Nutritional Regulation of Atherosclerosis and Hepatic Lipoprotein Metabolism in Primates

Lawrence Rudel, Mary Sorci-Thomas, Fred Johnson, and David Williams

Departments of Biochemistry and Comparative Medicine, Bowman Gray School of Medicine of Wake Forest University, Winston-Salem, North Carolina, and Department of Pharmacological Sciences, State University of New York at Stony Brook, Stony Brook, New York

ABSTRACT

Atherosclerosis in African green monkeys is induced by diets enriched in cholesterol. Animals fed cholesterol together with saturated fat have more atherosclerosis than animals fed the same amount of cholesterol with polyunsaturated fat. To investigate the potential mechanisms for such differences we have examined aspects of apolipoprotein gene expression for apolipoproteins A-I and B. Plasma lipoprotein and apolipoprotein concentrations, hepatic apolipoprotein production during liver perfusion, and hepatic mRNA abundance for apolipoproteins A-I and B were measured in groups of animals fed polyunsaturated and saturated fat. Animals fed diets enriched in polyunsaturated fat had lower plasma concentrations of total, LDL, and HDL cholesterol. ApoB and apoA-I concentrations were also generally lower in the polyunsaturated fat group. The average size of the plasma LDL was smaller in the polyunsaturated fat fed animals, and the cholesteryl esters were more polyunsaturated. While total HDL concentrations were lower in the polyunsaturated fat group, the intermediate size and density populations of HDL were present in higher concentration. The hepatic secretion rate for apoB was not different between dietary fat groups, while the apoA-I secretion rate was higher in the saturated fat group. The mRNA abundance in liver for apoB was not different between dietary fat groups, while the mRNA abundance for apoA-I was higher in the saturated fat group. Hepatic LDL receptor mRNA abundance was higher in animals fed cholesterol but was not different between animals fed saturated and polyunsaturated fat. In spite of the lower HDL concentrations, the polyunsaturated fat fed animals had significantly less atherosclerosis. Overall, these data suggest that the dietary fat-induced differences in plasma LDL and apoB concentrations that are related to atherosclerosis extent are not due to intrinsic effects of dietary fat on hepatic apoB production. Dietary influences on the metabolism of cholesterol in the liver and plasma compartment that determine LDL composition and concentration are more likely the important factors determining effects on atherosclerosis. On the other hand, direct effects of dietary polyunsaturated fat to decrease apoA-I production were demonstrated. However, this modification did not lead to more atherosclerosis since less atherosclerosis occurred in the animals fed polyunsaturated fat.

INTRODUCTION

The role of cholesterol in development of premature Coronary Heart Disease (CHD) has received a great deal of attention particularly in recent years. The transport system for cholesterol in plasma includes two families of lipoproteins, the low density lipoproteins (LDL) and the high density lipoproteins (HDL). Numerous epidemiologic

Published 1990 by Elsevier Science Publishing Co., Inc.
Molecular Biology of Atherosclerosis
A.D. Attie, Editor

studies have identified LDL cholesterol concentrations as strong positive risk factors and HDL cholesterol concentrations as strong negative risk factors for premature CHD (1,2). The role of dietary fat in atherosclerosis has also been increasingly recognized (3). The apparent paradox is that dietary polyunsaturated fat lowers LDL cholesterol concentrations, but also lowers HDL cholesterol concentrations and decreases atherosclerosis (4). Another potential paradox is that polyunsaturated fat-enriched diets increase the number of polyunsaturated fatty acids present in plasma lipoproteins and therefore would appear to increase the potential for oxidation of LDL, which is believed by some to be an atherogenic feature of lipoproteins (5).

Studies in animal models are useful in defining molecular mechanisms for the risk factor relationships in atherosclerosis. We have carried out studies in the African green monkey as a model for dietary interactions in atherosclerosis. This primate species was selected because the plasma lipoprotein responses to dietary cholesterol and saturated vs polyunsaturated fat were found to be remarkably similar to those described in human beings, and more similar than in other primate species (6,7). In addition, in the primate model, the marked individual animal variability allows us to correlate diet-induced lipoprotein modifications to the extent of atherosclerosis. This approach assures us that lipoprotein endpoints under study are important in the atherosclerotic disease process.

In the first studies completed (8,9), we have examined gene expression of the apolipoproteins apoA-I and apoB that are potentially involved in the regulation of plasma LDL and HDL, respectively. We studied both the mRNA abundance as well as the hepatic secretion rates of these apolipoproteins. These data suggest that regulation of apoB synthesis and secretion is not a major response variable in dietary-induced modifications of plasma LDL concentrations. On the other hand, dietary alteration of apoA-I gene expression was noted at the level of hepatic mRNA abundance and secretion, suggesting that diet-induced regulation of the production of this apolipoprotein may, at least in part, be controlling plasma HDL concentrations. We also examined the mRNA abundance in liver for the LDL receptor. The data suggest that regulation of clearance of LDL via this receptor is sensitive to dietary cholesterol, although in this monkey model, the LDL receptor mRNA abundance was not different in polyunsaturated vs saturated fat-fed animals.

MATERIALS AND METHODS

The animals used for atherosclerosis quantitation and measurement of apolipoprotein mRNA abundance in these studies were a subset of a larger study in African green monkeys (*Cercopithecus aethiops)* of the vervet subspecies that had been imported into this country from Kenya by a commercial importer. The animals were young adult males at the start of the study and were fed their diets for 5 years. The diet compositions have been published (10). Low cholesterol diets (LO) contained 0.03 mg of cholesterol per kcal and high cholesterol diets (HI) contained 0.74 mg cholesterol per kcal. All diets contained 40% of kcal as fat. Saturated fat diets (SAT) contained fatty acid compositions of 40%, 47% and 13% saturated, monounsaturated, and polyunsaturated fatty acids, respectively. Polyunsaturated fat diets (POLY) contained fatty acid distributions of 22%, 30, and 48%, respectively.

Blood samples were drawn from animals after an overnight fast and plasma lipoproteins were isolated and separated as described before (11). Cholesterol concentrations were measured for each major lipoprotein class (12), LDL size (13) and subfraction cholesterol distribution was determined using density gradient ultracentrifugation (14), and the distribution of cholesterol among HDL subfractions was determined using density gradient ultracentrifugation (15). For both LDL and HDL, six subfractions were collected. The lowest density LDL subfraction of d<1.025 g/ml was numbered I with LDL subfractions of progressively increasing density numbered II, 1.025-1.030; III, 1.030-1.035; etc. through VI, d>1.045 g/ml. For HDL density subfractions, the lowest density subfraction numbered I was d<1.09 g/ml, and sequentially increasing subfractions were II, 1.09-1.10; III, 1.10-1.11; IV, 1.11-1.12; V, 1.12-1.135; VI, d>1.135 g/ml. Plasma concentrations of apoA-I and apoB were measured using an enzyme-linked immunosorbent assay (ELISA) for quantitation of apolipoproteins (16) and apoA-II was measured using a radial immunodiffusion procedure (17). At termination, the extent and severity of atherosclerosis in the thoracic and abdominal aorta was determined using morphometric techniques as previously described (18). A portion of liver and sections of other tissues were taken and quick frozen in liquid nitrogen for measurement of mRNA abundance using the DNA excess solution hybridization assay (19). From a separate subset of male and female animals fed the HI diets for at least two years, livers were removed and perfusion was done using the procedures published previously (20). Apolipoprotein accumulation in perfusate was measured during liver perfusion by ELISA (16).

RESULTS AND DISCUSSION

The amount of atherosclerosis in the aorta after five years of diet induction was measured using morphometric techniques. Intimal area was measured as an indicator of the extensiveness of atherosclerotic lesions, since it indicates the average amount of involved intima across all sections evaluated for each tissue segment. The maximal intimal thickness was also measured for the aortic segments as an indication of the severity of the lesions; this endpoint is an indication of the largest lesion or the lesion most likely to project into the arterial lumen and affect blood flow. The data in Table I document the diet-related differences in the subset of animals used in these studies. There was significantly more abdominal aorta intimal area in the HISAT group than in the other groups, and the Maximal intimal thickness in the abdominal aorta of the HISAT group was significantly greater than in the HIPOLY group or in either of the LO groups. Together, these data demonstrate that more atherosclerosis occurred in the groups fed the higher cholesterol diet only when saturated fat was fed together with cholesterol. In general, the lesions in the thoracic aorta were smaller and less extensive, although similar dietary fat and cholesterol-related differences to those in the abdominal aorta were also seen in the measurements of intimal area for the thoracic aorta. No differences in maximal intimal thickness were found for the thoracic aorta.

TABLE I. Dietary fat and cholesterol effects on aortic atherosclerosis.

Diet		Intimal Area (mm^2)		Max IntimalThickness(mm)	
Group	N	Abdominal	Thoracic	Abdominal	Thoracic
LO SAT	4	0.19[a] ±0.11	0.06[a] ±0.02	0.11[a] ±0.04	0.06[a] ±0.00
LO POLY	5	0.09[a] ±0.03	0.07[a] ±0.02	0.07[a] ±0.01	0.10[a] ±0.05
HI SAT	8	1.42[b] ±0.64	0.52[b] ±0.13	0.49[b] ±0.13	0.16[a] ±0.03
HI POLY	8	0.32[a] ±0.07	0.19 [a,c] ±0.08	0.23[a,c] ±0.06	0.10[a] ±0.03

All values, mean ± SEM.
Values with different letters are significantly different, $p<0.05$, as determined using ANOVA with post-hoc Fisher Least Significant Differance test.

The average plasma cholesterol concentrations for each diet group are shown in Table II. The values were significantly lower in the LO groups and in the POLY groups. A similar pattern was seen for LDL cholesterol concentrations. In addition to LDL cholesterol concentration, we examined the average LDL particle size, estimated as LDL molecular weight during chromatographic separation of the lipoprotein classes (13). LDL particles were significantly smaller in the LO groups, and tended to be smaller in the POLY groups although the dietary fat-related difference was not statisticallysignificant. The particle concentrations for LDL were also evaluated. Particle concentrations were highest in the HISAT group and were also higher in the HIPOLY group than in the LO groups. The diet-related differences in LDL particle concentration were similar but more pronounced than those seen for LDL cholesterol concentrations. The data in Figure 1, which represent means for each diet group, show that the proportion of cholesterol in LDL of the lower density subfractions is greater in the HISAT group. The peak density among the LDL subfractions is higher in the HIPOLY (1.035-1.040) than in the HISAT (1.030-1.035), and is highest in the LO groups. In Figure 2, the data for cholesteryl ester fatty acid composition of LDL are summarized. The proportion of saturated cholesterol esters (as indicated by the ratio of the more saturated CE/polyunsaturated CE) is highest in the HISAT group and is progressively lower in LOSAT>HIPOLY>LOPOLY groups. This shift in core lipid composition is likely to have significant effects on the physical state of the LDL particle (21). In general the dietary effects on LDL particle concentration and size that seemed most remarkable were those induced by cholesterol. On the other hand, the dietary polyunsaturated fat-related difference in cholesteryl ester composition and on density distribution of LDL particles was also significant. At the same time, the effects of cholesterol in inducing atherosclerosis seem to be modulated by polyunsaturated fat. These findings suggest that the effects of polyunsaturated fat on LDL particle composition and/or concentration are important in limiting the development of atherosclerosis, i.e. fewer and smaller, relatively more dense LDL particles that contain a predominance of cholesteryl linoleate instead of cholesteryl oleate are apparently less atherogenic.

TABLE II. Dietary fat and cholesterol effects on plasma cholesterol, apo B and LDL.

Diet Group	N	TPC mg/dl	LDL Ch mg/dl	LDL MW g/μmole	Apo B mg/dl	LDL Particle (μM)
LO SAT	4	168.0 ±12.9	68.8 ±9.2	2.84 ±0.05	88 ±9	0.46 ±0.10
LO POLY	5	143.2 ±8.9	58.8 ±4.9	2.87 ±0.07	80 ±10	0.36 ±0.06
HI SAT	8	299.8 ±16.1	154.0 ±22.2	3.10 ±0.11	130 ±9	1.12 ±0.18
HI POLY	8	243.4 ±10.9	123.4 ±9.7	3.06 ±0.07	100 ±9	0.72 ±0.10
Significance determined by two-way analysis of variance						
Dietary Fat		p=0.041	NS	NS	p=0.099	NS
Dietary Cholesterol		p<0.001	p<0.001	p=0.006	p=0.001	p=0.001
Interaction		NS	NS	NS	NS	NS

All values are Mean ± SEM

In contrast to the effects on LDL, the average HDL cholesterol concentrations were significantly lower in the polyunsaturated fat group, but dietary cholesterol had no effect on the average HDL cholesterol concentrations (Table III). No statistically significant diet-related differences in plasma apoA-I concentrations were detected, and no statistically significant effects on plasma apoA-II concentrations were detected. Taken together, these data suggest that there is a difference in total HDL cholesterol to protein ratio which could represent a difference in subfraction distribution (10). The data in Table III also show that there is a difference in the HDL protein concentrations among density subfractions, with a higher HDL protein concentration being found in the intermediate density HDL subfractions of the POLY groups and a higher HDL protein concentration in the lowest density HDL subfractions of the SAT groups. Assuming that HDL concentration is inversely correlated to atherosclerosis extent in these animals, as has been found in other groups (22), this data suggests that the presence of a higher concentration of the intermediate density HDL may be more beneficial in limiting atherosclerosis development than the higher concentration of the larger, lower density HDL, since the polyunsaturated fat-fed animals had less atherosclerosis. On the other hand, it is difficult to know whether the dietary fat effects on HDL and LDL are separate or complimentary in their effects on atherosclerosis. For example, it is possible that the effect of polyunsaturated fat on LDL primarily determines the atherosclerosis outcome while the effect on HDL contributes little. Many more studies will be needed to determine which of these effects are the more important with multiple regression analysis used to determine the relative importance of each variable.

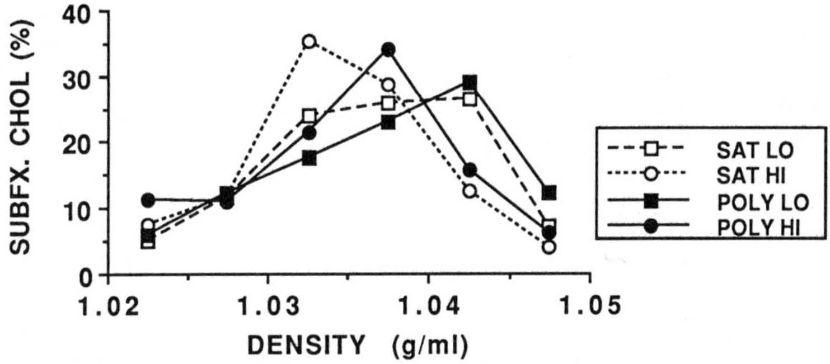

FIGURE 1. Density gradient distribution of LDL subfraction cholesterol. LDL from each of the 25 animals were fractionated by density gradient centrifugation into 6 subfractions as described in Materials and Methods. The percentage of cholesterol in each subfraction was determined and means for each diet group were determined. Mean values are plotted at the midpoint of the density range for the fraction, or at 1.0475 for the fraction of d>1.045.

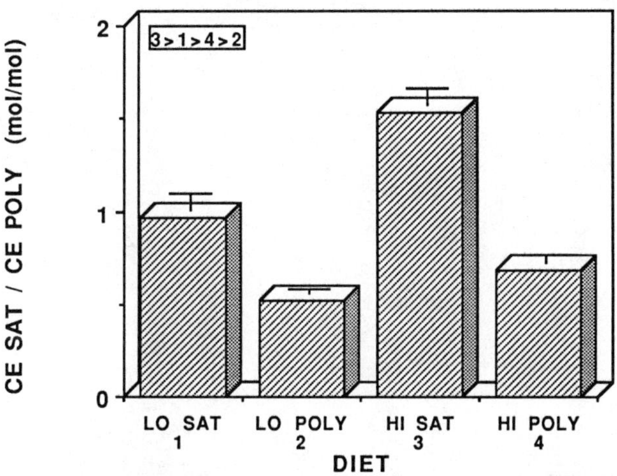

FIGURE 2. LDL Cholesteryl ester ratio for diet groups. The percentage distribution of individual cholesteryl esters was determined for LDL of each animal, and then the sum of the percents for all of the more saturated esters (myristate, palmitate, stearate, and oleate) was divided by sum of the percents for the polyunsaturated esters (linoleate, arachidonate, eicosapentenoate, etc) to give a ratio for each animal. Means (±SEM) for diet groups are plotted, and the significance ($p<0.05$), as determined by ANOVA and post hoc test, was determined as shown in the insert at upper left.

TABLE III. Dietary fat and cholesterol effects on plasma concentrations of HDL, apo A-I, apo A-II and HDL subfractions.

Diet Group	N	HDL Ch	ApoA-I	ApoA-II	HDL Protein					
					Frxn I	Frxn II	Frxn III	Frxn IV	Frxn V	Frxn VI
					[mg/dl]					
LO SAT	4	79 ±3	273 ±26	41 ±2	21.14 ±5.57	33.29 ±2.48	47.93 ±2.51	49.45 ±1.52	35.94 ±5.18	20.03 ±2.11
LO POLY	5	71 ±5	274 ±19	44 ±3	12.71 ±4.31	22.37 ±4.60	47.37 ±7.13	65.44 ±8.22	57.50 ±8.26	27.78 ±2.75
HI SAT	8	115 ±7	269 ±10	49 ±5	47.88 ±10.23	87.18 ±7.24	49.27 ±6.32	47.20 ±6.93	52.24 ±5.29	28.58 ±2.75
HI POLY	8	84 ±8	222 ±21	44 ±5	25.84 ±8.13	76.49 ±11.46	60.92 ±5.09	68.35 ±5.25	67.30 ±6.74	28.30 ±3.66
Significance determined by two-way analysis of variance										
Dietary Fat		p=0.003	NS	NS	p=0.07	NS	NS	p=0.002	p=0.003	NS
Dietary Cholesterol		p=0.001	NS	NS	p=0.01	p<0.001	NS	NS	p=0.023	p=0.08
Interaction		NS	NS	NS	NS	NS	NS	NS	NS	NS

All values are Mean ± SEM.

Given the dietary effects on plasma lipoproteins and atherosclerosis just described, it was of interest to determine the effects of these diets on the hepatic production of the apolipoproteins of the LDL and HDL. Apolipoprotein production is is a likely site of genetic regulation of lipoprotein particle metabolism. The data for mRNA abundance of apoB are shown in Table IV. No difference in hepatic apoB mRNA abundance was found although a dietary cholesterol-induced increase in intestinal apoB production was apparent. Since the intestine in the monkey produces only apoB-48, instead of apoB-100 which is the only apoB form produced in the liver (8), the increase in intestinal production of apoB mRNA induced by dietary cholesterol would not be expected to account for the increase in concentration of plasma LDL which contain only apoB-100. We also examined the rate of production of apoB-100 by using the isolated, perfused liver from a separate group of monkeys (8). The rate of apoB appearance during perfusion was linear and the same for animals fed either saturated or polyunsaturated fat plus cholesterol and no correlation was seen between the rate of apoB accumulation during perfusion and the concentration of LDL in plasma. Taken together, these data suggest that the rate of apoB-100 production (apoB gene expression) by the liver is not regulating the diet-induced difference in plasma LDL concentration.

Therefore, we examined the mRNA abundance for the LDL receptor in the liver, as a possible indicator of the extent of regulation of LDL clearance. The data are shown in Table IV. The HI groups had a lower LDL receptor mRNA abundance than the LO groups, showing that LDL receptor gene expression was apparently down-regulated in the livers of animals fed dietary cholesterol. However, there was no difference in POLY vs SAT groups for LDL receptor mRNA abundance, showing that no dietary fat-related difference in hepatic LDL receptor mRNA abundance occurs in this species. As a control, no difference among diet groups was seen in adrenal LDL receptor mRNA abundance. Significant inverse correlations were seen between the abundance of LDL receptor mRNA and plasma cholesterol and apoB concentrations (Figure 3), suggesting that regulation of expression of this gene was participating in the diet-induced regulation of plasma cholesterol concentrations in this species. Overall, these findings suggest that regulation of the LDL receptor in the liver, and its consequent effects on both LDL production and catabolism, are a more likely genetic site of diet modulation of plasma total and LDL cholesterol concentrations than any effect on hepatic apoB-100 production.

The expression of the apoA-I and apoA-II genes in the liver and intestine was also examined in these animals by measuring mRNA abundance and by measuring apoA-I and HDL particle mass accumulation during liver perfusion. The data in Table IV show that the mRNA abundance for apoA-I was equivalent between the LOSAT and LOPOLY groups, but was lower in the HIPOLY than in the HISAT group by about 20%. This 20% decrease was about the same as seen during liver perfusion studies in which the rate of apoA-I was lower in HIPOLY animals than in HISAT animals (9). The rate of accumulation of HDL mass was also lower in HIPOLY than in HISAT animals by about 20% (23). Finally, as shown in Figure 4, a strong positive correlation (r=0.7) across each of the diet groups was seen between the liver apoA-I mRNA abundance and plasma apoA-I concentrations for the animals of these studies, suggesting that hepatic production of apoA-I is a regulatory factor in determining plasma HDL levels. In contrast, no difference among diet groups in intestinal apoA-I mRNA abundance was seen, and no significant correlation between intestinal apoA-I mRNA and plasma apoA-I concentration was found. Thus, it appears that a tissue specific effect of dietary polyunsaturated fat to reduce apoA-I gene expression in the liver occurs which results in a lower plasma HDL and apoA-I concentration. Since approximately half of the apoA-I mRNA in the body of these animals appears to reside in the liver and half in the intestine (24), the dietary fat effect on plasma concentration of HDL and apoA-I could be completely explained by an effect on the liver but this would not represent an effect on all of the plasma HDL apoA-I. In contrast to the effects seen for apoA-I, no dietary effect on apoA-II gene expression in the liver was seen in these animals (Table IV) and undetectable levels of apoA-II mRNA in the intestine were found. Therefore, dietary regulation of apoA-II gene expression does not appear to be a primary site of diet-induced mediation of plasma HDL concentration in African green monkeys.

TABLE IV. Dietary fat and cholesterol effects on mRNA abundance.

DIET GROUP	N	LIVER mRNA pg/μg RNA				INTESTINE mRNA pg/μg RNA		ADRENAL mRNA pg/μg RNA
		Apo AI	Apo A II	Apo B	LDL recp	Apo AI	Apo B	LDL recp
LO SAT	4	66.0 ±12.8	50.2 ±6.1	167.7 ±45.5	2.42 ±0.46	136.0 ±17.0	75.5 ±24.4	11.88 ±4.19
LO POLY	5	75.0 ±8	41.6 ±11.6	185.0 ±17.1	1.85 ±0.38	121.3 (3) ±17.1	80.9 ±10.8	11.96 (4) ±2.07
HI SAT	8	78.0[a] ±4	46.0 ±5.5	147.5 (5) ±29.3	1.04 (5) ±0.12	136.6 (3) ±14.0	107.1 ±7.5	13.41 (7) ±3.70
HI POLY	8	61.0[a] ±4	48.8 (5) ±3.1	191.8 (5) ±15.6	1.18 ±0.06	134.8 (4) ±12.0	100.6 ±12.2	13.37 (5) ±5.74
Significance determined by two-way analysis of variance								
Dietary Fat		NS	NS	NS	NS	NS	NS	NS
Dietary Cholesterol		NS	NS	NS	$p=0.002$	NS	$p=0.03$	NS
Interaction		$p<0.02$	NS	NS	NS	NS	NS	NS

All Values are Mean ± SEM.
Values in parentheses indicate N for that group.
[a] Significance, $p=0.01$, as determined by Students t-test.

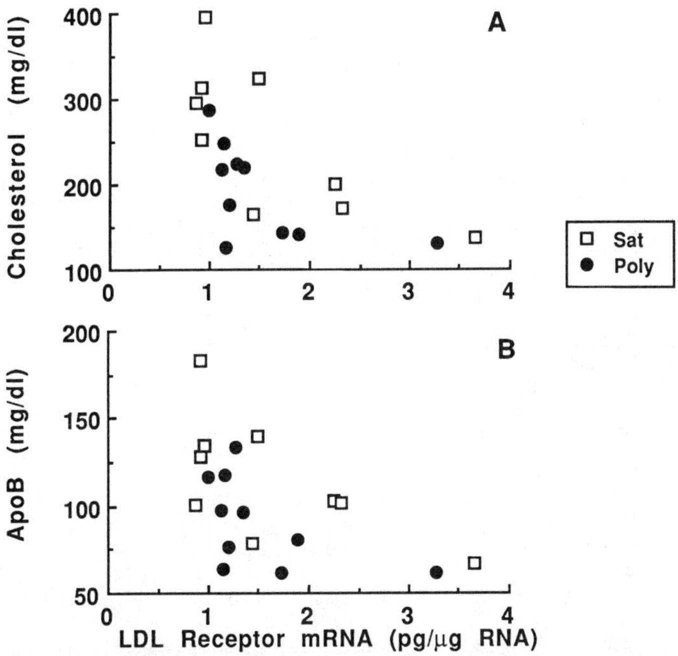

Figure 3. Liver LDL receptor mRNA abundance relationships with plasma cholesterol and apoB concentrations. *Panel B* shows the comparison of LDL receptor mRNA with plasma apoB concentration. Closed symbols represent the polyunsaturated fat diets and the open symbols represent the saturated fat diets. Linear correlation analysis showed this relationship to be significant, $p<0.02$ ($r=-0.52$). *Panel A* shows the comparison of LDL receptor RNA abundance with plasma cholesterol concentration. Linear correlation analysis showed this relationship to be significant $p<0.01$, ($r=-0.64$).

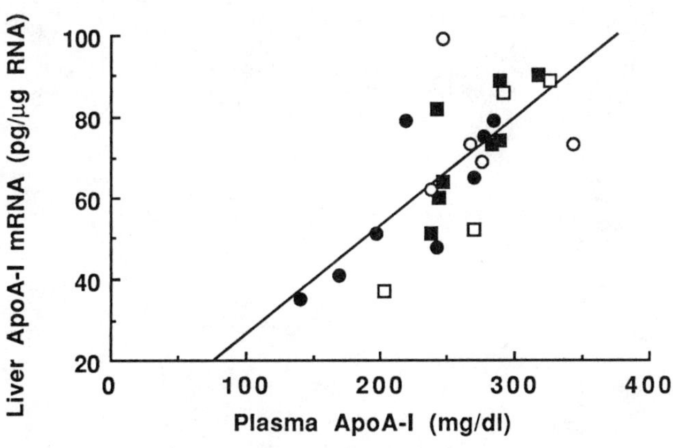

Figure 4. Correlation between hepatic apoA-I mRNA abundance and plasma apoA-I concentrations. Data points represent values from individual animals. Plasma apoA-I values are means from determinations on at least four plasma samples per animal. The correlation coefficient for the regression line, $r=0.70$, is significant, $p<0.001$. Open circles, LOPOLY; closed circles, HIPOLY; open squares, LOSAT; closed squares, HISAT.

REFERENCES

1. L.L. Rudel, Parks, J.S., Johnson, F.L. and J. Babiak, J. Lipid Res. 27, 465-474 (1986).
2. T. Gordon, W.P. Castelli, M.C. Hjortland, W.B. Kannel and T.R. Dawber, Am. J. Med. 62, 707-714 (1977).
3. S.M. Grundy and M.A. Denke, J. Lipid Res. 31, 1149-1172 (1990).
4. L.L. Rudel, J.S.Parks and M.G. Bond in: Current Topics in Nutrition and Disease. Nutritional Disease: Research Directions in Comparative Pathobiology, D.G. Scarpelli and G. Migaki, eds. (Alan R. Liss, Inc., New York 1986) pp. 501-523.
5. D. Steinberg, S. Parthasarathy, T.E. Carew, J.C. Khoo and J.L. Witztum, N. Eng. J. Med. 320, 915-924 (1989).
6. T.B. Clarkson, R.W. Prichard, B.C. Bullock, R.W. St. Clair, N.D.M. Lehner, D.C. Jones, W.D. Wagner and L.L. Rudel, Exp. Mol. Path. 24, 264-286 (1976).
7. L.L. Rudel, in: Use of Nonhuman Primates in Cardiovascular Research S.S. Kalter, ed. (University of Texas Press, Texas 1980) pp. 37-57.
8. M. Sorci-Thomas, M.D. Wilson, F.L. Johnson, D.L. Williams and L.L. Rudel, J. Biol. Chem. 264, 9039-9045 (1989).
9. M. Sorci-Thomas, M.M. Prack, N. Dashti, F. Johnson, L.L. Rudel and D.L. Williams, J. Lipid Res. 30,1397-1403 (1989).
10. J. Babiak, F. Lindgren and L.L. Rudel, Arteriosclerosis 8,22-32 (1988).
11. L.L. Rudel, C.A. Marzetta, F.L.Johnson, Methods Enz. 129,45-57 (1986).
12. L.L. Rudel and M.D. Morris, J. Lipid Res. 14,364-366 (1973).
13. L.L. Rudel, L.L. Pitts, II and C.A. Nelson, J. Lipid Res. 18,211-222 (1977).
14. C.A. Marzetta and L.L. Rudel, J. Lipid Res. 27,753-762 (1986).
15. L.L. Rudel, C.A. Nelson and K.R. Weiss, Arteriosclerosis 4,636-646 (1984).
16. D. L. Koritnik and L.L. Rudel, J. Lipid Res. 24,1639-1645 (1983).
17. J.J. Albers, P.W. Wahl, V.G. Cabana, W.R. Hazzard and J.J. Hoover, Metabolism 25,633-644 (1976).
18. T.B. Clarkson, M.G. Bond, B.C. Bullock and C.A. Marzetta, Exp. Molec. Path. 34,345-368 (1981).
19. D.L. Williams, T.C. Newman, G.S. Shelness and D.A. Gordon, Methods in Enz. 128:671-689 (1986).
20. F.L. Johnson, R.W. St.Clair and L.L. Rudel, J. Clin. Invest. 72,221-236 (1983).
21. A.R. Tall, D.M. Small, D. Atkinson and L.L. Rudel, J. Clin. Invest 62, 1354-1363 (1978).
22. L.L. Rudel, M.G. Bond and B.C. Bullock, Ann. NY Acad. Sci. US 454,48-253 (1985).
23. F.L. Johnson, J. Babiak and L.L. Rudel, J. Lipid Res. 27,537-548 (1986).
24. M. Sorci-Thomas, M.M. Prack, N. Dashti, F. Johnson, L.L. Rudel and D.L. Williams, J. Biol. Chem. 263,5183-5189 (1988).

APOLIPOPROTEIN STRUCTURE

The Crystal Structure of a Lipoprotein: Lipovitellin

Leonard Banaszak, Peter Timmins,* and Barbara Janik Poliks[†]

Department of Biochemistry, University of Minnesota, Minneapolis, Minnesota; Institut Laue Langevin, Grenoble, France; [†]Department of Biological Chemistry and Molecular Biophysics, Washington University, St. Louis, Missouri

ABSTRACT

The soluble lipoprotein, lipovitellin from lamprey oocytes, is a dimeric protein which contains about 70 molecules of bound phospholipid. Each subunit is made up of 3 polypeptide chains totalling about 1300 amino acids derived from a single chain precursor protein. Other workers have found amino acid sequence homology between human apoB100 and lipovitellin from other species. The conformation of the polypeptide portion of lipovitellin has been determined by x-ray crystallography. A large cavity appears in a central part of the structure surrounded mainly by β-strands. Although the β-sheet domains are adjacent to the cavity, the structure also contains a 17-membered α-helical domain.

INTRODUCTION

The protein components of soluble lipoproteins must have a unique conformation which permits them to bind variable numbers and types of lipid molecules. It is unknown what role the structure of serum lipoproteins play in the deposition and growth of arterial lipid plaques and therefore in atherosclerosis. However, conformational information would be useful in aiding the development of ideas on the mechanisms of assembly and recognition of lipoproteins. X-ray crystallography offers a powerful tool for deriving such structural information if crystals are obtainable. In general, the serum lipoproteins do not appear to be crystallizable probably because of compositional heterogeneity.

Lipovitellin is the principle lipoprotein found in oocytes from egg-laying animals. Unlike mammalian serum lipoproteins, lipovitellin appears far more homogeneous and amenable to crystallization. Moreover in many species, the lipovitellin granules found in these eggs are microcrystalline in vivo. The studies described below were carried out on specimens obtainable by re-crystallizing lipovitellin found in lamprey oocytes [1]. The

Published 1990 by Elsevier Science Publishing Co., Inc.
Molecular Biology of Atherosclerosis
A.D. Attie, Editor

resulting lattice is the same in the in vivo and in vitro forms of the crystals [2]. Low resolution studies have also been carried out on lipovitellin from X. laevis [3].

Biological Background

Unlike the serum lipoproteins, lipovitellin has two biological functions, transport and storage. Vitellogenin is synthesized in the liver, and is transported in the serum and eventually taken up by the ovaries. Within the yolk of the oocytes, it becomes the sole source of nutrients for the developing embryo. Important biochemical properties of lipovitellin are summarized in Table I, and the readers are referred to several review articles [4,5,6] for more details. Because it is a highy inducible protein and because ovaries have a mechanism for concentrating it, relatively large quantities of microcrystalline lipovitellin can be easily obtained. Note also in Table I, that with one exception, all post-translational modifications occur before secretion. The exception is the proteolytic cleavage which accompanies ovarian uptake. This modification seems to occur in a relatively consistent pattern throughout many species forming a large fragment (60-100kD) and several smaller proteins (20-40kD). One or more of the smaller protein chains is highly phosphorylated.

Table I
Summary Background Information for Lipovitellin

I. Source
- A. Liver in animals: birds, reptiles, fish
- B. Fat body in insects

II. Control of synthesis: Highly inducible protein
- A. Estrogens in animals
- B. Juvenile hormones in insects

III. Protein biosynthesis
- A. Single polypeptide chain of ≈200kD
- B. Multiple genes in some species

IV. Post-translational modification
- A. Glycosylation
- B. Phosphorylation
- C. Addition of lipids

V. Secretion and transport: precursor = vitellogenin
- A. Serum in animals
- B. Hemolymph in insects

VI. Ovarian uptake
- A. Specific receptor for vitellogenin
- B. Proteolytic modification
- C. Formation of microcrystals or granules of lipovitellin

The principal components of lamprey lipovitellin are listed in Table II. In the two instances where structural information is available, lipovitellin is generally found as a two-fold symmetrical dimer [3,7]. Therefore in terms of quaternary structure, lipovitellin behaves like any other globular protein oligomer. As can be seen in Table II, the proteolytic processing of lamprey vitellogenin results in three lipovitellin polypeptide chains in each subunit. Furthermore, each subunit is believed to contain about 35 molecules of lipid, mostly phospholipid [7,8].

Table II
Lamprey Lipovitellin

Molecular Weight	
Dimer	352000
Polypeptide-1	66800
Polypeptide-2	40750
Polypeptide-3	35200
Lipid w/w	16-19%
Molecules of lipid/monomer	≈35
^{31}P NMR phosphoserine/phospholipid molar ratio	2.8

Reference 7.

^{31}P NMR studies of lipovitellin from X. laevis indicated that the phospholipid bound to lipovitellin was present in a condensed phase resembling mono- or bilayer phases found in liposomes or membranes [11]. This was confirmed by using spin labelled phospholipids or fatty acids [12]. Based on the NMR and EPR studies, the phospholipid appears to be like a micro-domain of lipid bilayer confined to some internal region of the lipovitellin subunit. Small amounts of a variety of neutral lipids thought to be present, must be sequestered in regions defined by hydrophobic elements of the protein framework and the micro-domain of bilayer-like phospholipid.

Amino Acid Sequences

The amino acid sequence for lamprey vitellogenin or lamprey lipovitellin is being determined by Wm. Sharrock at the University of Minnesota but at this writing is not complete [Sharrock, personal communication]. From c-DNA data, the amino acid sequences of vitellogenin from chicken, X. laevis and C. elegans have been determined and compared in detail in a recent review article [4]. Particularly good amino acid sequence homology is observed between the chicken and X. laevis [4]. Vitellogenin from C. elegans however is missing the phosphoprotein portion, that is the amino acid sequence beginning about residue 1100 which contains mainly serine residues. Casual scanning of the amino acid sequence of the apoprotein reveals nothing unusual. There does not appear to be any long hydrophobic segments which is now thought to be associated with proteins containing a membrane spanning segment.

Of more relevance to this symposium is the question of whether or not there is any relationship between the serum lipoproteins and lipovitellin. A comparison of the amino acid sequences of the vitellogenins and apoB100 suggests that the two are homologous [4,9]. The extent of the homology is poorly defined but significant in the first 1000 residues [4,9]. This suggests that there is a common ancestor for the two proteins. Furthermore since they both form lipoproteins, it seems reasonable that some common structural motifs must exist in the two proteins. The amino acid sequence homology noted for apoB100 includes about 40% of apoB48, a polypeptide which is associated with chylomicrons [9]. In the case of C. elegans vitellogenin, a small segment of the amino acid sequence also appears to be homologous to human von Willebrand factor [10] and a segment of the Drosophila yolk protein has weak homology with lipoprotein lipase [9].

CRYSTAL STRUCTURE

Crystals of lamprey lipovitellin suitable for x-ray study were grown in citrate solutions at pH 6.2 [1]. They contain one lipovitellin subunit per asymmetric unit, the dimer having crystallographic twofold rotational symmetry. An electron density map to a nominal resolution of 2.8Å could be partially interpreted in terms of the overall conformation. The original crystallographic model was subsequently improved using density modified maps [7,13]. It is shown in cartoon form in Figure 1 below [7].

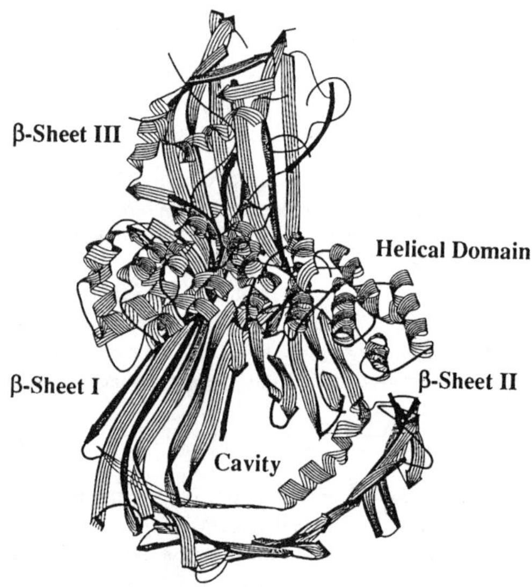

FIGURE 1: Conformation of Crystalline Lipovitellin
The schematic drawing of lipovitellin was prepared from the α-carbon coordinates by a computer program [14,15]. β-strands are described by pointed ribbons, α-helices by coiled ribbons and interconnecting random coils by solid curved lines.

The cartoon shown in Figure 1 is derived from a polyalanine model fitted to the electron density map at 2.8Å resolution. We have omitted 41 residues which were crudely fitted to weak electron density visible in part of the region labelled *cavity* in Figure 1. The model therefore contains 1011 amino acids in 11 different segments. Recall from Table II that 3 polypeptide chains are present in lipovitellin. One of these chains must belong to the *helical domain* where we are certain about the connectivity and polarity of the chain direction in the model. In the β-structure, we are less certain about the chain direction and in some instances we were unable to make all connections. This explains the 11 rather than 3 model segments. However, we believe the electron density map has sufficient information to fit an amino acid sequence when it becomes available. The fore-mentioned problems related to the present model are therefore solvable.

For descriptive purposes, the crystal structure of lipovitellin can be divided into several domains. The topmost third of the molecule, β-*sheet III*, as displayed in Figure 1 contains both α-helix and β-structure. The lower part of this domain is surrounded by the *helical domain* itself comprised of 17 α-helices arranged in a superhelical motif [7]. This form of super-secondary structure has not been observed in other proteins [7]. Only two of the 17 α-helices appear to be in contact with the *cavity*. The *cavity* has two β-sheet elements in immediate proximity. β-*sheet I* has seven strands and is most interesting because the strands extend upwards and lie parallel to several β-strands in β-*Sheet III* in Figure 1. In a very crude manner, the connections between β-*Sheet I and* β-*Sheet III* appear to form a possible hinge like region.

Work in progress includes the use of contrast variation and neutron diffraction to determine whether lipid or solvent is present in the *cavity*. Measurements of the volume of this space in the crystal structure indicates that it is of sufficient size to contain the approximately 35 molecules of lipid known to be present in lipovitellin [7].

DISCUSSION

The x-ray studies of lipovitellin cannot be completed until the amino acid sequence is available. However the preliminary crystal structure along with other biophysical experiments suggest that this lipoprotein molecule contains a microdomain of lipid partially surrounded by protein. The phospholipid in lipovitellin is in an anisotropic condensed phase which resembles bilayer- or monolayer-like forms found in membranes [11,12].

Assuming that the cavity region visible in Figure 1 contains the bound lipid, it is surrounded mainly by β-structure. In several places, the cavity also appears to be in direct contact with surrounding solvent. This may be somewhat misleading. The present model although accounting for all the visible electron density, is still missing about 300 amino acids. The latter are apparently disordered in the crystal lattice and most likely include most of the phosphoprotein portion of lipovitellin. The disordered segment could be located in a region which would provide additional shielding separating the lipid microdomain from solvent. The seventeen membered α-helical domain is in contact with all three of the β-sheets. Its function is obscure although it could be the framework which ties the sheet domains together.

Finally, the contacts between the β-*Sheet I and* β-*Sheet III* are sufficiently unusual, that it is tempting to speculate about their purpose. If the apo-form of vitellogenin is in a folded state prior to lipid incorporation, then some flexibility must be present in the conformation. The contacts between the fore-mentioned sheet structures could allow for conformational adjustments which must accompany the uptake of lipid.

The x-ray analysis at its present stage does not explain the homogeneity and ease of crystallization which are a property of lipovitellins from a variety of species. But, because of this property, it has been possible to partially determine its crystal structure. Other workers have shown some amino acid sequence homology between the polypeptide component of lipovitellin and apoB100. This suggests that the two lipoproteins may have some structural similarities as well. However, apoB100 provides the protein for LDL which has a much higher lipid content. This makes it very difficult to reconcile the structure of lipovitellin with any hypothetical model of LDL.

REFERENCES

1. T. Meininger, R. Raag, S. Roderick and L. Banaszak, J.Mol.Biol.179,759-764 (1984).

2. R.H. Lange, J.Mol.Biol. 179,765-768 (1984).
3. D.H. Ohlendorf, R.F.Wrenn and L. Banaszak, Nature 272,28-32 (1978).
4. B.M. Byrne, M. Gruber and G. AB, Prog.Biophys.Molec.Biol. 53,33-69 (1989).
5. J.R. Tata and D.F. Smith, Rec. Prog. in Hormone Res. 35,47-95 (1979).
6. R.A. Wallace in The Vertebrate Ovary ed. by R.E.Jones (Plenum, New York, 1978) 469-502.
7. R. Raag, K. Appelt, N.-H. Xuong and L. Banaszak, J. Mol. Biol.200, 553-569 (1988).
8. D. Ohlendorf, G. Barbarash, A. Trout, C. Kent and L. Banaszak, J. Biol. Chem. 252, 7992-8001.
9. M.E. Baker, Biochem. J. 255, 1057-1060 (1988).
10. M.E. Baker, Biochem. J. 256, 1059-1063 (1988).
11. L. Banaszak and J. Seelig, Biochemistry 21, 2436-2443 (1982).
12. G. Birrell, P. Anderson, P. Jost, O. Griffith, L. Banaszak and J. Seelig, Biochemistry 21, 2444-2452 (1982).
13. B.C. Wang in Methods of Enzymology Vol. 115 ed. by H.W. Wyckoff (Academic Press, New York,1985) 90-111.
14. J. Priestle, J.Appl.Crystl. 21,572-576 (1988).
15. T. Callahan, W. Gleason and T. Lybrand, J.Appl.Crystl. (in press, 1990)

Structural Studies of Lipid Binding Proteins

Deborah R. Breiter, Matthew M. Benning, Michael R. Kanost,* Michael A. Wells,* John H. Law,* Ivan Rayment, and Hazel M. Holden

*Departments of Chemistry and Biochemistry and the Institute for Enzyme Research, University of Wisconsin-Madison, Madison, Wisconsin; *Department of Biochemistry, University of Arizona, Tucson, Arizona*

ABSTRACT

The three-dimensional structures of two different insect lipid transport proteins have been solved by x-ray crystallographic analyses: apolipophorin-III (apoLp-III) isolated from *Locusta migratoria* and insecticyanin isolated from *Manduca sexta* L..

In the case of insecticyanin, its molecular structure has been solved and refined to a nominal resolution of 2.0 Å. Interestingly, the overall three-dimensional architecture of the molecule shows remarkable similarity to the structural motifs exhibited by bovine β-lactoglobulin and human serum retinol-binding protein. The three-dimensional fold of insecticyanin devoid of its biliverdin chromophore has also been determined to 2.2 Å resolution.

With respect to apoLp-III, its structure has recently been solved to a nominal resolution of 2.5 Å. As predicted from amino acid sequence studies, the secondary structure of this protein is almost entirely α-helical with five long amphiphilic helices. The preliminary structural investigation of apoLp-III described here is of special importance since it represents the first successful high resolution x-ray analysis of an apolipoprotein.

Taken together, the x-ray crystallographic investigations described in this chapter have provided important structural information on two very different classes of insect lipid binding proteins. Furthermore, while the focus is on insect models, the knowledge gained from these studies will undoubtedly provide valuable insight into mammalian lipid transport pathways as well.

INTRODUCTION

Lipids serve both structural and metabolic roles in all living systems. Consequently, the effective transport of such water insoluble molecules is of central biochemical importance. Both vertebrate and invertebrate species have evolved a variety of methods to overcome the problem of shuttling hydrophobic molecules within an aqueous environment. For example, in both mammals and insects, there exist soluble lipoprotein particles specifically designed for the transport of lipids in the blood or hemolymph. These large lipoprotein complexes are believed to be composed of a lipid core surrounded

© 1990 by Elsevier Science Publishing Co., Inc.
Molecular Biology of Atherosclerosis
A.D. Attie, Editor

by a "coat" of protein. Another type of lipid transport in both mammalian and insect systems are the small proteins, such as retinol binding protein, fatty acid binding protein and insecticyanin, that bind only one lipid molecule thereby rendering it soluble in an aqueous medium.

In lipoprotein complexes, the lipids and proteins are held together primarily by hydrophobic effects and their geometric relationship may not be rigidly defined. In contrast, proteins such as insecticyanin bind one lipid molecule in a precise and specific manner. We are presently investigating, by x-ray crystallographic techniques, the molecular structures of two insect lipid binding proteins; apolipophorin-III (apoLp-III) from *Locusta migratoria* and insecticyanin from *Manduca sexta* L.. These proteins were chosen for study because they represent specific examples of the above-mentioned classes. ApoLp-III is part of a lipoprotein complex whereas insecticyanin belongs to the category of small lipid-binding proteins. As will be described, these two proteins differ markedly in their three-dimensional architecture and thus provide excellent models for understanding the different structural elements involved in protein:lipid interactions. Insect models were chosen for these structural studies because their lipid transport systems are somewhat less complicated than their mammalian counterparts. However, it is important to note that insects use lipids for many of the same processes as do vertebrates and consequently what is learned from these x-ray investigations will also yield valuable insight into the mammalian lipid transport pathways.

I. INSECTICYANIN

Insecticyanin is a blue biliprotein isolated from the tobacco hornworm, *Manduca sexta* L.. Although its biological role is not entirely clear, insecticyanin is believed to play a key role in the camouflage coloration of the insect [1]. The protein was first isolated and purified by Cherbas [2] and the amino acid sequence subsequently determined by Riley *et al.,* [3]. Each subunit of insecticyanin contains 189 amino acid residues with two disulfide bridges. In terms of quaternary structure, insecticyanin is a tetramer with 222 symmetry as seen in the crystalline lattice [4]. The chromophore responsible for giving insecticyanin its intense blue coloration is the γ-isomer of biliverdin IX as first proposed by Cherbas [2] and demonstrated by crystallographic analyses [4].

The molecular structure of insecticyanin was initially solved to a resolution of 2.6 Å using the techniques of multiple isomorphous replacement and molecular averaging [4]. Least squares refinement of the model to a nominal resolution of 2.0 Å resolution has now been completed with a final crystallographic R-factor of 15.7% using x-ray data from 5.0 Å to 2.0 Å resolution. Details of the refinement will be published elsewhere. An α-carbon trace of one subunit of insecticyanin, along with the biliverdin, is shown in stereo on the following page.

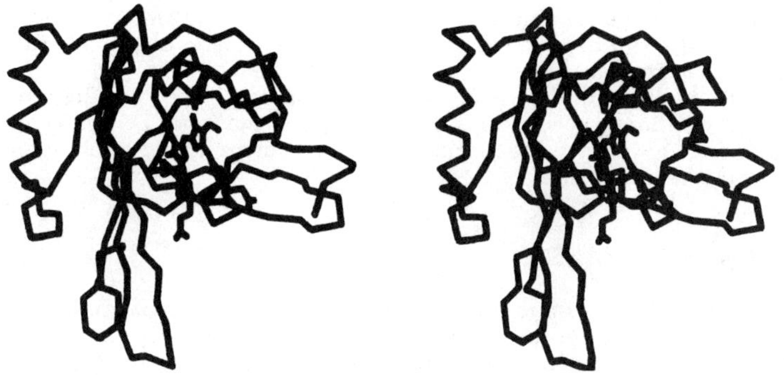

FIG. 1. α-carbon trace of insecticyanin.

The individual subunit shown above has overall dimensions of 44 Å x 37 Å x 40 Å and consists primarily of an eight-stranded anti-parallel β-barrel flanked on one side by a 4.5-turn α-helix. The biliverdin lies towards the open end of the β-barrel with its two propionate side chains pointing towards the solvent and it adopts a rather folded conformation, much like a heme.

As the initial polypeptide model for insecticyanin was being built, it became apparent that the overall three-dimensional fold of the molecule was remarkably similar to the structures of bovine β-lactoglobulin [5], and human serum retinol-binding protein [6]. Dr. Terry Meyer at the University of Arizona has carried out amino acid sequence alignments of these proteins based on three-dimensional considerations and has found there to be less than a dozen common residues (personal communication). Yet, when considering only the positions of the alpha carbons, insecticyanin and human serum retinol binding protein superimposed with an RMS value of approximately 1.6 Å for 93 structurally equivalent atoms. For the superposition of bovine β-lactoglobulin and insecticyanin, the RMS value for a total of 86 structurally equivalent α-carbon positions is approximately 2.0 Å.

Within the last several years it has become increasingly apparent that this molecular fold seen in insecticyanin, bovine β-lactoglobulin, and human serum retinol binding protein may be more common than was originally thought. A variant of this structural motif has now been crystallographically demonstrated in rat intestinal fatty acid binding protein [7], bovine P2 myelin protein [8] and photoreceptor protein [9]. These proteins contain a ten-stranded rather than eight stranded anti-parallel β-barrel. Amino acid sequence studies have further suggested that a variety of proteins with quite different physiological functions may have three-dimensional structures similar to that observed in insecticyanin, examples of which include human α_1-microglobulin [10], olfactory binding protein [11,12], rat α_{2u}-globulin, [13], human α_1-acid glycoprotein [14], human placental protein 14 [15], rat androgen-dependent secretory protein [16], purpurin [17] and human apolipoprotein D [18]. Apolipoprotein D is of particular interest since it has been assumed that this apolipoprotein binds and transports cholesterol [18,19]. Recent model building and binding studies of Peitsch and Boguski

[20], however, suggest that apolipoprotein D binds bilirubin and other heme-related metabolites. Clearly, the structural motif seen in insecticyanin is ideally suited for the binding and transport of small, hydrophobic molecules and undoubtedly will be found in still other proteins whose biological role is to transport such ligands.

In an effort to understand on a molecular level the specificity of the insecticyanin binding pocket as well as the conformational flexibility of the protein fold we have solved the structure of the protein devoid of biliverdin as described in the next section.

II. APOINSECTICYANIN

The biliverdin chromophore is tightly bound to insecticyanin and can only be removed under denaturing conditions such as treatment with formamide [2] or guanidine hydrochloride [3]. Following the procedure of Cherbas [2], apoinsecticyanin was prepared by treatment with 50% formamide, followed by column chromatography to separate the protein and ligand. The formamide was removed by extensive dialysis against 10 mM N-2-hydroxyethylpiperazine-N'-2-ethanesulfonic acid (HEPES), 150 mM NaCl and 5 mM sodium azide, pH 7.5. Details of the protein preparation, crystallization, x-ray structure determination and least squares refinement will be published elsewhere. In summary, the apoinsecticyanin structure was solved by the technique of molecular replacement and the model is presently being refined to a nominal resolution of 2.2 Å. The current R-factor is 22.0% with good overall molecular geometry. An α-carbon trace of one subunit of apoinsecticyanin superimposed on the native structure is shown in stereo below.

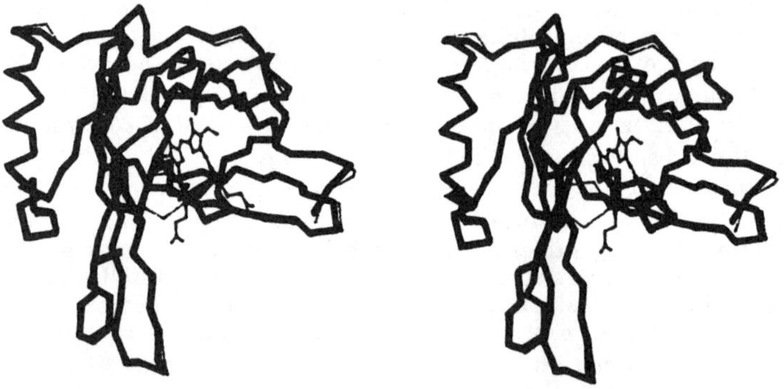

FIG. 2. Superposition of insecticyanin and apoinsecticyanin.

The apo-structure is shown above in bold lines; the native insecticyanin model along with the biliverdin ligand is shown in thin lines. As can be seen the overall molecular fold has changed very little except for one loop region near the opening of the binding pocket. While a detailed comparison of these two models must await completion of the refinement of apoinsecticyanin, it can be concluded that their overall three-dimensional architecture is very similar.

As a continuing effort to understand the conformational flexibility of this protein fold, experiments have been initiated to substitute the biliverdin with other small hydrophobic ligands. Small amber-colored crystals of insecticyanin in which the biliverdin has been replaced by heme have now been grown. Experiments designed to bind other molecules in the insecticyanin pocket are in progress.

III. APOLIPOPHORIN III

Insecticyanin is one of the major hemolymph proteins found in the tobacco hornworm as well in the adult sphinx moth. There is another major component in the hemolymph of the adult moth referred to as lipophorin. Lipophorin is a lipoprotein particle and depending on the metabolic state of the insect, is typically comprised of 60% protein and 40% lipid [21]. The protein portion of the lipophorin particle consists of two apolipoproteins referred to as apolipophorin I and apolipophorin II. Both apolipophorin I and apolipophorin II are integral constituents of lipophorin and have molecular weights of approximately 250,000 and 80,000 respectively [22,23]. In some insects there exists another apolipoprotein referred to apolipophorin III (apoLp-III). This protein typically has a molecular weight of approximately 20,000 and exists as a soluble monomer in the hemolymph. During flight, however, when lipophorin is loaded with diacylglycerol, apoLp-III associates with the lipoprotein particle and it has been suggested that this smaller apoprotein serves to stabilize the lipid-enriched complex [24,25,26].

ApoLp-III has been isolated from several insect species but the most extensively studied proteins are those isolated from *Manduca sexta* and *Locusta migratoria*. It has been suggested that the *M. sexta* protein is a prolate ellipsoid with an axial ratio of approximately 3 based on its hydrodynamic properties and its behavior during gel permeation chromatography [25]. In addition, the circular dichroic spectrum of apoLp-III indicates a helical content of approximately 50%. The amino acid sequence of the sphinx moth apoLp-III, deduced from the cDNA sequence, shows the presence of repeating tetradecapeptide units, each having the potential to form amphiphilic helices [27]. A sequence homology study of apoLp-III with mammalian apolipoproteins suggests considerable functional but little amino acid sequence identity [27].

Locust apoLp-III was first studied by Van der Horst *et al.,* [28] and subsequently purified to homogeneity by Chino and Yazawa [29]. Unlike the *M. sexta* protein, however, this apoLp-III is glycosylated with a total sugar content of approximately 12%. A cDNA coding for the locust protein has recently been cloned and the amino acid sequence determined based on the cDNA sequence [30]. The protein contains 161 amino acid residues and sequence comparisons with the *M. sexta* molecule have revealed a homology of approximately 30%.

Although there is little amino acid sequence identity between apoLp-IIIs isolated from different insects, the surface properties of these small apolipoproteins may be more critical than the actual sequence identity in fulfilling their physiological function. Support for this view is found in the studies of Van der Horst *et al.,* [28]. Their experiments demonstrate that the uptake of lipids by lipophorin in an *in vitro* fat body preparation from *L. migratoria* is supported equally well using apoLp-III from either *L.*

migratoria or *M. sexta*. Clearly, speculations about similar surface properties can only be confirmed when the three-dimensional structures of the various proteins are known.

Due to the small size of apoLp-III and the fact that during certain metabolic states it exists as a soluble hemolymph protein, it seemed an ideal apolipoprotein for crystallization trials. Small micro-crystals of apoLp-III isolated from the adult sphinx moth were grown but all attempts to prepare larger crystals for an x-ray analysis were unsuccessful. However, the apolipoprotein isolated from the African locust, *Locusta migratoria*, crystallized readily and in a form suitable for a high resolution structural analysis [31].

The molecular structure of locust apoLp-III described here was determined by multiple isomorphous replacement using six heavy atom derivatives. Details of the structure determination will be described elsewhere (manuscript in preparation). An electron density map calculated to a nominal resolution of 3.0 Å was used to build the initial model and the structure is presently being refined to a resolution of 2.5 Å. The first six amino acid residues as well as residues 157 to 161 are not clear in the electron density map. Otherwise, the amino acid sequence has been fitted unambiguously into the electron density. A ribbon drawing of this apolipoprotein is shown below.

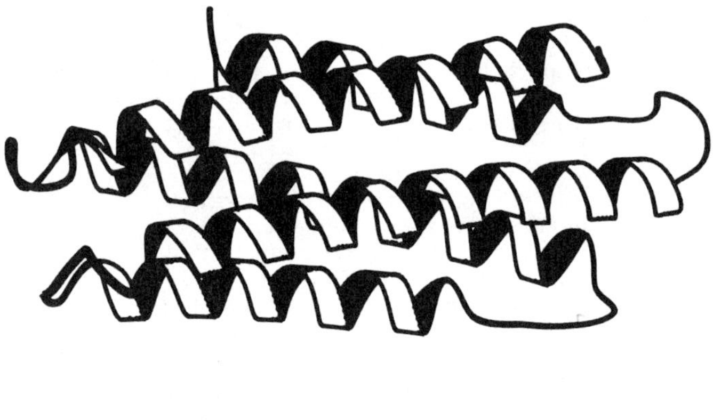

FIG. 3. *Ribbon drawing of apoLp-III.*

As can be seen from the figure, the protein contains five long amphiphilic helices. Three of these helices order up to 30 amino acid residues while the other two helices contain approximately 20 amino acid residues. The molecule is indeed elongated as first suggested by Kawooya *et al.*, [25] with an approximate length of 53 Å and a width of 22 Å.

Locust apoLp-III can exist as either a soluble monomer in the hemolymph of the insect or bound to lipophorin. Numerous biophysical and biochemical studies indicate that apoLp-III undergoes a profound conformational change upon binding to the lipoprotein complex [25]. Since the crystals used in this investigation were grown in the absence of any lipid [31], the next step in the structural analysis of locust apoLp-III is to grow crystals in the presence of lipids and/or detergents. These experiments are presently underway.

There have been many investigations within recent years directed toward understanding the structural elements of apolipoproteins that allow them to interact with lipid surfaces. It has been suggested that amphiphilic helices play a key role in such protein:lipid interactions [32]. To date, however, there has been a lack of three-dimensional structural information concerning apolipoproteins and these putative helices. The molecular structure of apoLp-III described here is the first apolipoprotein structure to be solved by x-ray crystallographic techniques and represents the first direct three-dimensional evidence for the presence of amphiphilic helices in this class of lipid transport proteins. Also, while the primary sequence homology between insect apolipoproteins and mammalian apolipoproteins is low, as in the case of insecticyanin and human serum retinol binding protein, it is likely that their overall three-dimensional structures are quite similar.

In conclusion, the molecular structures of two insect proteins involved in lipid transport have been solved by x-ray crystallographic techniques. Insecticyanin represents one class of lipid transport proteins that binds a hydrophobic ligand in a well defined 1:1 ratio. The overall molecular structure of this molecule can be described simply as an eight-stranded anti-parallel β-barrel flanked on one side by a 4.5 turn α-helix. ApoLp-III belongs to another class, the apolipoproteins, which interact with a lipoprotein particle in a still not well understood manner. Unlike insecticyanin which contains predominantly β-sheet, apoLp-III is almost entirely α-helical. These two different structural motifs have clearly evolved to overcome the problem of shuttling hydrophobic molecules within the aqueous milieu of the organism.

ACKNOWLEDGMENTS

This work was supported by grants from the NIH (HL42322, GM29238, and HL39116). Deborah R. Breiter is supported by an NIH pre-doctoral training grant (GM08293). Ivan Rayment and Hazel M. Holden are Established Investigators of the American Heart Association. We thank Janet Dewane for her excellent assistance in the preparation of this manuscript. We also gratefully acknowledge the computing expertise of Dr. Gary Wesenberg.

REFERENCES

1. J.K. Kawooya, P.S. Keim, J.H. Law, C.T. Riley, R.O. Ryan and J.P. Shapiro. *ACS Symp. Ser.* 276, 511-521 (1985).
2. P.K. Cherbas. *Ph.D. Thesis*, Harvard University.
3. C.T. Riley, B.K. Barbeau, P.S. Keim, F.J. Kezdy, R.L. Heinrikson and J.H. Law. *J. Biol. Chem.* 259, 13159-13165 (1984).
4. H.M. Holden, W.R. Rypniewski, and I. Rayment. *The EMBO Journal* 6, 1565-1570 (1987).
5. H.L. Monaco, G. Zonitti, P. Spadon, M. Bolognesi, L. Sawyer and E.E. Eliopoulos. *J. Mol. Biol.*, 197, 695-706 (1987).
6. M.E. Newcomer, T.A. Jones, J. Aquist, J. Sundelin, U. Eriksson, L. Rask and P.A. Peterson. *The EMBO Journal* 3, 1451-1454 (1984).
7. J.C. Sacchettini, J.I. Gordon and L.J. Banaszak. *J. Mol. Biol.* 208, 327-339 (1989).
8. T.A. Jones, T. Bergfors, J. Sedzik, and T. Unge. *The EMBO Journal* 7, 1597-1604 (1988).

9. D.E. McRee, J.A. Tainer, T.E. Meyer, J. Van Beeumen, M.A. Cusanovich and E.D. Getzoff. *Proc. Natl. Acad. Sci., USA* 86, 6533-6537 (1989).
10. S. Pervaiz and K. Brew. *Science* 228, 335-337 (1985).
11. K-H. Lee, R.G. Wells and R.R. Reed. *Science* 235, 1053-1056 (1987).
12. J. Pevsner, R.R. Reed, P.G. Feinstein, and S.H. Synder. *Science* 241, 336-339 (1988).
13. R.D. Unterman, K.R. Lynch, H.L. Nakhasi, K.P. Dolan, J.W. Hamilton, D.V. Cohn, and P. Feigelson. *Proc. Natl. Acad. Sci. USA* 78, 3478-3482 (1981).
14. S. Pervais and K. Brew. *FASEB J.* 1, 209-214 (1987).
15. M. Julkunen, M. Seppala, and O.A. Janne. *Proc. Natl. Acad. Sci., USA* 85, 8845-8849 (1988).
16. D.E. Brooks, A.R. Means, E.J. Wright, S.P. Singh, and K.K. Tiver. *J. Biol. Chem.* 261, 4956-4961 (1986).
17. P. Berman, P. Gray, E. Chen, K. Keyser, D. Erlich, H. Karten, M. LaCorbiere, F. Esch, and D. Schubert. *Cell* 51, 135-142 (1987).
18. D. Drayna, C. Fielding, J. McLean, B. Baer, G. Castro, E. Chen, L. Comstock, W. Henzel, W. Kohr, L. Rhee, K. Wion and R. Lawn. *J. Biol. Chem.* 261, 16535-16539 (1986).
19. O.L. Francone, A. Gurakar and C. Fielding. *J. Biol. Chem.* 264, 7066-7072 (1989).
20. M.C. Peitsch and M.S. Boguski. *The New Biologist* 2, 197-206 (1990).
21. H. Chino, R.G.H. Downer, G.R. Wyatt, and L.I. Gilbert. *Insect Biochem.* 11, 491 (1981).
22. R.O. Ryan, J.O. Schmidt and J.H. Law. Arch. *Insect Biochem. Physiol.* 1, 375-383 (1984).
23. J. P. Shaprio, P.S. Keim, and J.H. Law. *J. Biol. Chem.* 259, 3680-3685 (1984).
24. J.K. Kawooya, P.S. Keim, R.O. Ryan, J.P. Shapiro, P. Samaraweera, and J.H. Law. *J. Biol. Chem.* 259, 10733-10737 (1984).
25. J.K. Kawooya, S.C. Meredith, M.A. Wells, F.J. Kezdy, and J.H. Law. *J. Biol. Chem.* 261, 13588-13591 (1986).
26. M.A. Wells, R.O. Ryan, J.K. Kawooya and J.H. Law. *J. Biol. Chem.* 262, 4172-4176 (1987).
27. K.D. Cole, G.J. P. Fernando-Warnakulasuriya, M.S. Boguski, M. Freeman, J.I. Gordon, W.A. Clark, J. H. Law, and M.A. Wells. *J. Biol. Chem.* 262, 11794-11800 (1987).
28. D.J. Van Der Horst, J.M. Van Doorn, and A.M.Th. Beenakkers. *Insect Biochem.* 14, 495-504 (1984).
29. H. Chino and M. Yazawa. *J. Lipid Res.* 27, 377-385 (1986).
30. M.R. Kanost, M.S. Boguski, M. Freeman, J.I. Gordon, G.R. Wyatt, and M.A. Wells. *J. Biol. Chem.* 263, 10568-10573 (1988).
31. H.M. Holden, M.R. Kanost, J.H. Law, I. Rayment, and M.A. Wells. *J. Biol. Chem.* 263, 3960-3962 (1988).
32. J.P. Segrest, R.L. Jackson, J.D. Morrisett, A.M. Gotto, Jr. *FEBS Lett.* 38, 247-253 (1974).

Role of Amphipathic Helixes in HDL Structure/Function

G.M. Anantharamaiah, C.G. Brouillette, J.A. Engler, H. De Loof, Y.V. Venkatachalapathi, J. Boogaerts, and J.P. Segrest

Departments of Medicine, Biochemistry and the Atherosclerosis Unit, UAB Medical Center, Birmingham, Alabama

ABSTRACT

In a recent analysis we classified amphipathic α helix domains into a minimum of seven distinct classes. Four amphipathic helix classes are found in lipid-associating proteins: apolipoproteins, certain polypeptide hormones, polypeptide venoms and antibiotics, and certain complex transmembrane proteins. Three amphipathic helix classes are involved in both intra- and intermolecular protein-protein interactions: calmodulin- regulated protein kinases, coiled-coil containing proteins that include the so-called leucine zipper, and globular α helical proteins.

Three central hypothesis have been developed in our studies of the apolipoprotein class of amphipathic helixes: 1) The "Snorkel" hypothesis proposes that when the amphipathic helix is associated with phospholipid, amphipathic basic residues extend toward the polar face of the helix to insert their charged residues into the aqueous milieu: thus the entirety of the uncharged van der Waals' surface of the amphipathic helix is buried within the lipid. 2) We have formulated a hypothesis that Glutamyl residues located at positions 78 and 111 in apolipoprotein A-I on the nonpolar face of two amphipathic helical domains are critical to LCAT activation. 3) The hinged-domain hypothesis was proposed to explain the structural basis for the quantization of HDL subspecies, protein-protein interactions in HDL, and the HDL disc to sphere transformation.

INTRODUCTION

The amphipathic α helix is an often encountered secondary structural motif in biologically active peptides and proteins. The amphipathic helix was first described as a unique structure/function motif involved in lipid interaction by Segrest et al. in 1974 (1). Amphipathic helical domains have been described for other lipid associating proteins, including polypeptide hormones such as endorphins, polypeptide venoms such as bombolitin, polypeptide antibiotics such as the meganins, and certain complex transmembrane proteins, such as bacteriorhodopsin (2). Based upon a detailed analysis of their physical-chemical and structural properties, we have grouped amphipathic helixes into seven classes (A, H, L, G, K, C, and M; Fig. 1) (2).

The exchangeable apolipoproteins from plasma lipoproteins (apo A-I, A-II, A-IV, C-I, C-II, C- III and E) belong to the class A amphipathic helixes. They differ from the rest of the classes in that they possess positively charged residues at the polar-nonpolar interface and negatively charged residues at the center of the polar face. The most striking feature of these exchangeable apolipoproteins is the presence of internal 22-residue-long repeats (3). More

Published 1990 by Elsevier Science Publishing Co., Inc.
Molecular Biology of Atherosclerosis
A.D. Attie, Editor

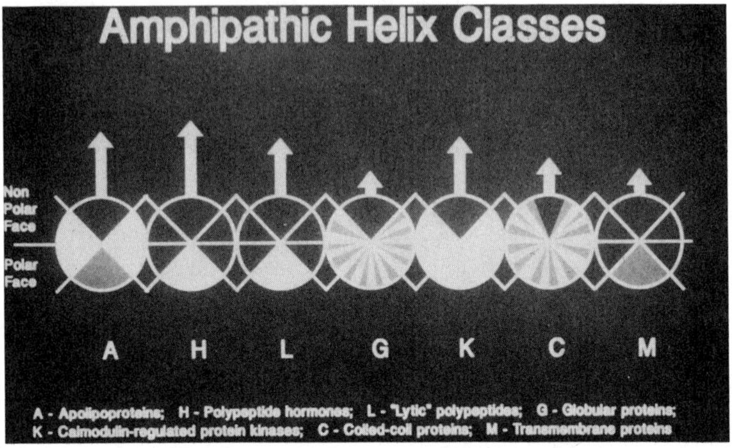

Fig. 1. Schematic representation of seven different classes of the amphipathic helix. Different circles represent each class. Arrows above each class indicate the relative mean hydrophobic moment.

importantly, this repeating unit has the periodicity of an amphipathic α helix. These observations form a major basis for the investigations of the structure and functions of the apolipoproteins in our laboratory.

THE "SNORKEL HYPOTHESIS":

Our approach to understanding the factors responsible for the lipid association of the apolipoprotein class of amphipathic helix was the synthesis of model peptide analogs of this class. Our initial studies of peptide analogs involved two sets of peptides (4–7). One set of model peptides were designed to mimic the class A amphipathic helix: i.e., positively charged residues at the polar–nonpolar interface and negatively charged residues at the center of the polar face. The second set of analogs had a reverse charge distribution (Fig. 2). Examination of the lipid–associating properties of these peptide analogs showed that the class A mimicking peptide analogs interacted much more effectively to form stable discoidal peptide:lipid complexes than the analogs with the reverse charge distribution. These analogs for the class A amphipathic helix were also able to competitively displace apo A–I from HDL compared to the analogs with reverse charge distribution. From these studies we recognized that the positively charged residues at the interface, because of their longer acyl chainlength, may be playing an important role in increasing the lipid affinity of the peptide analogs of class A amphipathic helix.

As part of a study to understand the molecular properties of apo A–I we synthesized analogs for the 22mer consensus lipid-associating domain with the sequence PVLDEFREKLNE X EEALKQKLK. As can be seen in Fig. 3, the 13th position (denoted by X in the sequence) is located at the nonpolar face, 40° from the polar–nonpolar interface of the amphipathic helix. Amino acid substitutions were therefore carried out in this position to see the effect of the acyl chain length on lipid affinity. Three peptide analogs were synthesized with X at the 13th position substituted by Glu, Lys and L–homoaminoalanine (Haa). The peptide containing Haa served as a control peptide to study the effect of acyl chain length on lipid affinity because this amino acid has the same acyl chainlength as Glu but a positively charged side chain, similar to Lys. Thus the effect of the longer acyl chain length of Lys on lipid affinity when it is close to the polar–nonpolar interface was studied.

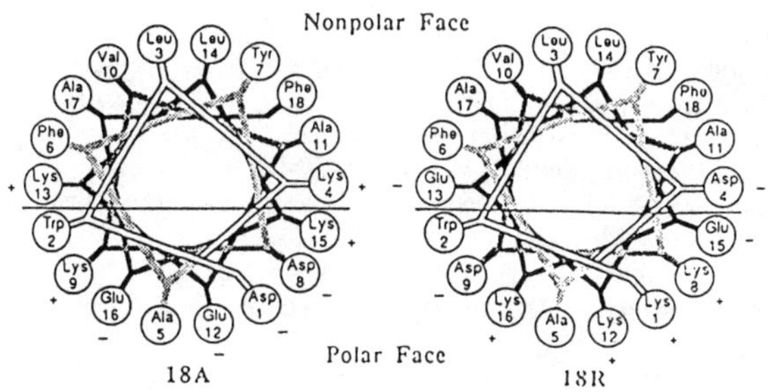

37aA = 18A - Ala - 18A

37pA = 18A - Pro - 18A

Fig 2. Helical wheel representation of model 18A and 18R peptide analogs.

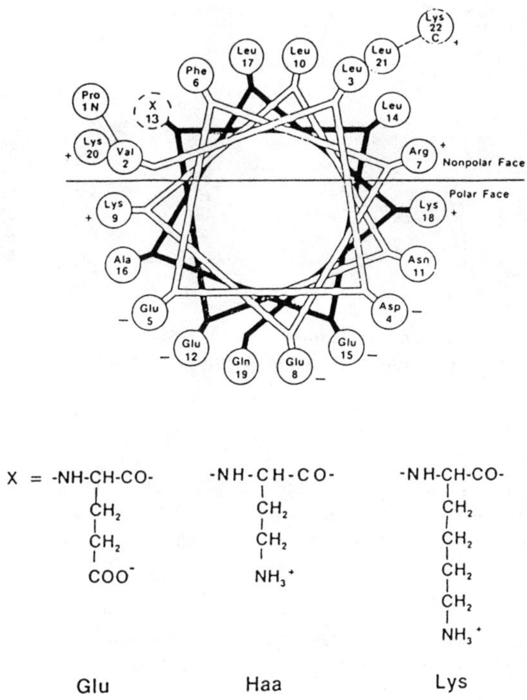

Fig. 3 Helical wheel representation viewed from the amino terminal end of the consensus 22mer peptide for the 22mer repeating units of apo A-I. X = Glu, Lys or Haa.

The peptides were compared for their ability to interact with multilamellar vesicles of dimyristoyl phosphatidylcholine (DMPC): the extent of interaction was estimated by their ability to clarify turbid multilamellar vesicles of DMPC and to form stable discoidal complexes. Turbidity clarification studies showed that the Lys analog was the only peptide which clarified the multilamellar vesicles of DMPC. The Lys analog formed the smallest discoidal complex of the three peptides (Stokes diameters: [Lys^{13}]A–I_{con}, 110 ± 30 A; [Glu^{13}]A–I_{con}, 200 ± 50 A; and [Haa^{13}]A–I_{con}, 310 ± 30 A). We have shown previously that the size of the discoidal complexes varies inversely with the lipid affinity of the peptide. Thus, based on these studies, the Lys analog has a greater lipid affinity than the other two.

Dye leakage experiments using fluorescence–entrapped egg PC liposomes also suggested that the Lys analog possesses increased lipid affinity compared to the other two analogs. The results of the fluorescence leakage are shown in Fig. 5. The results show that [Lys^{13}]A–I_{con} at 200 µg equals Triton X–100. The other two analogs at the same peptide concentration released only about 50% of the entrapped dye.

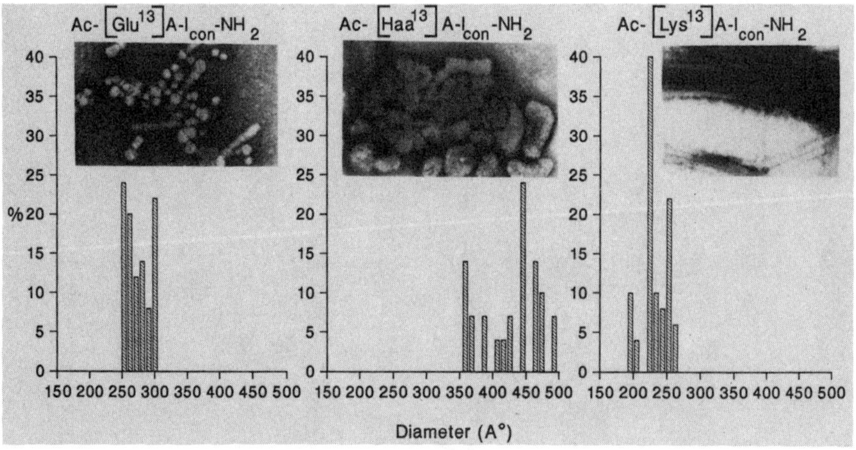

Fig. 4. (A) Negative stain electron microscopy of peptide DMPC complexes at 1:1 weight ratio. (B) Morphographic analysis of diameters of discoidal complexes.

Based on these results we propose the "Snorkel" model shown in Fig. 6 for the lipid association of apolipoprotein class amphipathic helix. The bulk of the van der Waals surface areas of the positively charged residues are hydrophobic. We propose that the amphipathic basic residues, when associated with phospholipid, extend toward the polar face of the helix to insert their charged moieties into the aqueous milieu for solvation. We suggest that essentially all of the uncharged van der Waals surface of the amphipathic helical domains of the apolipoproteins can be buried within the interior of a phospholipid monolayer. Compared to the other classes of the amphipathic helix, the arrangement of the charged residues found in the apolipoproteins provides for a deeper helix insertion into a monolayer and thus a greater lipid affinity.

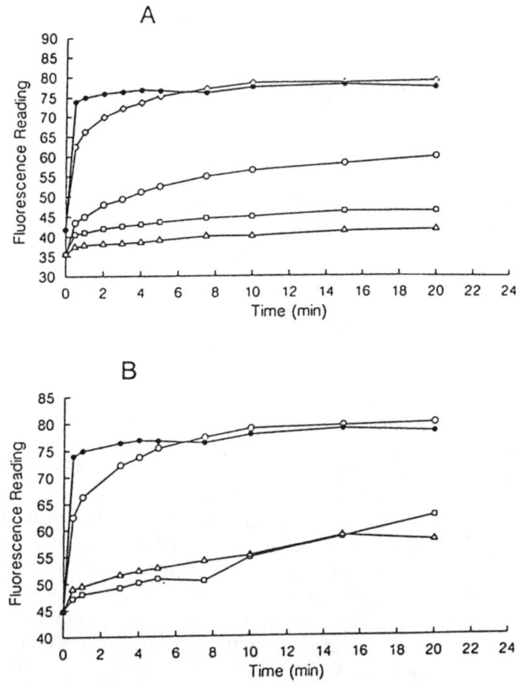

Fig. 5. Fluorescence dye leakage from egg PC entrapped vesicles: Carboxy fluorescein was trapped in small unilamellar egg PC vesicles. Perturbation by the protein of the lipid bilayer was monitored by the rate of leakage and dequenching of fluorescent dye into the media. A. Triton X-100 ●--● and ◆—◆ 200 ug. ○--○ 100 ug. □--□ 50 ug and ▲--▲ 25 ug of A-I_{con} Lys[13]. B. ○--○ A-I_{con} Lys[13]. □--□ A-I_{con} Haa[13] and ▲--▲ A-I_{con} Glu[13].

MECHANISM OF LCAT ACTIVATION BY APO A-I:

Apolipoprotein apo A-I is the major co-factor for activation of the plasma enzyme lecithin:cholesterol acyl transferase (LCAT). LCAT is thought to mediate reverse cholesterol transport by trapping cholesterol in the form of cholesteryl ester in the HDL particle for removal by the liver. Many apolipoproteins also can serve as co-factors for the enzyme LCAT. However, the extent of activation for these proteins is similar to that of the nonspecific activators such as non-homologous synthetic peptides (5). Human apo A-I has therefore been studied extensively to localize the LCAT activating domain(s) in its sequence (6,7). Based on studies of the CNBr fragments and the synthetic peptides corresponding to the CNBr fragmentation products the LCAT activating domain(s) could not be localized. We therefore examined the repeating 22mer units of apo A-I to attempt to understand the structure and function of apo A-I.

There are eight 22mer tandem repeats at the C-terminal end of apo A-I. In every case but one, the eight tandem 22mer repeats are punctuated by a single proline. Each tandem 22mer repeat in apo A-I is an amphipathic helix. Because each tandem 22mer in apo A-I appears

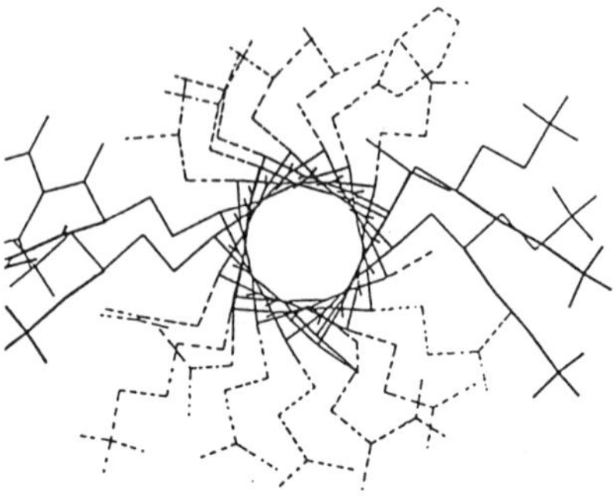

Fig. 6. Computer model of an amphipathic peptide indicating features of the "Snorkel" model. The consensus class A apolipoprotein amphipathic helical peptide (apo A–I_{con}) was modeled using the "SYBYL" program package (TRIPOS Associates Inc.). An idealized α helix was built with backbone dihedral angles $Y = 58°$ and $F = -47°$. One side chain dihedral angle of each of the four positively charged residues was changed from the trans to gouche conformation so as to bring the end of the side chains closer to the hydrophilic side of the helix. Both the initial and the "snorkel" structure were subsequently energy minimized with SYBYL using AMBER force–field parameters. A superposition of the two minimized helixes is shown in the figure. The energy difference between them was very small, showing the "snorkel"–configuration is possible without bad intramolecular steric constraints. Positively charged residues are shown in solid light (initial) and dark (snorkel).

to represent a duplication of a primordial gene sequence (8). as part of our studies on the molecular properties of amphipathic helixes, a consensus sequence approximation of the primordial 22mer was derived. The sequence, called A–I_{con}, is as follows: Pro Val Leu Asp Glu Phe Arg Glu Lys Leu Asn Glu X Leu Glu Ala Leu Lys Gln Lys Leu Lys (Fig. 3). This sequence represents the most prevalent amino acid residue at each position of the eight 22mers. Although the 13th residue is positioned at the nonpolar face of the consensus sequence, six out of the eight tandem repeats of apo A–I have a charged residue at this position. The anamolous nature of this residue suggested to us the possibility that this position might play a role in the LCAT–activating properties of apo A–I. To investigate this possibility we synthesized four 22mer peptide analogs differing only in the 13th position. Three homo and one heterodimeric combinations were synthesized (Table 1).

TABLE I.

E	PVLDE FREKL NEELE ALKQK LK
R	PVLDE FREKL NERLE ALKQK LK
K	PVLDE FREKL NEKLE ALKQK LK
H	PVLDE FREKL NEHLE ALKQK LK
EE	PVLDE FREKL NEELE ALKQK LK PVLDE FREKL NEELE ALKQK LK
RE	PVLDE FREKL NERLE ALKQK LK PVLDE FREKL NEELE ALKQK LK
RR	PVLDE FREKL NERLE ALKQK LK PVLDE FREKL NERLE ALKQK LK
HH	PVLDE FREKL NEHLE ALKQK LK PVLDE FREKL NEHLE ALKQK LK

These peptides were studied for their ability to activate the enzyme LCAT using two different assay systems: i) the egg PC vesicular assay, and ii) the discoidal assay method using the cholate dialysis procedure (10, 13). The results were compared with the ability of apo A-I to activate LCAT in these two assay systems. The results of the LCAT activation using the dimer peptide analogs are shown in Fig.7. In both assay systems the homodimer analog containing Glu at the 13th position equaled apo A-I in its ability to activate LCAT.

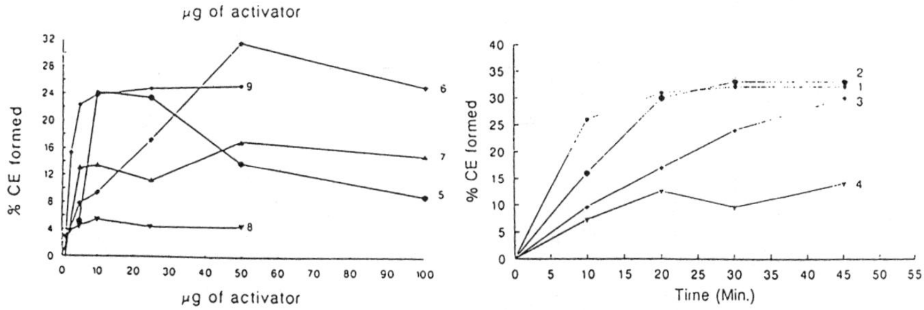

Fig 7. Activation of LCAT by synthetic peptide analogs as measured by: (A) egg lecithin small unilamelar vesicle procedure: (B) egg lecithin discoidal particle prepared by the cholate dialysis procedure (10, 13).

Examination of the order of distribution of 13th amino acid in the eight tandem repeats of apo A-I (Fig. 8) shows that residues 66-121 of apo A-I are similar to the Glu-dimer analog. We therefore propose that the major LCAT activating domain of apo A-I resides in 66-121 region of apo A-I. These results thus explain the reason for failure in localizing the LCAT activating domain of apo A-I. The 66-121 region of apo A-I contains three Methionyl residues. CNBr cleavage would thus fragment this region of apo A-I and the fragments would be devoid of 66-121 apo A-I sequence. Recent studies by Jonas et al. 12) provide additional support for this hypothesis.

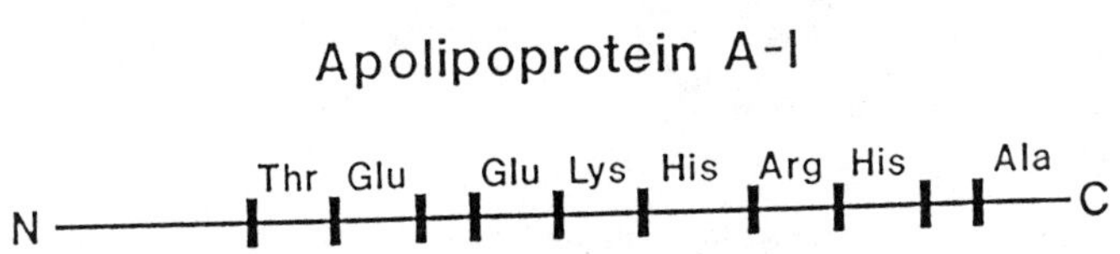

Fig. 8. Order of distribution of 13th amino acid in the eight tandem 22mer repeats of apo A-I. Two vertical lines between the amino acid residues represent 22mer. The peptide ([Glu 13]A-I_{con}) 2 is similar to the two glutamic acid-containing 22mers in having glutamic acid residues at the same position as the two 22mers.

These results led us to believe that glutamic acids at residues 78 and 111 of apo A-I are critical for the LCAT activating ability of apo A-I. With a view to test this we have prepared recombinant apo A-I and a mutant apo A-I in which the 78th Glu residue is changed to Ala. These two proteins were compared with human apo A-I for their ability to activate the enzyme LCAT following the assay systems used for synthetic peptide analogs. Results from these preliminary LCAT studies are shown in Fig. 9. These results indicate that the Glu^{78} —> Ala apo A-I is half as effective in activating the enzyme LCAT as the recombinant apo A-I with the sequence identical to that of plasma apo A-I. These results support the hypothesis that sequence specific glutamic acid residues are important for the LCAT activation by apo A-I.

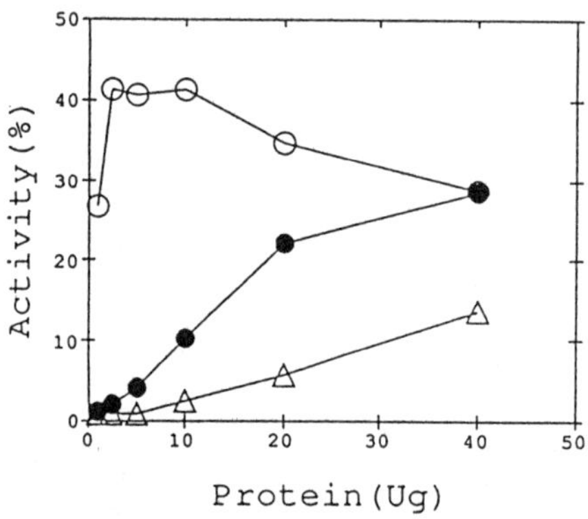

Fig. 9. Activation of LCAT by: (1) plasma apo A-I, (2) recombinant apo A-I and (3) mutant (Glu^{78} ---> Ala) apo A-I as measured by the egg lecithin small unilamellar vesicles assay method.

THE "HINGED-DOMAIN" HYPOTHESIS:

Analysis of the complexes formed between apo A-I and DMPC has shown the formation of a highly controlled stoichiometric class of particles of discrete size containing 2 apo A-I molecules (R-2 complexes) and three apo A-I molecules (R-3 complexes) (11). Variation of the molar ratio of lipid to protein produced discoidal complexes which varied in diameter by a uniformly spaced increment. These observations led to the proposal that the size of the disc produced by this reaction is controlled by conformational changes in apo A-I that result in the all-or-none binding of complete α helical (hinged) domains (11). Recently, this hypothesis has been supported by the preliminary studies of apo A-I/POPC micellar subspecies (12).

Using affinity columns containing anti-apo A-I or anti-apo A-II, nine plasma HDL subpopulations were isolated and characterized using single vertical spin centrifugation (13, 14), electronmicroscopy and nondenaturing gradient gel electrophoresis (8). These were designated as $HDL_{1, 2, 3, 4, 5, 6, 7a, 7b, 7c, 8,}$ and $_9$. The difference in surface area of HDL_4 compared to HDL_3, HDL_5 compared to HDL_4, and HDL_6 compared to HDL_5 averaged 26000 ± 300 Å ^{2}, the differences in surface area of HDL_{7b} compared to HDL_{7a}, and HDL_{7c} compared to HDL_{7b} average 3400 ± 100 Å ^{2}, while the difference in surface area of HDL_{7a} compared to HDL_6 was 56000 A 2. This is reminiscent of the results of apo A-I:DMPC recombinants described earlier (11) in which incremental changes in discoidal diameter between several discrete R-2 and R-3 recombinant particles were observed. The quantized changes observed in the HDL populations and apo A-I:DMPC discoidal structures could be best explained by the stoichiometric and conformational changes to apo A-I in the hinged-domain.

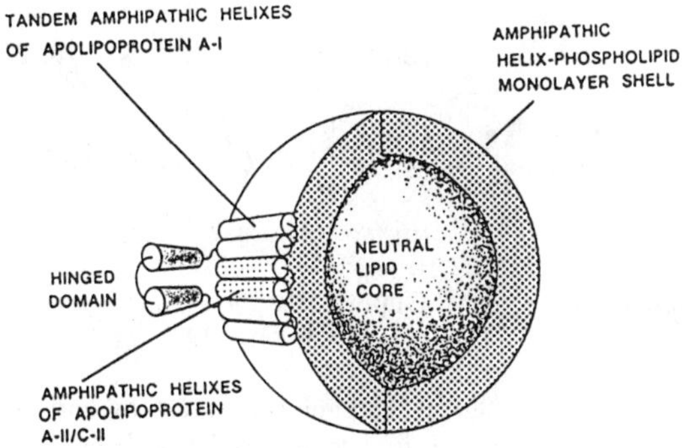

The mechanism of subspecies formation in HDL based on the "hinged domain" hypothesis is illustrated in Fig 10.

CONCLUSIONS

1. Class A amphipathic helixes, via the Lys/Arg "snorkel" process, mediate strong lipid affinity without damage or alteration to cell membranes. (Class H and L amphipathic helixes mediate strong lipid affinity but damage or alter cell membranes.)

2. Amphipathic helical repeats 2 and 3 represent the major LCAT-activating domain in apoA-I. This domain activates LCAT in a 2-step process:

> Step 1. The amphipathic helix produces a protein-lipid cleft recognized by the active site of LCAT, allowing the enzyme to get at the Sn-2 bond of phosphatidylcholine.
>
> Step 2. Sequence- and structure-specific glutamyl residues in repeats 2 and 3 create an activated cholesterol intermediate.

3. There are one, or probably two, hinged-domains in apo A-I that have an amphipathic α-loop-α helical motif. These domains possess two reversible states (lipid-bound and lipid-unbound) that mediate the following:

   a. A low free energy mechanism for reorganization of the amphipathic helical arrays on the edge of discoidal HDL to an array that covers the surface of spheroidal HDL.
   b. Interactions of apo A-I with other apos (e.g., apo A-I).
   c. HDL subspecies (including size quantization).

REFERENCES

1. Segrest. J.P.. Jackson. R.L.. Morrisett, J.D.. Gotto. A.M. .Jr. *FEBS lett.* **38**:247–253. 1974.

2. Segrest. J.P.. DeLoof. H.. Dohlman. J.G.. Brouillette. C.G.. and Anantharamaiah. G.M. *Proteins*. In Press. 1990.

3. Luo. C–C.. Li. W–H.. Moore. M.N., and Chan. L. *J. Mol. Biol.* **187**:325–340. 1986.

4. Anantharamaiah. G.M.. Jones. J.L.. Brouillette. C.G.. Schmidt. C.F.. Chung. B.H.. Hughes. T.A.. Bhown. A.S.. and Segrest. J.P. *J. Biol. Chem.* **260**: 10248–10255. 1985.

5. Anantharamaiah. G.M. Methods *Enzymlo*. **128**:628–248. 1986.

6. Epand. R.M.. Gawish. A.. Iqbal. M.. Gupta. K.B.. Chen. C.H.. Segrest. J .P.. and Anantharamaiah. G.M. *J. Biol. Chem.* **262**:9389–9396. 1987.

7. Venkatachalapathi. Y.V.. Gupta. K.B.. DeLoof. H.. Segrest. J.P. and Anantharamaiah. G.M. In *Peptides*. ESCOM press. (J. Rivier. Ed.) 672–674. 1990.

8. Fielding. C.J.. Shore. V.G.. Fielding P.E. *Biophys. Biochem. Res. Commun.* **46**:1493–1498. 1972.

9. Albers. J.J.. Lin. J.T.. Roberts. G.P. *Artery* **5**:61–75. 1979.

10. Anantharamaiah. G.M.. Venkatachalapathi. Y.V.. Brouillette. C.G.. and Segrest. J.P. *Arteriosclerosis* **10**:95–105 1990.

11. Brouillette. C.G.. Jones. J.L.. Ng. T.C.. Kercert. H.. Chung. B.H.. and Segrest. J.P. *Biochemistry* **23**:359–367. 1984.

12. Jonas. A.. Kezdy. K.E.. and Wald. J.H. *J. Biol. Chem.* **264**:4818–4824. 1989.

13. Cheung. M.C.. Segrest. J.P.. Albers. J.J.. Cone. J.T.. Brouillette. C.G.. Chung. B.H.. Kashyap. M.. Glasscock. A. and Anantharamaiah. G.M. *J. Lipid Res.* **28**:913–924. 1987.

14. Chung. B.H.. Segrest. J.P.. Ray. M.J.. Brunzell. J. D.. Hokanson. J.E.. Krauss. R.M.. Beaudrie. K. and Cone. J.T. *Methods Enzymol.* **128**:181–209. 1986.

Investigation of Lysine Residues in Apolipoprotein B100 by NMR

Sissel Lund-Katz

Department of Biochemistry, Medical College of Pennsylvania, Philadelphia, Pennsylvania

ABSTRACT

The Lysine (Lys) residues of apo B in normal human LDL have been examined by high resolution [^{13}C]NMR to further characterize the conformation of apoB-LDL. [^{13}C]-Formaldehyde was used to reductively methylate apo B to form [^{13}C]dimethyl Lys from 3-65% of the Lys residues. The exposed [$^{13}CH_3$]$_2$ Lys residues of apo B in LDL showed two chemical shifts (δ) at 42.8 and 43.2 ppm while random coil apo B gave a single [^{13}C]Lys resonance. It follows that the two Lys environments in LDL reflect the native conformation of apo B. The pH-dependencies of δ indicated that the two pools of Lys have different pK values; there are about 50 Lys with pK8.9 (active) and 170 Lys with pK10.5 (normal). Addition of paramagnetic shift reagents indicated that the normal and active Lys have different exposures to the aqueous phase; this presumably is a reflection of folding of the apo B molecule. The Lys residues of apo B in familial defective apo B100 subjects have also been characterized by NMR. Familial defective apo B100 is a genetic mutation that is characterized by abnormal LDL and moderate hypercholesterolemia. The mutation that disrupts binding is Gln for Arg substitution at apo B residue 3500. Examination of the mutant LDL from 5 patients shows that about 7 Lys are redistributed from the active to the normal pool. The CD spectra of mutant and normal LDL are identical. Therefore, substitution of Gln for Arg at position 3500 induces a change in local conformation which disrupts the receptor binding domain of apo B. The properties of Lys in apoB in pig LDL have been examined by similar techniques.

INTRODUCTION

The low density lipoprotein (LDL)[1] particle is the principal carrier of cholesterol in human plasma and delivers exogenous cholesterol to cells by endocytosis via the LDL receptor (Goldstein and Brown, 1977). The ligand on LDL which is recognized by the receptor is apo B-100. To understand this interaction at the molecular level, it is necessary to know the tertiary structures of both the apo B and receptor protein molecules. The recent application of molecular genetics techniques has provided a great deal of detail about both proteins. The primary structure of the LDL receptor is known, and the functional contributions of the various domains of the molecule are being elucidated (for a review, see Goldstein et al., 1985). Similarly, the amino acid sequence of the apo B-100 molecule has been determined by several laboratories (Cladaras et al., 1986; Knott et al., 1986; Law et al., 1986; Yang et al., 1986). The mature apo B-100

[1]ABBREVIATIONS

apo, apolipoprotein; FDB, familial defective apo B-100; LDL, low density lipoprotein; mAb, monoclonal antibody; SDS, sodium dodecyl sulfate.

Published 1990 by Elsevier Science Publishing Co., Inc.
Molecular Biology of Atherosclerosis
A.D. Attie, Editor

molecule comprises a single polypeptide chain of 4536 amino acid residues, and there is one copy of the protein on an LDL particle. The secondary and tertiary structures of apo B-100 molecule are not known, and this information is required before structure-function relationships can be elaborated in detail.

The conformation of the apo B molecule on the surface of low density lipoproteins is sensitive to the size of the particle and the lipid environment, because different epitopes are expressed as a function of these parameters (for a review, see Schonfeld and Krul, 1986). Chemical modification of functional groups in the apo B-100 molecule have shown that basic Lys and Arg residues are involved in binding to the LDL receptor (Mahley et al., 1977; Weisgraber et al., 1978). The exact structure and location of the receptor binding domain(s) in the apo B-100 molecule are unresolved at present.

In humans, the binding of the low density lipoprotein particle to its cell surface receptor is critical for the determination of the plasma cholesterol level (Brown and Goldstein, 1986). For this interaction to be effective, the conformations of both the LDL receptor and apo B-100 molecule on the LDL particle must be correct. Mutations in the structure of either molecule can lead to hypercholesterolemia. The structure and conformations of normal and mutant forms of the LDL receptor and the ligands of the LDL receptor, apo B-100 and apo E, are being studied intensely. For the LDL receptor, site-directed mutations have identified key amino acids in certain cys-containing, repeat domains as essential for binding to apo B-100 and apo E (Russell et al., 1989). Monoclonal antibodies (mAb) have been used to identify the apo B-100 region(s) responsible for LDL binding to the receptor (e.g. Innerarity et al., 1987b; Milne et al., 1989). This approach has suggested that sequences of residues near the C-terminal of the apo B-100 molecule are critical for receptor binding (Knott et al., 1985, 1986). The idea that the receptor binding domain is in this region is also supported by the discovery of a mutation in this region of the molecule that abolishes the binding of LDL to the LDL receptor (for a review, see Innerarity et al., 1990).

This mutation gives rise to the genetic disorder known as familial defective apo B-100 (FDB) which is characterized by abnormal LDL that binds defectively to the LDL receptor (Innerarity et al., 1987a; Weisgraber et al., 1988; Soria et al., 1989). The subjects are moderately to severely hypercholesterolemic and those characterized so far are heterozygous for the disorder. These individuals possess two populations of LDL, one with normal receptor binding and the other which has almost no binding activity. The mutation that disrupts binding is a substitution of Gln for Arg at residue 3500 of apo B-100. The current lack of detailed information about the conformation of the apo B-100 molecule and the mechanism of its interaction with the LDL receptor makes it difficult to understand this dramatic effect of a single amino acid substitution.

It is known that Lys residues in the apo B-100 molecule are involved in the binding of LDL to the receptor (Weisgraber et al., 1978). ^{13}C-NMR characterization of these residues has suggested that a subset of Lys with pK 8.9 are particularly involved in this binding (Lund-Katz et al., 1988). The NMR spectra of ^{13}C-labelled Lys residues are sensitive to apo B molecules in different conformations (Aviram et al., 1988) and we have employed this approach to compare normal and familial defective apo B-100 (Lund-Katz et al., 1990). The spectroscopic data suggest that the receptor binding domain of the apo B-100 molecule is disrupted by the substitution of Gln for Arg at position 3500.

EXPERIMENTAL

Materials

Plasma was obtained from either normal subjects or subjects known to be heterozygous for familial defective apo B-100 and who have been described previously (Innerarity et al., 1987a; Weisgraber et al., 1988; Soria et al., 1989). The LDL (d=1.02-1.05g/ml) was isolated by sequential ultracentrifugation and washed by recentrifugation at d=1.05 g/ml (Innerarity et al., 1987a; Weisgraber et al., 1988). The purities of the LDL fractions were assessed by agarose gel electrophoresis (Nobel, 1968). The LDL isolated from FDB subjects in this fashion contained two allelic populations of particles. The first population (about 30% of the total LDL) bound to the LDL receptor normally and to mAb 19 (Young and Hubl, 1989) with high affinity. The second population (about 70% of the total LDL) exhibited defective receptor binding and bound to mAb 19 with low affinity. The two types of LDL particle were separated by immunoaffinity chromatography on a mAb 19 column using a pH gradient (Innerarity et al., 1988). The LDL fraction exhibiting defective receptor binding eluted from the column and was about 93-94% pure and had about 92% of normal receptor binding activity. The protein content and the LDL receptor-binding activity of LDL preparations were determined as described previously (Innerarity et al., 1987a; Weisgraber et al., 1988).

Labeling of LDL--The reductive methylation procedure of Jentoft and Dearborn (1983) was employed to introduce $^{13}CH_3$ groups into the amino groups of Lys residues of apo B-100 on LDL. Conditions described previously (Lund-Katz et al., 1988) were used to convert about 10% of the Lys residues to the ^{13}C dimethyl derivative. When the degree of labelling of Lys residues was <15%, there was no detectable change in the electrophoretic mobility of the LDL on agarose gels. In addition, there was no degradation of apo B-100 as monitored by electrophoresis on SDS-3% polyacrylamide/1% agarose gels. It should be noted that as long as the degree of modification is such that no more than about 15% of the Lys residues are converted to the ^{13}C dimethyl derivative, so that they can be visualized by ^{13}C-NMR spectroscopy, there is no significant change in the conformation of the apo B-100 molecule (cf. Lund-Katz et al., 1988).

Methods

^{13}C NMR spectra at 126 MHz of the ^{13}C-labelled LDL preparations were obtained using a Bruker AM 500 spectrometer. The conditions employed to determine chemical shifts (δ) and resonance intensities have been described previously (Lund-Katz et al., 1988). Circular dichroism (CD) spectra were obtained on a Jasco J-41 A spectropolarimeter as described previously (Reijngoud and Phillips, 1984).

RESULTS

The ^{13}C NMR spectrum of human LDL (Fig. 1A) is dominated by lipid resonances (cf. Hamilton and Morrisett, 1986; Lund-Katz and Phillips, 1986).

A.

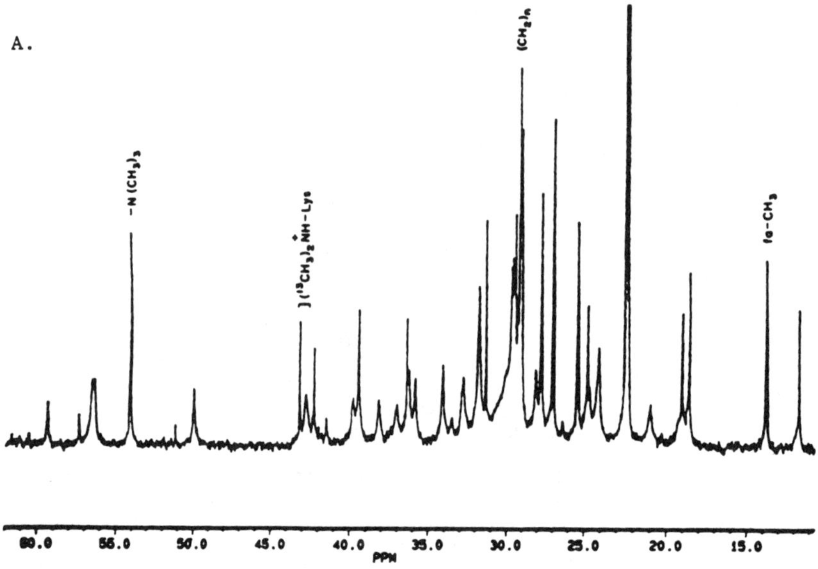

FIG 1A. Proton-decoupled ^{13}C NMR spectrum (126 MHz) of human LDL from a normal subject in which 8.5% of the lysine residues have been converted to $(^{13}CH_3)_2$ Lys by reductive methylation. The spectrum was obtained at 37°C on a Brüker AM500 and was accumulated using 90° pulses of 8 us duration and a recycling time of 1.08 s (23422 acquisitions). The spectrum was processed with 2.0 Hz exponential filtering.

However, the conversion of about 10% of the Lys residues to the $(^{13}CH_3)_2$Lys derivative gives rise to the two well-defined resonances at δ 42.8 and 43.2 ppm. These chemical shifts are sensitive to pH and titration shows that the dimethyl-Lys residues which resonate at $\delta = 42.8$ ppm at pH 7.6 have pK = 10.5. The dimethyl-Lys with $\delta = 43.2$ ppm at pH 7.6 have pK = 8.9 (Lund-Katz et al., 1988). These pK values apply to the unmodified lysine sidechain because the titration characteristics of the dimethylated and unmethylated Lys ε-amino groups are essentially identical. The electrophoretic mobilities on agarose gels and the CD spectra between 184-260 nm of normal and familial defective apo B-100 samples labelled $\leq$ 15% are the same as those of unmodified LDL. The fact that the surface charge density on the LDL particle and the average secondary structure of the apo B-100 molecule are unaltered (data not shown) indicates that the conformation of the protein molecule is not significantly perturbed by low degrees of labelling.

The fact that Lys residues can be converted to dimethyl derivatives without significant alteration in their pK means that, as long as the modification does not alter the conformation of the apo B, ^{13}C NMR spectral analysis of ^{13}C-labeled LDL provides an essentially nonperturbing procedure for visualizing the distribution of Lys with different titration characteristics.

Integration of the $(^{13}CH_3)_2$Lys resonances in Fig. 1A under conditions where the nuclear Overhauser effect is suppressed gives the number of labelled Lys contributing to the signals. For this sample in which 9% of the Lys are visualized by conversion to the dimethyl derivative, there are about 16 dimethyl Lys with pK 8.9 and 16 with pK 10.5 (cf. Lund-Katz et al., 1988). The sizes of the pK 8.9 and pK 10.5 pools of dimethyl Lys of normal LDL at different degrees of methylation are shown by the continuous lines in Fig. 2. It is apparent that the pK 8.9 Lys are preferentially methylated at low degrees of labelling while, at higher degrees of modification, the number of pK 10.5 Lys increases dramatically. At the maximum level of modification, the NMR method visualizes 53 Lys which titrate with pK 8.9 and 172 Lys which titrate with pK 10.5.

The distributions of pK 8.9 and pK 10.5 dimethyl Lys residues in normal and familial defective LDL labelled to 11 $\pm$ 2% are compared in the NMR spectra depicted in Fig. 1B-D.

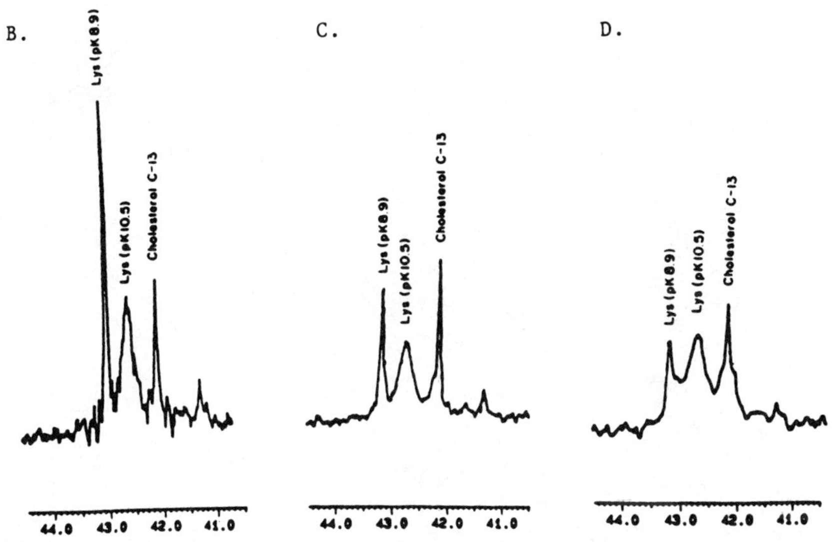

FIG. 1B-D. Proton-decoupled ^{13}C NMR spectra (126 MHz) of human LDL from normal (B) and familial defective apo B-100 subjects (C, D) in which lysine residues have been converted to $(^{13}CH_3)_2$Lys by reductive methylation. B) $(^{13}CH_3)_2$Lys resonances of human LDL from a normal subject in which 11.1% of the lysine residues were labeled (64368 acquisitions). C) $(^{13}CH_3)_2$Lys resonances of total LDL from a familial defective apo B-100 subject in which 8.9% of the lysine residues were labeled (36352 acquisitions). D)

$(^{13}CH_3)_2$ Lys resonances of pure familial defective apo B-100 LDL particles, obtained by mAb 19 immunoaffinity chromatography, in which 12.5% of the lysine residues were labeled (42535 acquisitions).

The normal LDL (Fig. 1B) contains 18 pK 8.9 and 22 pK 10.5 dimethyl Lys. It is apparent from the spectrum in Fig. 1C that the total LDL from a familial defective apo B-100 proband has a decreased ratio of pK 8.9 to pK 10.5 dimethyl Lys. This LDL sample is approximately a 70/30 mixture of familial defective apo B-100 and normal apo B-100 particles.

The NMR spectrum of a preparation of purified familial defective apo B-100 particles (92% pure) obtained by mAb 19 immunoaffinity chromatography of the LDL of a FDB heterozygote is also presented in Fig. 1D. In this case, the number of pK 8.9 dimethyl Lys is 13 and the number of pK 10.5 dimethyl Lys is 32; passage of normal LDL through the mAb 19 immunoaffinity chromatography column did not alter the distribution of pK 8.9 and pK 10.5 Lys (data not shown). The chemical compositions and physical properties of normal and familial defective apo B-100 LDL particles are indistinguishable (Innerarity et al., 1987a). The CD spectra of the LDL preparations described in Fig. 1 are identical (data not shown) indicating that the average secondary structures of normal and familial defective apo B-100 are not significantly different.

The numbers of pK 8.9 and pK 10.5 dimethyl Lys in various preparations of LDL obtained from familial defective apo B-100 and normal subjects are compared in Fig. 2.

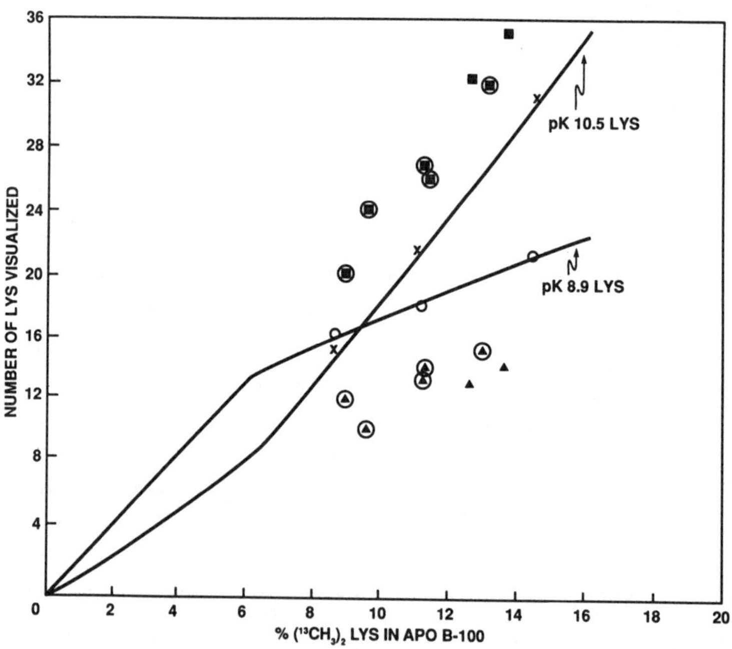

FIG. 2. Lysine pools in apo B-100 of human LDL from normal and familial defective apo B-100 subjects. The degree of methylation is an average of

the values computed from the incorporation of [^{14}C]formaldehyde (scintillation counting and of [^{13}C]formaldehyde (NMR); for a given sample the values agreed to $\pm$ 0.1%. The number of visualized Lys was derived by integration of the ($^{13}CH_3)_2$Lys resonances at δ = 43.2 and 42.8 ppm of NMR spectra of the type shown in Fig. 1 and rounding to the nearest whole number. The nuclear Overhauser effect was suppressed so that the integrals reflect the number of ^{13}C nuclei contributing to each resonance; the integrals for each type of Lys are accurate to $\pm$ 10%. The sizes of the pK 8.9 and pK 10.5 pools of dimethyl Lys of normal LDL at different degrees of methylation are shown by the continuous lines (data taken from Lund-Katz et al., 1988). ○, pK 8.9 Lys and X, pK 10.5 Lys in apo B-100 from normal human LDL samples used in this study as controls. Ⓐ and Ⓑ are pK 8.9 and pK 10.5 Lys of total LDL from familial defective apo B-100 subjects, respectively. ▲ and ■ are pK 8.9 and pK 10.5 Lys of purified familial defective apo B-100 LDL particles obtained by mAb 19 immunoaffinity chromatography.

It is apparent that, relative to normal apo B-100, familial defective apo B-100 (obtained from five different FDB heterozygotes) contains a decreased number of pK 8.9 dimethyl Lys and the same number more of pK 10.5 dimethyl Lys. Relative to normal apo B-100 labeled to the same degree, there is an average decrease of 7 $\pm$ 1 pK 8.9 dimethyl Lys in familial defective apo B-100. This number was obtained either directly from the NMR spectra of the purified familial defective apo B-100 LDL or after correction for the 30% of normal LDL particles present in the total LDL obtained from familial defective apo B-100 probands.

DISCUSSION

Current understanding of the way the apo B-100 molecule is accommodated in the human LDL particle is relatively limited. The protein molecule is apparently extended on the particle surface (cf. Yang et al., 1986) and seems to be composed of multiple domains (Phillips and Schumaker, 1989). The apo B-100 molecule on LDL contains about 45% α-helix, some of which has the potential to be amphiphilic (Cladaras et al., 1986). In addition, analysis of the primary structure suggests that regions of amphiphilic β-structure also exist in the molecule (Knott et al., 1986). The native conformation of apo B-100 contains three types of microenvironments for Lys residues (Lund-Katz et al., 1988). About one-third of the Lys are shielded and not available for labelling by the relatively mild reductive methylation procedure used here.

The 172 normal (pK 10.5) Lys residues which are exposed at the LDL surface titrate like free lysines indicating that they are hydrated normally and that their local environment is not significantly perturbed by interaction with other groups. In contrast, the 53 active (pK 8.9) Lys exposed at the LDL surface are situated so that the affinity of the ε-amino group for protons is decreased (the $-N^+H_3$ groups are 50% deprotonated at pH 8.9 rather than pH 10.5). In principle, this destabilization of the $-N^+H_3$ group could arise because the Lys residues are located in either a basic or a nonpolar microenvironment. In either case, the free energy would be reduced by formation of the uncharged $-NH_2$ group. The fact that active Lys resonate downfield from normal Lys at 43.2 compared to 42.8 ppm (at pH 7.6) is consistent with the polarity of the microenvironment of the active Lys being greater than that of the normal Lys. On this basis, the most probable explanation for the existence of the active Lys with unusually low pK values in apo B-100 of LDL is that they occur in a basic microenvironment. Since several domains which are enriched in basic residues are known to be exposed on the surface of LDL it is a reasonable postulation that these domains contain many, if not all, of the exposed, active Lys. There is NMR evidence for differential exposure of pK 8.9 and 10.5 Lys to ions in the aqueous phase; this implies that there is some local folding of the apo B-100 molecule to form pockets in which pK 8.9 Lys are situated (Lund-Katz et al., 1988). Without more information about the tertiary structure of the apo B-100 molecule on LDL it will not be possible to know the spatial arrangement of the pK 8.9 Lys residues.

It is likely that there are rather precise steric requirements for effective binding of LDL to the receptor. This arises from the need to accommodate the folded Lys-containing basic domain(s) with the appropriate site on the LDL receptor. Upper limits of 21 pK 8.9 and 31 pK 10.5 Lys in the entire apo B-100 molecule are involved in the binding of the LDL to the receptor (Lund-Katz et al., 1988). Since monoclonal antibodies specific for a region that spans a thrombin cleavage site at apo B-100 residue 3249 totally block LDL binding to the receptor (Innerarity et al., 1987b; Milne et al., 1989), it is believed that the receptor binding domain(s) is located around residues 3000-3600. On this basis, it can be inferred that an upper limit of 10 pK 8.9 Lys may be particularly involved in the binding of normal apo B-100 to the receptor. In light of this, the reduction in the number of pK 8.9 Lys in familial defective apo B-100 (Fig. 2) would be expected to have a major effect on the receptor binding affinity. The removal of at least seven Lys residues from the basic microenvironment where they titrate with pK 8.9 to a microenvironment where they titrate normally with pK 10.5 is sufficient to reduce the binding of familial defective apo B-100 to the LDL receptor to 2-4% of the normal level (Innerarity et al., 1990).

Arg 3500 in the amino acid sequence of normal apo B-100 must be a critical structural residue for the native folding of the region of the molecule comprising the LDL receptor binding domain(s). Substitution of Gln at this position causes a conformational change so that the micro-environment of at least seven pK 8.9 Lys is altered. The reorganization of the basic microdomain is sufficient to abolish binding to the 5 acidic, 40-amino acid Cys-rich, repeats which are required for LDL to bind to the LDL receptor (Russell et al., 1989). The structural rearrangement does not involve a major change in the average secondary structure of the apo B-100 molecule because the CD spectrum is unaltered. The loss of the positive Arg residue at position 3500 which slightly reduces the electrostatic attraction between familial defective apo B-100 and the acidic domains of the LDL receptor could be a factor. However, conformational changes induced by the single amino acid substitution and the concomitant disruption of the LDL-receptor binding domain(s) are most likely the predominant reason for the abnormal interaction of familial defective apo B-100 with the LDL receptor.

REFERENCES

1. Aviram, M., Lund-Katz, S., Phillips, M.C. and Chait, A., J. Biol. Chem. 263, 16842-16848 (1988).
2. Brown, M.S. and Goldstein, J.L., Science 232, 34-47 (1986).
3. Cladaras, C., Hadzopoulou-Cladaras, M., Nolte, R.T., Atkinson, D. and Zannis, V.I., EMBO J. 5, 3495-3507 (1986).
4. Goldstein, J.L. and Brown, M.S., Annu. Rev. Biochem. 46, 897-930 (1977).
5. Goldstein, J.L., Brown, M.S., Anderson, R.G.W., Russell, D.W. and Schneider, W.J., Annu. Rev. Cell Biol. 1, 1-39 (1985).
6. Hamilton, J.A. and Morrisett, J.D., Methods Enzymol. 128, 472-515 (1986).

7. Innerarity, T.L., Weisgraber, K.H., Arnold, K.S., Mahley, R.W., Krauss, R.M., Vega, G.L. and Grundy, S.M., Proc. Natl. Acad. Sci. USA 84, 6919-6923 (1987a).
8. Innerarity, T.L., Weisgraber, K.H., Rall, S.C. and Mahley, R.W., Acta Med. Scand. Suppl. 715, 51-59 (1987b).
9. Innerarity, T.L., Balestra, M.E., Arnold, K.S., Mahley, R.W., Vega, G.L., Grundy, S.M. and Young, S.G., Arteriosclerosis 8, 551a (1988).
10. Innerarity, T.L., Mahley, R.W., Weisgraber, K.H., Bersot, T.P., Krauss, R.M., Vega, G.L., Grundy, S.M., Friedl, W., Davignon, J., and McCarthy, B.J., J. Lipid Res. (1990) in press.
11. Jentoft, N. and Dearborn, D.G., Methods Enzymol. 91, 570-579 (1983).
12. Knott, T.J., Rall, S.C., Innerarity, T.L., Jacobson, S.F., Urdea, M.S., Levy-Wilson, B., Powell, L.M., Pease, R.J., Eddy, R., Nakai, H., Byers, M., Priestley, L.M., Robertson, E., Rall, L.B., Betsholtz, C., Shows, T.B., Mahley, R.W. and Scott, J., Science 230, 37-43 (1985).
13. Knott, T.J., Pease, R.J., Powell, L.M., Wallis, S.C., Rall, S.C., Innerarity, J.L., Blackhart, B., Taylor, W.H., Marcel, Y., Milne, R., Johnson, D., Fuller, M., Lusis, A.J., McCarthy, B.J., Mahley, R.W., Levy-Wilson, B. and Scott, J., Nature 323, 734-738 (1986).
14. Law, S.W., Grant, S.M., Higuchi, K., Hospattankar, A., Lackner, K., Lee, N., and Brewer, H.B., Proc. Natl. Acad. Sci. USA 83, 8142-8146 (1986).
15. Lund-Katz, S., Ibdah, J.A., Letizia, J.Y., Thomas, M.T. and Phillips, M.C., J. Biol. Chem. 263, 13831-13838 (1988).
16. Lund-Katz, S. and Phillips, M.C., Biochemistry 25, 1562-1568 (1986).
17. Lund-Katz, S., Innerarity, T.L., Arnold, K.S., Curtiss, L.K. and Phillips, M.C. Submitted.
18. Mahley, R.W., Innerarity, T.L., Pitas, R.E., Weisgraber, K.H., Brown, J.H. and Gross, E., J. Biol. Chem. 252, 7279-7287 (1977).
19. Milne, R., Theolis, Jr., R., Maurice, R., Pease, R.J., Weech, P.K., Rassart, E., Fruchart, J.-C., Scott, J. and Marcel, Y.L., J. Biol. Chem. 264, 19754-19760 (1989).
20. Nobel, R.P., J. Lipid Res., 9, 693-700 (1968).
21. Phillips, M.L. and Schumaker, V.N., J. Lipid Res. 30, 415-422 (1989).
22. Reijngoud, D.-J. and Phillips, M.C., Biochemistry 23, 726-734 (1984).
23. Russell, D.W., Brown, M.S. and Goldstein, J.L., J. Biol. Chem. 264, 21682-21688 (1989).
24. Schonfeld, G., and Krul, E.S., J. Lipid Res. 27, 583-601 (1986).
25. Soria, L.F., Ludwig, E.H., Clarke, H.R.G., Vega, G.L., Grundy, S.M. and McCarthy, B.J., Proc. Natl. Acad. Sci. USA 86, 587-591 (1989).
26. Weisgraber, K.H., Innerarity, T.L. and Mahley, R.W., J. Biol. Chem. 253, 9053-9062 (1978).
27. Weisgraber, K.H., Innerarity, T.L., Newhouse, Y.M., Young, S.G., Arnold, K.S., Krauss, R.M., Vega, G.L., Grundy, S.M. and Mahley, R.W., Proc. Natl. Acad. Sci. USA 85, 9758-9762 (1988).
28. Yang, C.-H., Chen, S.-H., Gianturco, S.H., Bradley, W.A., Sparrow, J.T., Tanimura, M., Li, W.-H., Sparrow, D.A., DeLoof, H., Rosseneu, M., Lee, F.-S., Gu, Z.-W., Gotto, A.M. and Chan, L., Nature 232, 738-742 (1986).
29. Young, S.G. and Hubl, S.T., J. Lipid Res. 30, 443-449 (1989).

ACKNOWLEDGEMENTS

We thank Maria Davidson for expert technical assistance and Dr. R.M. Krauss for providing plasma from FDB subjects. This research was supported by National Institutes of Health grant HL22633.

Secondary Structure of the Exon 3 Encoded Portion of Apolipoprotein E

Demetrios T. Braddock, Peter G. Kovatsits, and Stephen C. Meredith

Departments of Pathology and Biochemistry and Molecular Biology, University of Chicago, Chicago, Illinois

ABSTRACT

The exon 3 encoded portion of human apolipoprotein E (apoE), residues 1-61, is not predicted to contain 22 amino acid amphiphilic α helical domains like those of apo A-I or the exon 4 encoded portion of apoE. Predictive algorithms suggest the presence of other amphiphilic structures, however. We synthesized two peptides, NH_2-VETEPEPELRQ-COOH (residues 6-16 of human apo E, Peptide I) and NH_2-QTLSEQVQEELLSSQVTQEL-COOH (residues 40-60 of guinea pig apoE, Peptide II). Peptide I forms an amphiphilic ß strand, of which the ß content by CD spectroscopy increases upon self-association or binding to lipid surfaces. An anomalous effect is seen as guanidine hydrochloride is added to concentrations up to 0.5 M: the apparent ß content of the peptide increases. The same phenomenon has been observed (23) for intact apoE. Peptide II displays helicity by CD spectroscopy, but the minima, at 217.5 and 204 nm, are atypical of α helices. The ellipticity increases in the presence of phospholipid vesicles or calcium ions, and the effects of vesicles and Ca^{++} are somewhat additive. Peptide II is also amphiphilic as shown by its force-area isotherm in monolayers at the air-water interface. Two possible structures are considered for Peptide II: the amphiphilic π helix, and α helix with twisted hydrophobic face.

INTRODUCTION

Apolipoprotein E (apoE) is unique among the apolipoproteins in several important respects. While most other apolipoproteins are synthesized mainly or exclusively in hepatocytes and enterocytes, apo E is synthesized by hepatocytes, macrophages, ovarian and testicular cells, microglia, and numerous other cell types (1). Another distinctive feature of apo E is that it is a constituent of lipoproteins across the spectrum of sizes and densities (2). It is most abundant in VLDL, chylomicrons, chylomicron remnants, and the HDL_c subpopulation of HDL, but can also be found in smaller quantities in 6the other classes of lipoproteins. Human preapoE consists of a mature peptide of 299 amino acids plus a signal peptide of 18 amino acids. Unlike apo A-I and apo A-II, which are secreted as proapoproteins, there is no proapoE. Rodent apoEs are

© 1990 by Elsevier Science Publishing Co., Inc.
Molecular Biology of Atherosclerosis
A.D. Attie, Editor

shorter than human apo E; guinea pig apoE, for example, has a mature peptide of only 280 amino acids, with deletions confined to the N- and C-terminal extremes of the molecule (3). More striking than these differences, however, is the conservation of apo E sequences, on the order or 70% homology between rodent and human apoE on both amino acid and nucleotides levels. The amino acid sequences of apo E from seven species is shown in Table 1 (3-10). Apo E cDNAs structures have been reported for the human and several other species, and the structure of the human apoE gene is known. The gene is about 3.7 kB long, and has 4 exons and 3 introns. Intron 1 is about 700 bases long and occurs in the 5' untranslated region between bases 23 and 24 upstream of the initiation codon for methionine. Intron 2 is about 1100 bases long, and interrupts the codon of amino acid -4, i.e., in the apo E prepeptide. Intron 3 is about 600 bases long and interrupts the codon for amino acid 61 of the mature protein. The intron locations are similar to those occurring in the genes for apo A-I, apo C-I and apo C-III. The cDNA structure and gene structure of apo Es have been reviewed recently.

The domains of apo E reflect the structure of the apo E gene. Only three of the four exons encode the amino acids of preapoE, while the first is untranslated. The second exon encodes all but the last four of the amino acids of the prepeptide. This prepeptide appears to be a lipophilic α helix, like most prepeptides. The remaining two exons encode most of the protein, and the two exons appear to be so distinct structurally that on is tempted to view apo E as a fusion protein of two virtually unrelated parts.

The domains encoded by exon 4, amino acids 62-299 in human apo E, have been discussed extensively, and will be mentioned only in passing. Apo E, like apo A-I, appears to have amphiphilic α helical segments, each about 22 amino acids long, though different authors disagree as to whether there are six, seven or eight of such units. The potential amphiphilic α helices show homology with each other, and with amphiphilic α helical domains in apo A-I and other apolipoproteins, but within apo E the eight potential helical units differ widely in their helical potentials, and in their predicted amphiphilicity, as defined by predictive algorithms.

The amino acids encoded by the third exon do not share the foregoing traits. They do not appear to contain amphiphilic α helices by the analyses for secondary structures (13,14) nor are these sequences strongly homologous with those encoded by exon 4. The domain encoded by the third exon contains the most highly conserved region of apo E, and the second least conserved region. The extreme N-terminal portion of apo E, approximately the first 20-30 amino acids, is quite variable among species and shows many deletions; only the C-terminal amino acids are more variable. A portion of this domain can be arrayed as an amphiphilic ß strand. Amino acids 40-61 are the most highly conserved of apo E, both at the amino acid and nucleotide level. In order to probe the secondary structural characteristics of the exon 3 encoded domain of apo E, we have studied synthetic peptide fragments of this region, which will be described in the remainder of this paper. The work is divided into two sections: one on a potential amphiphilic ß strand near the N-terminus of apo E; the other on the highly conserved domain corresponding to residues 41-60 of human apo E.

MATERIALS AND METHODS

Peptide Synthesis and Purification: Segments of apolipoprotein E were synthesized by the solid phase method, using an Applied Biosystems Peptide Synthesizer Model 120. Solvents and reagents used in the synthesis were prepared as per the manufacturer's recommendations. The resin used was tBOC-o-benzyl-L-threonine-PAM and tBOC-L-glutamine-PAM, each substituted to 0.68 mmol/g resin. The sequences synthesized were residues 35 through 55 of guinea pig apo E, NH_2-QTLSDQVQEELLSNQVTQELT-COOH, and residues 6 through 16 of human apo E, NH_2-AVETEPEPELRQ-COOH. Residues were added to the resin using the method of asymmetric anhydrides, as recommended by Applied Biosystems. Yields were checked using a quantitative ninhydrin test and were found to exceed 99% in all steps, except for the one arginine residue for which the yield was >98%. Peptides were cleaved from the resin using anhydrous hydrogen fluoride/p-cresol/p-thiocresol = 95/5/5 (v/v/v) at 0°C for one hour. After the cleavage, the resin was washed with ethyl acetate and dichloromethane to remove the radical scavengers and reaction byproducts. The peptides were eluted from the resin with water/trifluoroethanol/ammonium bicarbonate = 80/20/1 (v/v/w). The peptides were purified in batches of 50 mg, first by gel permeation chromatography using Sephadex G-25 superfine; the column (0.9 x 90 cm) eluant was 1% (w/v) ammonium bicarbonate, pH 8.0. Column effluent was monitored by absorbance at 220-240 nm; the peaks eluting just after the void volume was collected and lyophilized. The peptides were redissolved and further purified by reverse phase HPLC using a Vydac C4 silane column (4.6 x 250 mm), and a one hour gradient from 0.1% (v/v) trifluoroacetic acid in water to 0.1% (v/v) trifluoroacetic acid in acetonitrile; flow rate was 1 mL/min. Column effluent was monitored by absorbance at 230 nm. A single major peak comprising approximately 85% of the UV absorbing material eluted at an acetonitrile concentration of 44% (v/v)for the longer peptide, and 24% for the shorter one. The identity of the peaks were ascertained by amino acid analysis (13) and N-terminal sequencing by Edman degradation (14). Peptide concentrations were measured by amino acid analysis.

Circular Dichroic Spectroscopy: Circular dichroic (CD) spectra of the synthetic peptides were measured using a Jasco-600 spectropolarimeter. Spectra were the averaged results of 10 scans. Solvents were 0.02 M MOPS, pH 7.40, containing 0.16 M KCl; the same solvent also containing 0.05 M $CaCl_2$; and water/trifluoroethanol, 1/1 (v/v). In some experiments with the peptide of residues 6-16 of human apo E, 0.05 M sodium phosphate, pH 7.40, 0.10 M NaCl was used as the solvent. The CD spectrum of peptides mixed with egg lecithin single bilayer vesicles in 0.02 M MOPS, pH 7.40, containing 0.16 M KCl, was also measured. Vesicles were prepared as previously described (15). For spectra of samples containing vesicles, the contributions made by the lipids to the ellipticities were subtracted from the spectra. Peptide concentrations for these measurements ranged between 10^{-5} and 10^{-4} M.

Monolayers at the Air-Water Interface: Monolayers of the synthetic peptides were formed at the air-water interface by allowing a solution of the peptide to slide down a slightly inclined glass coverslip onto the surface. Surface pressure measurements were made using either a Lauda automated Langmuir trough or a Nima surface balance equipped with a Wilhelmy plate. Data were digitized and stored, and then analyzed using nonlinear least squares methods (16). Monolayers were compressed and expanded at a rate of 0.3 cm^2/sec. Water and buffers used in these experiments were previously ascertained to have no detectable surface pressure; all solvents were foamed immediately prior to use, and the surface of the solvents were vacuum-cleaned to remove traces of surfactants. Surface isotherms were analyzed using a two-dimensional gas equation for surface pressures $\leq$ 1 dyn/cm: $\pi(A - nA_o) = nRT$, where π = surface pressure, A = surface area, Ao = area excluded by peptide molecules in the monolayer, n = number of moles of peptide in the monolayer, R = 8.3 x 10^7 erg/mole°K, and T = absolute temperature. For surface pressures above 1 dyn/cm, the equation was: $\pi(A - A_{oo}(1 - \kappa\pi)) = nRT$, where A_{oo} = area excluded by the peptide molecules in the monolayer when π = 0, and κ = compressibility in cm/dyn (17). From the mass of the peptide spread onto the surface and the value of n obtained, the apparent number-average molecular weight of the peptide at the interface could be calculated.

A POSSIBLE AMPHIPHILIC ß STRAND NEAR THE N-TERMINUS OF HUMAN APO E

In addition to their role as ligands for cell surface receptors, the apolipoproteins stabilize the lipoprotein surface through the binding of numerous, short, amphiphilic peptide segments of defined secondary structure. Unlike the small exchangeable apolipoproteins A-I, A-II, C-I, C-II, C-II, and the carboxy-terminal two-thirds of apo E, which contain amphiphilic α helices, apo B appears to have many short amphiphilic ß strands as its prominent secondary structure (18-23). An important result of this difference in secondary structure is the segregation of the apoproteins to particles of different size. We have calculated the spacing of phospholipid headgroups as a function of particle radius. The shape of the curve suggests that there is much more splaying of headgroups in HDL than in LDL, though there is not much difference in the splay of LDL and larger particles. The wider grooves between headgroups of HDL can accomodate the wider α helical structure of apo A-I, whereas the narrower grooves between the headgroups of LDL and larger particles are ideally suited for accomdating the ßstrands of apo B. In this light, apo E is of particular interest because of its unique ability to associate with lipoproteins across the size spectrum (19). One would expect, then, that apo E might contain domains suitable for binding both HDL and LDL -- i.e., both α helical and ß strand domains -- and that these domains would be segregated into distinct portions of the polypeptide. Indeed, predictive algorithms, monolayer studies, and circular dichroic spectra by Chen et al. suggest that lipid-free apo E has both α helix and ß strand (49% and 10%, respectively (22)). Moreover, Wetterau et al. have shown that denaturation of apo E in guanidine hycdrochloride is biphasic, and characteristic of a protein having two structural domains (23).

Examination of the amino acid sequence of apo E suggests that there is a potential amphiphilic ß strand near the amino terminus, amino acids 6 through 16 of human apo E. Typically amphiphilic ß strands have alternating hydrophilic and lipophilic amino acids; in a peptide with such a sequence, the amino acids side chain project towards opposite sides of the planes of the peptide bonds when the peptide is in the ß conformation. Amino acids 6 through 16 of human apo E display this property, though the presence of proline residues suggests that a ß strand in this region either would be kinked or interrupted by a turn. To ascertain whether this segment of apo E might be an amphiphilic ß strand, and, on the more theoretical level, to test whether a sequence containing prolines would be capable of forming an amphiphilic ß strand, we synthesized the peptide of the sequence, NH_2-AVETEPEPELRQ-COOH. The peptide was studied in three ways: 1) CD spectrum of the peptide, including denaturation of the peptide in GuHCl since amphiphilic ß strands have a characteristic resistance to denaturation by GuHCl (20); 2) the effects of egg lecithin single bilayer vesicles on the secondary structure of peptide; and 3) the properties of peptide monolayers at the air-water interface. In this paper, we propose to show that apo E does indeed have an amphiphilic ß strand domain, somewhat similar to those in apo B.

CD spectra between 210 and 250 nm are consistent with a mixture of ß strand and random coil, and were analyzed using the procedure of Greenfield and Fasman. The molar ellipticity at 217 nm of a solution of peptides at 5 X 10^{-5}M at 217nm was -4700 deg cm^2 $dmol^{-1}$ from which one calculates a ß strand content of 40%. The mean residue ellipticity of the peptide varied with peptide concentration, however, as shown in Figure 1 in which the slope of the line changes with peptide concentration. Thus, the mean residue ellipticity, which can be calculated from the slope, increases with increasing peptide concentration. These results suggest that the ß strand structure is stabilized by self-association of the peptide, as has been observed for both amphiphilic α and ß peptides (23). To calculate an aggregation number, the self-association was analyzed using the equations:

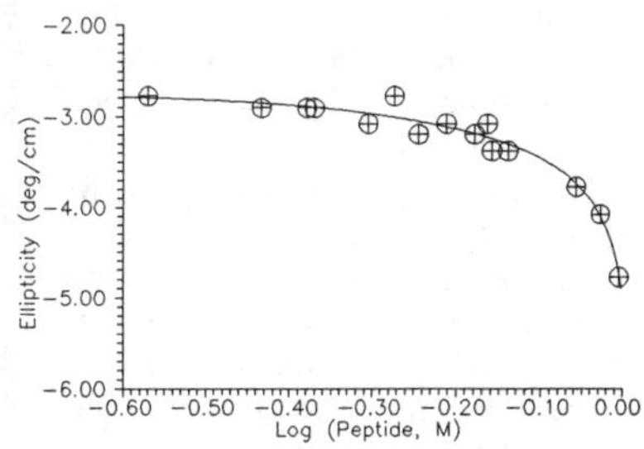

$$nM \rightarrow A_n$$

$$K_d = M^n/A_n$$

$$T = M + nA_n$$

where M = monomer concentration, A = aggregate concentration, T= total (analytical) concentration, n = aggregation number, and K_d = dissociation constant. In the figure, the points are data, and the line is the least squares fit to these equation. The data were found to be consistent with a monomer-dimer equilibrium.

The denaturation of the peptide in guanidine hydrochloride (GuHCl) was studied next (Figure 4). Surprisingly, increasing the GuHCl concentrations up to 0.75M actually made the mean residue ellipticity more negative, -7240 deg cm^2 $dmol^{-1}$ at 0.75 M GuHCl. With further increments in the GuHCl concentration, the molar ellipticity at 217 nm became less negative exhibiting a typical denaturation curve. The transition midpoint occurred at about 3M GuHCl, which is typical of other amphiphilic ß strand peptides. This unusual multiphasic denaturation curve was also observed by Wetterau et al. (24, 25) for intact apo E , and suggests that there may be stable intermediates induced by low concentrations of GuHCl.

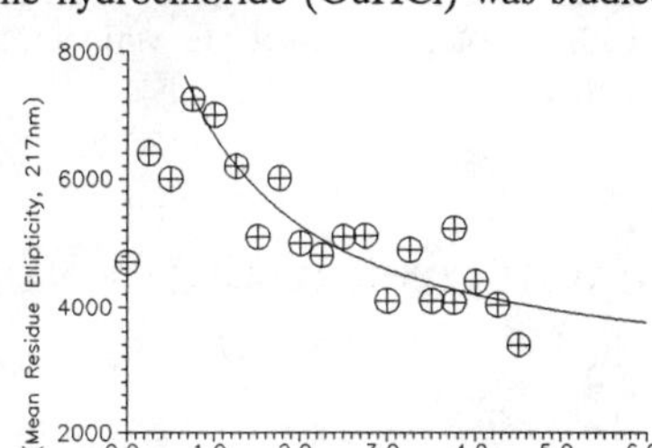

The peptide readily forms monolayers at the air-water interface with a collapse pressure of 28 dyn/cm and a limiting area of 16.1 Å^2/amino acid. Both the collapse pressure and low limiting area are characteristic of amphiphilic secondary structures. The calculated molecular weight from the data was 1014 g/mole which approximates the actual molecular weight of 1684.8 g/mole suggesting that the peptide was monomeric at the surface.

A characteristic of many amphiphilic peptides is that their secondary structure is stabilized by adsorption onto an amphiphilic interface. The CD spectrum of the peptide was measured in the presence of egg lecithin single bilayer vesicles. Peptide concentration was 10 μM; vesicles were at 1 mM lecithin. Thus, in order to favor complete binding of peptide to the vesicles, there was a great excess of potential binding sites on the vesicles compared to peptide molecules. The spectrum showed a marked increase in ellipticity, to -11,500 deg cm^2/dmol, corresponding to an increase in the ß content to 70%. Such an increase strongly suggests the peptide binds to lipid surfaces as an amphiphilic ß strand.

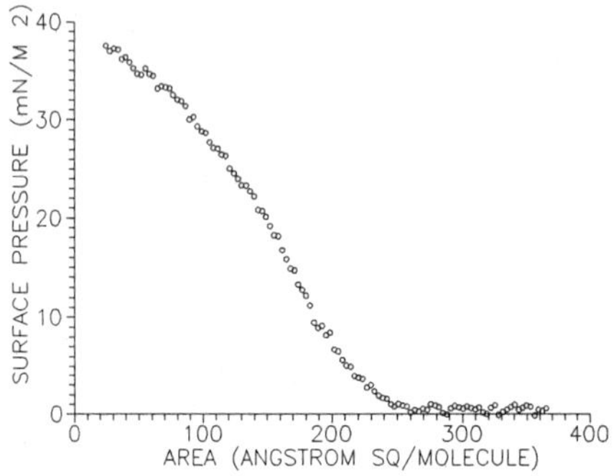

In summary, the above studies describe the synthesis and characterization of a putative amphiphilic ß strand segment of apo E. The peptide had several properties typical of amphiphilic ß strands, as well as some more unusual properties. Like other amphiphilic ß strands, this peptide has a CD spectrum consistent with a mixture of ß structure and random coil. Significantly, like other amphiphilic ß strand peptides, the ß content increased upon self-association or binding to a lipid surface. The peptide resists denaturation by guanidine hydrochloride, as do other amphiphilic ß strand peptides. The surface isotherm was also typical of amphiphilic ß strand peptides, e.g., those from apo B. An unusual feature, and one atypical of amphiphilic ß strands, is the apparent increase in ß content induced by low concentrations of GuHCl. This property is also seen in intact apo E. Finally, these findings underscore the difference between the exon 3 and exon 4 encoded domains of apo E, and are consistent with the hypothesis stated above that the multiple structural domains in apo E uniquely allow this protein to associate with lipoprotein particles across the size and density spectrum.

THE MOST CONSERVED REGION OF APOLIPOPROTEIN E -- BUT WHAT IS IT?

The most highly conserved region of apo E, even more conserved than the LDL receptor binding region, is amino acids 40-61 of human apo E. In eight species, from rodents (guinea pig, mouse, rat, rabbit) to primates (human, cynomolgus, and baboon), there is remarkable conservation: generally only one conservative difference occurs in these domains between one species and the next, and some distant species, the guinea pig and the baboon for example, have identical sequences. There is 90.5% homology for the corresponding domains of rat, rabbit, mouse and guinea pig apoE, and 95.2%

homology for the corresponding regions of baboon apoE. The genomic DNA sequence of rat and human apoE and the location of introns have been reported (9,10). In both the human and rat sequences, the third intron is between the second and third nucleotide of the codon for amino acid 61 (or, in the rat, the residue corresponding to residue 61 of human apoE). Among all species for which the sequence of apo E is known, there is only one amino acid in one species with a nonconservative variation.

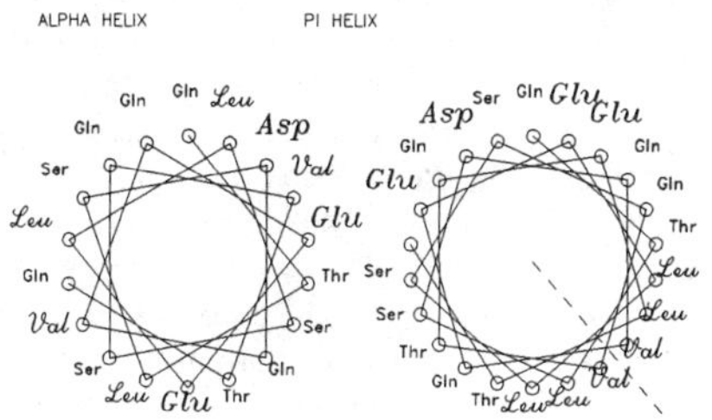

The function of this domain is not known, and when the amino acid sequence of apo E is analyzed for potential secondary structures using the algorithms of Chou and Fasman (11), or Garnier et al. (12), there is no strong indication that this region possesses a particular secondary structure. While the C-terminal domain of the protein contains the well-known amphiphilic α helices, and the extreme N-terminal domain discussed above contains the putative amphiphilic ß strand, the highly conserved region does not appear to be amphiphilic if the sequence is arrayed as an α helix or a ß strand -- i.e., it does not show segregation of hydrophilic and lipophilic amino acids. On the other hand, as shown in figure 4, when residues 41 through 60 of human apoE, or any of the corresponding regions of apoE from the other species, are arrayed as a π-helix, there is a perfect segregation of the hydrophilic and lipophilic residues to separate faces of the helix. This pattern of segregation of hydrophiles and lipophiles is conserved in all species for which the sequence of apo E is known. Indeed, analysis of the sequence for possible amphiphilic structure using the algorithm of Finer-Moore and Stroud (38), indicates that this region may in fact be amphiphilic, but the amphiphilic periodicity identified in this part of the protein by this algorithm is 4.5 amino acids per turn -- i.e., the periodicity of a π helix.

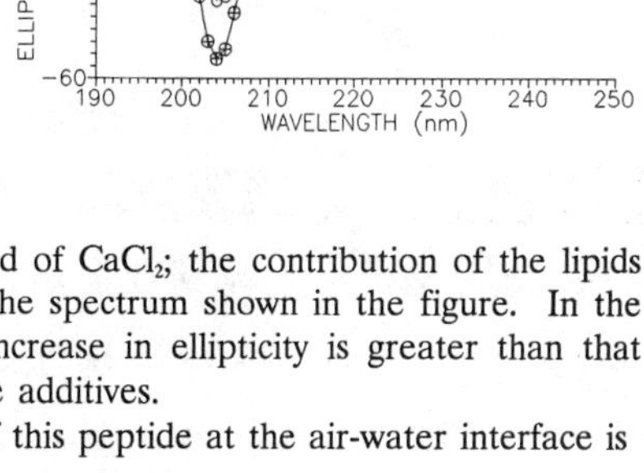

In view of this notable putative secondary structural organization, we have synthesized the peptide corresponding to residues 35 through 55 of guinea pig apolipoprotein E. Figure 5 shows the circular dichroic spectra of the synthetic peptide in aqueous buffer (*), and in the same buffer in the presence of either egg lecithin single bilayer vesicles (o), $CaCl_2$ (---) or both vesicles and $CaCl_2$ (⊕). From 190 to 250 nm, the peptide shows negative ellipticity with two minima: a smaller trough at 217.5 nm, and a larger one at 204 nm. The ellipticity of the peptide is increased in the presence of the vesicles and of $CaCl_2$; the contribution of the lipids to the ellipticity has been subtracted from the spectrum shown in the figure. In the presence of both vesicles and $CaCl_2$, the increase in ellipticity is greater than that caused by the presence of only one of these additives.

The surface isotherm of a monolayer of this peptide at the air-water interface is shown in figure 6. The peptide formed stable monolayers, with a collapse pressure of 24 dyn/cm. The exclusion area, A_{∞}, was calculated to be 24 A^2/ amino acid, and the apparent molecular weight of the peptide at the surface was 2450, i.e., the peptide was monomeric at the surface and the spreading was essentially quantitative. The monolayer was highly compressible; the value of κ was calculated to be 150 cm/dyn.

The unanswered question remains: what is the structure of this domain? Is it a π helix? In fact, one might well ask: do π helices exist? The π helix has been proposed as a possible secondary structure (39-41), with 4.4 residues per turn and 22 amino acids in a full cycle of the helix. Ramachandran plots suggest that this structure has a higher energy than the common secondary structures, but is still a "permitted" structure. A π helical peptide, Poly(ß phenethyl L-aspartate), has been synthesized (42), but the existence of naturally occurring π helices in proteins has never been demonstrated. If π helices exist in globular proteins, they must be extremely rare. More recently, this structure has been proposed as one which might occur in the amphiphilic form (43), i.e., though the π helix is of marginal stability in aqueous media, the amphiphilic form of the π helix might become a stable structure within an amphiphilic environment. Growth hormone releasing factor and ß endorphin were proposed to possess such an amphiphilic π helical structure. When amino acids 34 through 54 of guinea pig apoE, or residues 40 through 60 of human apoE are arrayed as a π helix on a helical wheel, there is perfect segregation of the six lipophilic amino acids to one face of the helix. A further intriguing characteristic of this putative π helix is that there is a plane of symmetry through the lipophilic amino acids which extends through two hydrophilic amino acids on both sides of the lipophiles.

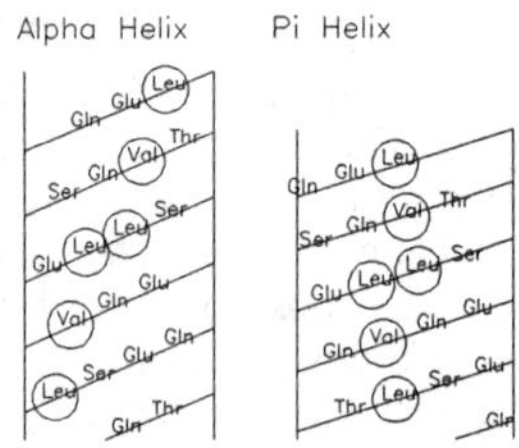

Given the lack of precedent for the occurrence of π helices, as well as theoretical arguments against this structure, one needs to consider alternative structures for the highly conserved domain of apo E. The alternative must be consistent, however, with the observations presented above that the peptide is both amphiphilic in its monolayer properties and helical by circular dichroic spectroscopy, and that the spectral minima are atypical of α helices. One possibility is that the domain is an α helix in which the lipophilic face of the helix twists around the helical surface. The two alternate structures -- π helix and twisted α helix -- are shown in Figure 6. Although the sequence of ß-endorphin is consistent with either a π helix or a twisted α helix, critical experiments on D-amino acid-containing models of ß-endorphin favor the latter structure (44). A similar approach is currently under investigation for the conserved region of apo E.

REFERENCES

1. RW Mahley (1988), Science 240:622-630.
2. AM Scanu, and AA Spector, 1986, Biochemistry and Biology of Lipoproteins, Marcel Dekker Inc., N.Y.
3. T Matsushima, GS Getz, and SC Meredith, Nucleic Acid Res. 18:202.
4. JW McLean, C Fukazawa and JM Taylor (1983), J. Biol. Chem. 258:8993-9000.
5. TB Rajavashisth, JS Kapstein, KL Reue, and AJ Lusis (1985), Proc. Natl. Acad. Sci. USA 82: 8085-8089.
6. Q-L Hao, T-T Yamin, T-C Pan, S-L Chen, B-S Chen, PA Kroon and Y-S Chao (1987)

Atherosclerosis 66:125-130.
7. JH Hixson, LA Cox and S Borenstein (1988), Genomics 2:315-323.
8. JW McLean DJ Chang, RW Mahley and JM Taylor (1984), J. Biol. Chem. 259:6489-6504.
9. HK Das, J McPherson, GAP Bruns, SK Karathanasis and JL Breslow (1985), J. Biol. Chem. 260:6240-6247.
10. WP Feng, GJ Howlett, and G Schreiber (1986), J. Biol. Chem. 261:13777-13783.
11. PY Chou and GD Fasman (1978), Ann. Rev. Biochem. 47:251-276.
12. J Garnier, DJ Osguthorpe and B Robson (1978), J. Mol. Biol. 120:97-120.
13. RL Heinrikson and SC Meredith (1982), Anal. Biochem. 138:65-74.
14. WP Levy (1981), Methods in Enz. 79:27-31.
15. S Batzri and ED Korn (1973), Biochim. Biophys. Acta 298:1015-1019.
16. K Yamaoka, Y Tanigawa, T Nakagawa and T Uno, J. Pharm. Dyn. 4:879-885.
17. BW Shen, AM Scanu, and FJ Kezdy (1973), Circulation 48, Suppl. IV:48.
18. AM Gotto Jr (1969), Proc. Natl. Acad. Sci. USA 64:1199-1127.
19. JA Reynolds (1980), Ann. NY Acad. Sci 348: 174-186.
20. JCH Steele Jr. and JA Reynolds (1979), J. Biol. Chem. 254:1633-1638.
21. JCH Steele Jr. and JA Reynolds (1979), J. Biol. Chem. 254:1639-1643.
22. TJ Knott, SC Rall Jr., TL Innerarity, SF Jacobson, MS Urdea, B Levy-Wilson, LM Powell, RJ Pease, R Eddy, H Nakai, M Byers, LM Priestly, E Robertson, LB Rall, C Betsholtz, TB Shows, RW Mahley, and J Scott (1985), Science 230:37-43.
23. D Osterman, R Mora, FJ Kezdy, ET Kaiser, and SC Meredith (1984), J. Am. Chem. Soc. 106:6845-6847.
24. RW Mahley, TL Innerarity, SC Rall Jr., and KH Weisgraber (1984), J. Lipid Res. 25:1277-1294.
25. GC Chen, LSS Guo, RL Hamilton, V Gordon, EG Richards, JP Kane (1984), Biochem. 23:6530-6538.
26. JR Wetterau, LP Aggerbeck, SC Rall Jr., KH Weisgraber (1988), J. Biol. Chem. 263:6240-6248.
27. LP Aggerbeck, JR Wetterau, KH Weisgraber, C-SC Wu, and FT Lindgren (1988), J. Biol. Chem 263:6249-6258.
28. WB Rippon, HH Chen, AG Walton (1973), J. Mol. Biol. 75:369-375.
29. G Seipke, H-A Arfman, and KG Wagner (1974), Biopolymers 13:1621-1633.
30. A Brack and A Caille (1978), Int. J. Peptide Protein Res. 11:128-139.
31. S St. Pierre, RT Ingwall, MS Verlander, and M Goodman (1978), Biopolymers 17:1837-1848.
32. H Yamamoto and T Hayakawa, (1983) Macromolecules 16:1058-1063.
33. B Barbier, A Caille, and A Brack (1984), Biopolymers 23:2299-2310.
34. J Vives, F Azorin and JA Subirana (1985), Biopolymers 24:1801-1808.
35. S Yokoyama, D Fukushima, JP Kupferberg, FJ Kezdy, and ET Kaiser (1980), J. Biol. Chem. 255:7333-7339.
36. YK Paik, DJ Chang, CA Reardon, GE Davies, RW Mahley, and JM Taylor (1985), Proc. Natl. Acad. Sci. U.S.A. 82:3445-3449.
37. WP Feng, GJ Howlett, and G Schreiber (1986), J. Biol. Chem. 261:13777-13783.
38. J Finer-Moore and RM Stroud (1984), Proc. Natl. Acad. Sci. USA 81: 155-159.
39. Pauling L. and R.B. Corey, (1950), J. Am. Chem. Soc. 72: 5349.
40. BW Low and RB Baybutt (1952), J. Am. Chem. Soc. 74:5806-5807.
41. C Ramakrishnan and GN Ramachandran (1965), Biophys. J. 5:909-933.
42. S Sasaki, Y Yasumoto, and I Uematsu (1981), Macromolecules 14: 1797-1801.
43. ET Kaiser and F.J. Kezdy (1984), Science 223:249-255.
44. JP Blanc and ET Kaiser (1984), J. Biol. Chem. 259:9549-9556.

Table 1 -- Comparison of Amino Acid Sequences of Apolipoprotein E

	-1	1									
HUM	KVLWAALLVT	VFLAGCQA	KVEQAVETEP	EPELRQQTEW	QSGQRWELAL	GRFWDYLRWV	QTLSEQVQEE	LLSSQVTQEL	RALMDETMKE	LKAYKSELEE	80
BA	----------	--------	----P--P-T	--DV---A--	----P-----	----------	----------	---P------	TT--------	----------	80
CM	----------	--------	----P--P-T	-------A-G	----P-----	----------	----------	---P------	TT--------	----------	80
GP	--------V-	-L----RA	******DV--	-V-V-EPAV-	----P-----	S---------	----D-----	---N------	TL-IED----	V----A---K	74
RT	--A---L---	PL-T--LA	********-G	-L-VTD-LPG	--D-P--Q--	N---------	----D-----	-Q--------	TV--ED--T-	V----K----	72
MO	--A---V---	-L-T--LA	********-G	---VTD-L--	--N-P--Q--	N---------	----D-----	-Q--------	T---ED--T-	V----K----	74
RB	---W--V-AA	AI----RA	******---Q	-V-VPE-AR-	KA--P-----	----------	-S--D-----	----------	TM--E-----	V---------	74

HUM	QLTPVAEETR	ARLSKELQAA	QARLGADMED	VRGRLVQYRG	EVQAMLGQST	EELRVRLASH	**LRKLRKRLLR**	DADDLQKRLA	VYQAGAREGA	ERGLSAIRER	180
BA	--S-------	----------	----------	--S------S	----------	----A-----	----------	----------	----------	---V------	180
CM	--S-------	----------	----------	--S------S	----------	----A-----	----------	----------	----------	---V------	180
GP	E-G---D-K	---A------	---------E	--N--S---S	---------S	----A--T--	**P--M----Q-**	-I-E----M-	--K---Q---	---V------	174
RT	--G-------	---A--V--T	----------	L-N--G---N	--NT------	D---S--ST-	**---M---M-**	----------	--K---Q---	---V------	172
MO	--G-------	---G--V---	----------	L-N--G---N	--HT------	--I-A--ST-	**---M---M-**	----------	--K-------	---V------	172
RB	--S-M-Q-H-	--------V-	G-*-E-----	-CN--A----	-A--------	---ARAFS--	----------	--E-----M-	--G-------	---V--V---	173

HUM	LGPLVEQGRV	RAATVGSLAG	QPLQERAQAW	GERLRARMEE	MGSRTRDRLD	EVKEQVAEVR	AKLEEQAQQI	RLQAEAFQAR	LKSWFEPLVE	DMQRQWAGLV	280
BA	----------	---------S	---------L	----------	----------	----------	----------	S---------	----------	----------	280
CM	----------	---------S	---------L	----------	----------	----------	----------	S---------	----------	----------	280
GP	--S-I----L	Q-*****--S	----------	--QM-G-L-K	V--QA----E	--R--ME---	V-V----***	****------	-------MM-	--R----E-I	262
RT	---------Q	-T-NLRWRRP	A-*RD----L	SD-I-G-L--	V-NQA----E	--R--ME---	S-M---T---	-----I----	I-G-------	-------N-M	272
MO	---------Q	-T-NL-AG-A	---RD----F	-D-I-G-L--	V-NQA----E	--R-HME---	S-M---T---	-----I----	--G---I--	--H----N-M	272
RB	--SRL-R--L	-V----T---	R--R------	-----GHL--	V---A----N	--R---E---	V-V----P-M	----------	----------	----------	273

HU	EKVQAAVGTS	AAPVPSDNH•		299
BA	--------A-	T--------•		299
CM	--------A-	T----I---•		299
GP	Q---V---A-	TS*A--QEP•		280
RT	--I--S-A-N	SIASTTVPWR	NQ•	292
MO	--I--S-A-N	PIIT-VAQE*	NQ•	292
RB	--L---MPSK	-PAAAPIE**	NQ•	291

Amino acid sequence of apolipoprotein E from seven species: sequences from guinea pig (3), rat (6), mouse (7), rabbit (8), baboon (9), and cynomolgus (10), are aligned with that of the human protein (11,12). The species are identified as follows: HU=human, BA=baboon, RT=rat, CM=cynomolgus monkey, MO=mouse, GP=guinea pig, RB=rabbit. Sequences of human apo E are in upper case letters, other sequences in lower case letters. A dash (-) represents conservation of the human apo E sequence. An asterisk (*) is a deletion of an amino acid. Highly conserved segment, which was synthesized and is discussed in this paper, is underlined; receptor binding region is in boldface. Termination codon is represented by •.

ARTERIAL WALL, CELL GROWTH

The Effect of Minimally Modified Low-Density Lipoprotein on the Expression of Cytokines and Adhesion Molecules in Endothelial Cells

Ali Andalibi,*† Susan Imes,† Judith A. Berliner,** Alan M. Fogelman,† and Aldons J. Lusis*†

*Department of Microbiology, University of California, Los Angeles, California; †Department of Medicine, University of California, Los Angeles, California; **Department of Pathology, University of California, Los Angeles, California

ABSTRACT

Minimally modified low-density lipoprotein is a mildly oxidized molecule capable of inducing the expresssion of a variety of growth factors as well as chemaotactic and adhesion molecules in endothelial cells. Due to its low level of oxidation it is more likely to be the molecule involved in the early stages of atheroscleosis. Experimental data lend support to this hypothesis.

INTRODUCTION

Epidemiological studies have shown that a high level of low density lipoprotein (LDL), the major cholesterol-carrying particle in the blood, appears to be a prerequisite for most forms of atherosclerosis [for example, see 1 and 2]. The degree of variation, however, in the clinical manifestation of disease, even in homozygous patients with familial hypercholesterolemia, suggests that other factors must also be contributing to the clinical expression of atherosclerosis.

Recent studies have implicated oxidative modification of LDL as a major contributor to the formation of atherosclerotic lesions. For example, studies of atherosclerotic lesions isolated from humans, as well as those isolated from Watanabe heritable hyperlipidemic (WHHL) rabbits, have shown that oxidized lipoproteins and products of lipoprotein oxidation are indeed present within the lesions [3, 4]. Furthermore, the observations that the administration of antioxidants such as probucol can prevent progession of atherosclerosis in WHHL rabbits suggest that oxidation of LDL is, in fact, an important event during atherogenesis [5,6]. The highly oxidized LDL which is found in advanced lesions is no longer capable of binding to the LDL receptor and appears to result from oxidative modification by endothelial cells, smooth muscles cells and macrophages [7, 8, 9, 10, 11, 12]. Such a high degree of oxidation, however, is unlikely to occur during the initial stages of lesion formation, during which the subendothelial space appears to be acellular and there are no visible damage-induced structural changes in the endothelium that could, in turn, provide microenvironments where LDL oxidation could

© 1990 by Elsevier Science Publishing Co., Inc.
Molecular Biology of Atherosclerosis
A.D. Attie, Editor

take place without interference from the antioxidant property of the plasma [13]. A low steady-state level of peroxidation occurs in cultured mammalian cells, but it probably does not occur at a high enough level to give rise to significant amounts of highly oxidized LDL [14]. Thus, the initial atherogenic events are unlikely to be caused by highly oxidized LDL molecules. It has been known for some time that even freshly isolated LDL can be cytotoxic to both smooth muscle cells and endothelial cells [15, 16]. Hence, we have hypothesized that a minimally modified LDL (MM-LDL) may be responsible for the subtle changes in the endothelium during the initial phase of atherogenesis. MM-LDL, unlike highly oxidized LDL (10-50 nmol TBARS per mg cholesterol), is recognized by the LDL receptor and shows only minimal oxidation (2-5 nmol TBARS per mg cholesterol) [17]. The studies summarized below show that MM-LDL induces the expression of a set of cytokines and adhesion molecules that may contribute to the early stages of atherosclerosis.

RESULTS AND DISCUSSION

One of the earliest detectable events in atherosclerosis is the binding of circulating monocytes to the endothelium [18, 19]. This enhanced interaction of endothelium with monocytes is seen in areas with propensity towards lesion formation but not in nonpredisposed regions, suggesting expression of molecules that would facilitate monocyte-endothelium interaction in the regions of predilection. When cultured rabbit aortic endothelial cells were exposed to MM-LDL, a three-fold increase in the adhesion of monocytes to the endothelial cells was seen. Futhermore, monocyte binding was markedly reduced upon treatment of the endothelial cells with cycloheximide prior to addition of MM-LDL. No increase in monocyte binding was seen with native LDL even at a concentration exceeding, by twenty fold, that used for MM-LDL. Moreover, the enhanced adhesion was specific for monocytes only. Neutrophil adhesion to the endothelial cells was not stimulated by MM-LDL treatment [17].

Another requirement for endothelium-monocyte interaction is the localized recruitment of monocytes by a chemotactic factor. Endothelial cells treated with MM-LDL showed a seven-fold increase in the amount of the monocyte chemotactic protein, MCP-1 ([17, 20]; Cushing et al., in press). Antibodies to a chemotactic factor isolated from baboon smooth muscle cells [21], which appears to be identical to the MCP-1 protein,isolated from U105 GM glioma cell line, inhibited the chemotactic activity secreted by MM-LDL treated endothelial cells. Furthermore, MM-LDL treatment of endolthelial cells resulted in a time and dose dependant increase in the mRNA levels for MCP-1, with maximal induction occuring after 4 hours (Cushing et al., in press).

Once monocytes have been recruited and adhere to an area of the endothelium, they must be sustained by the monocyte-macrophage colony stimulating factor (M-CSF). This growth factor is required for the survival, proliferation, and differentiation of the cells of the monocyte-macrophage lineage [for a reveiw see 22]. A significant increase in the mRNA levels for M-CSF was seen in both rabbit and human endothlial cells treated with MM-LDL. Moreover, the supernatants from the MM-LDL treated endothelial cells showed a marked increase in the amount of active M-CSF secreted, as assayed by the colony formation assay. The MM-LDL stimulated increase in M-CSF mRNA levels was both time and dosage dependent, with maximal induction occuring at approximately four hours (Figure 1).

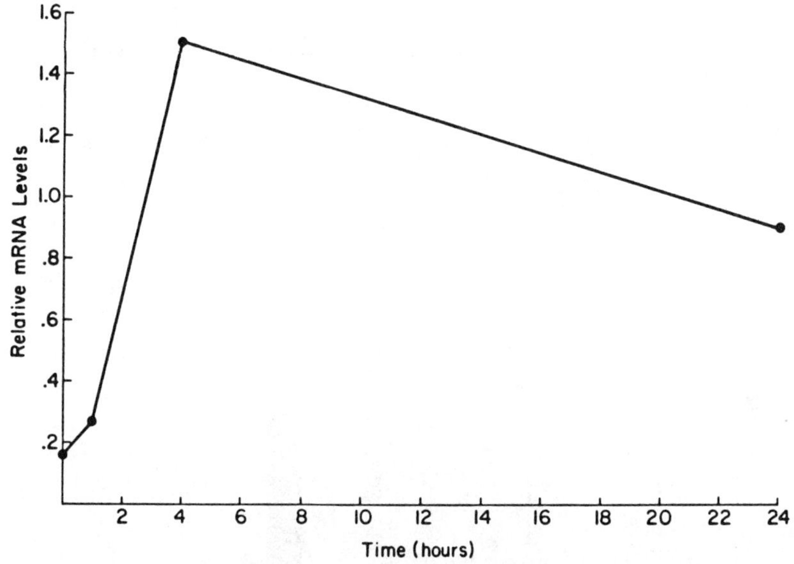

FIG. 1. Time course of induction of M-CSF by MM-LDL in rabbit aortic endothelial cells. Cells were either untreated or were treated with 2.0 μg per ml of MM-LDL for the times indicated, after which they were lysed and total RNA was extracted. Northern blots were autoradiographed and signals were quantitated by densitometric scanning.

The mRNA levels for two other growth factors, GM-CSF and G-CSF, were also increased, but those of TGF-ß, and IL-1ß remained unchanged, suggesting that the action of MM-LDL was, indeed, specific. Treatment of endothelial cells with native LDL, or MDA-LDL had no effect on CSF induction [23]. Furthermore, higher levels of M-CSF mRNA were observed in the areas with atherosclerotic lesions from both WHHL and cholesterol-fed normal rabbits as compared to nonatherosclerotic aortas from normal rabbits. The presence of heightened M-CSF mRNA levels in atherosclerotic lesions suggests that it is, in fact, produced in vivo and may account, in part, for the accumulation of monocyte-macrophages in the subendothelial space of the lesion (Figure 2). This is perhaps not surprising, as the macrophages within the subendolthlial space would require M-CSF in order to survive. What is of interest is the possibility that, in vivo, MM-LDL stimulates the production of M-CSF, a molecule whose presence is necessary for the survival of the macrophages within the lesion. To address this question, we injected MM-LDL into mice. This treatment resulted in a rapid and significant increase in the plasma M-CSF activity, as assayed by the colony formation assay. Injection of native LDL, however, did not induce M-CSF activity (Liao et al., manuscript in preparation). The results of this set of experiments suggest that a minimally modified LDL molecule is in fact capable of stimulating M-CSF production in vivo, and that the increased M-CSF production is not confined to areas of atherosclerotic lesions.

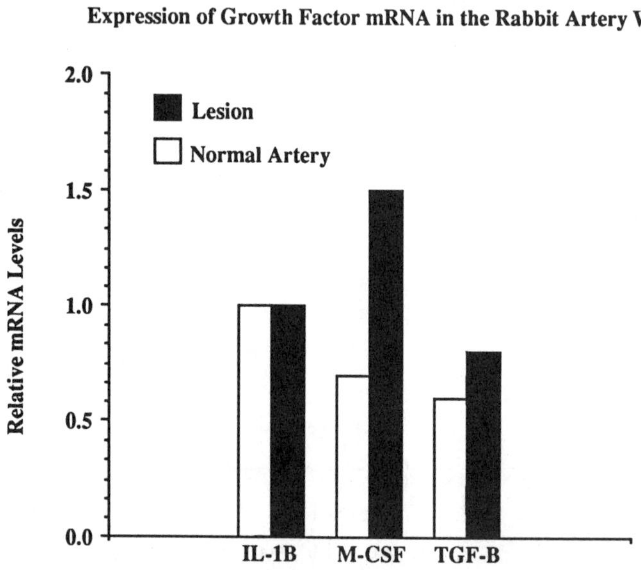

FIG. 2. Expression of the mRNA's for growth factors in normal and lesioned regions of the aorta in a rabbit maintained on a high-cholesterol diet for 2 months. Total RNA was extracted from the respective tissues and subjected to northern analysis. The blots were probed with the cDNA's for IL-1B, TNF-α, and M-CSF. The autoradiograms were quantitated by densitometric scanning.

The above mentioned mouse studies suggest that M-CSF production can be stimulated, in vivo, upon MM-LDL treatment. Furthermore, in vitro studies showed that MM-LDL was capable of inducing M-CSF mRNA and protein in both human and rabbit aortic endothelial cells. It has been demonstrated by Gerrity and coworkers that certain regions of the aorta are more susceptible to lesion formation than others [24]. This alludes to the possibility that cells from different regions of the aorta may be differentially susceptible to damage. Consistent with this hypothesis is the observation that MM-LDL treatment did not cause CSF induction in human umbilical vein endothelial cells (HUVEC) [23]. HUVEC have been shown to be resistant to MM-LDL toxicity. Treatment of HUVEC with cycloheximide abolishes this resistance, suggesting that an actively translated protective protein confers the observed resistance to cytotoxicity of MM-LDL [17]. Thus, the observed disparity of response between

RAEC and HUVEC may be pertinent to the large variation in susceptibility to atherosclerosis that is observed between different regions of the artery. The fact that resistance of HUVEC to MM-LDL toxicity was dependant on protein synthesis suggests that MM-LDL treatment causes induction of a protective mulecule(s) in HUVEC which then renders the cells resistant to the toxic effect of MM-LDL.

Many of the above mentioned effects of MM-LDL can be explained by LPS contamination of the MM-LDL preparation. As almost all biological preparations contain some degee of contamination by LPS, we conducted a series of experiments to rule out the possibility of LPS involvement in the observed effects. Measurement of LPS levels in the MM-LDL preparations used indicated that less than five picograms of LPS was present per milligram of LDL protein, an amount much lower than that needed to stimulate the effects seen by MM-LDL ([23]; Andalibi et al., manuscript in preparation). As shown in figures 3 and 4 , only concentrations of LPS greater than or equal to 1 ng per ml are capable of inducing CSF mRNA in either HAEC or RAEC.

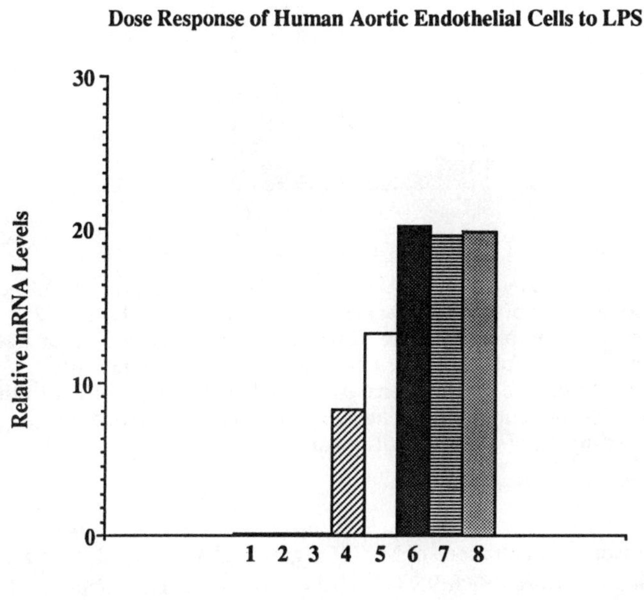

FIG. 3. Dose response of human aortic endothelial cells to LPS. Lanes 1, 2, 3, 4, 5, 6, 7, and 8 represent samples that were treated with 0, 0.01, 0.1, 1, 5, 50, 100, and 1000 ng of LPS respectively. Total RNA was extracted from the cells 4 hours after treatment and subjected to northern analysis. The blots were hybridized to the cDNA for GM-CSF and the autoradiograms were quantitated by densitometric scanning.

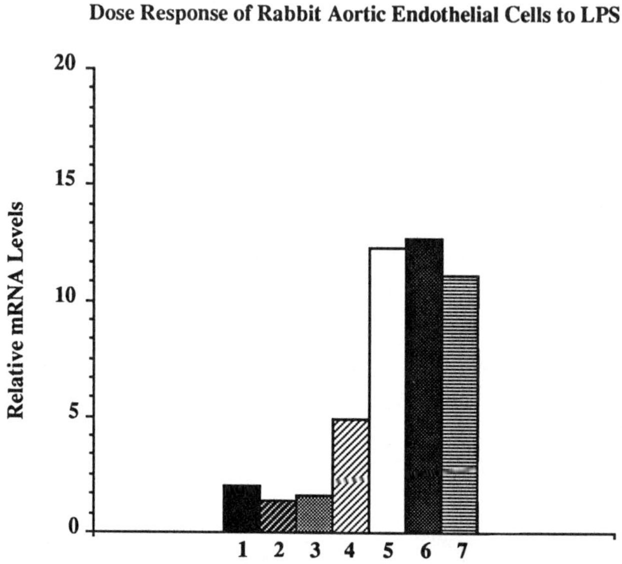

FIG. 4. Dose response of rabbit aortic endothelial cells to LPS. Lanes 1, 2, 3, 4, 5, 6, and 7 represent samples that were treated with 0, 0.01, 0.1, 1, 5, 10, and 1000 ng of LPS respectively. Total RNA was extracted from cells 4 hours after treatment and subjected to northern analysis. The blots were probed with the cDNA for GM-CSF and autoradiographed. Signals were quantitated by densitometric scanning of the autoradiograms.

By comparison, concentrations of MM-LDL greater than or equal to 5 µg per ml are required to induce CSF mRNA in HAEC (Figure 5). Thus 10 µg of MM-LDL, which was the total amount of MM-LDL used in the experiments, would only contain 0.05 picograms of LPS, several orders of magnitude less than the amount required to induce the CSF mRNA's. Furthermore, injection of LPS into the LPS-resistant C3H/HeJ mice resulted in no increase in M-CSF activity, whereas injection of MM-LDL into these animals caused a significant increase in the levels of M-CSF. Moreover, incubation of endothelial cells with a mixture of LPS and MM-LDL did not show a superinduction as is seen upon coincubation of TNF-α and LPS (Andalibi et al., manuscript in preparation, Liao et al., manuscript in preparation). Thus, it is clear that the effects of MM-

LDL cannot be attributed to contaminating LPS. The polar lipids fraction of MM-LDL has been shown to contain the active moeity (Berliner et al., 1989). It is still unclear, however, which component of this polar lipids fraction is the actual active component (Berliner et al., 1989), although conjugated dienes are a likely candidate (G. Popjack unpublished data).

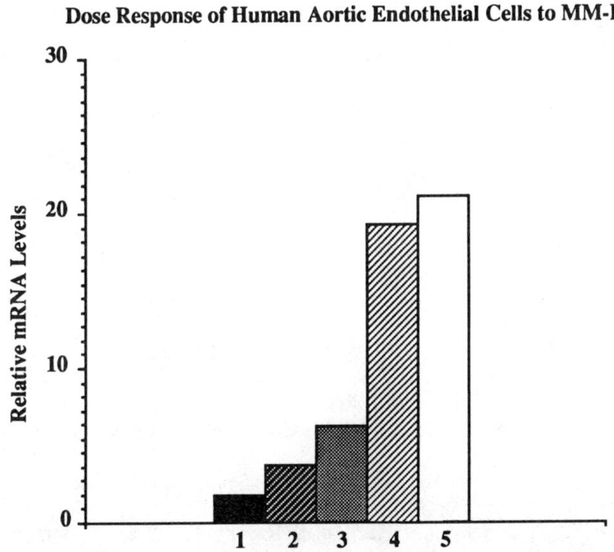

FIG. 5. Dose response of human aortic endothelial cells to MM.LDL. Lanes 1, 2, 3, 4, and 5 represent samples that were treated 0, 0.5, 2, 5, 20, and 40 µg per ml of MM-LDL respectively. Total RNA was extracted 4 hours after treatment and subjected to northern analysis. The blots were probed with the cDNA for M-CSF and autoradiographed. The autoradiograms were quantitated by densitometric scanning.

The above set of experiments suggest that MM-LDL may indeed play a major role in the initiation of the cascade of events that finally culminates in the atherosclerotic lesion. The mechanism by which it triggers the process, however, remains unclear, although involvement of oxygen free radicals is a likely possibility. Understanding the mechanisms involved in the early stages of atherosclerosis should enable us to devise new strategies for the prevention and treatment of this disease.

RERERENCES

1. J.L. Goldstein and M.S. Brown, Annu. Rev. Biochem. 46 , 897-930 (1977).
2. D. Steinberg, Arteriosclerosis. 3, 283-301 (1983).

3. W. Palinski, M.E. Rosenfeld, S. YLA-Herttuala, G. Gurtner, S.S. Socher, S.W. Butler, S. Parthasarathy, T.E. Carew, D. Steinberg, and J.L. Witztum, Proc. Natl. Acad. Sci. USA. 86, 1372-1376 (1989).
4. M.E. Haberland, D. Fong, and L. Cheng, Science. 241, 215-218 (1988).
5. T.E. Carew, D.C. Schwenke, and D. Steinberg, Proc. Natl. Acad. Sci. USA. 84, 7725-7729 (1987).
6. T. Kita, Y. Nagano, M. Yokode, K. Ishii, N. Kume, S. Narumiya, and C. Kawai, Am. J. Cardiol. 62, 13B-19B, (1988).
7. T. Henriksen, E.M. Mahoney, and D. Steinberg, Proc. Natl. Acad. Sci. USA. 78, 6499-6503 (1981).
8. T. Henriksen, E.M. Mahoney, and D. Steinberg, Arteriosclerosis. 3, 149-159, (1983).
9. J.W. Heinecke, H. Rosen, and A. Chait, J. Clin. Invest. 74, 1890-1894, (1984).
10. D.W. Morel, P.E. DiCorleto, and G.M. Chisolm, Arteriosclerosis. 4, 357-364, (1984).
11. M.D. Cathcart, D.W. Morel, and G.M. Chisolm III, J. Leukocyte Biol. 38, 341-350, (1985).
12. S. Parthasarathy, D.J. Printz, D. Boyd, L. Joy, and D. Steinberg, Arteriosclerosis. 6, 505-510, (1986).
13. D. Steinberg, S. Parthasarathy, T.E. Carew, J.C. Khoo, and J.L. Witztum, N. Engl. J. Med. 320, 915-924, (1989).
14. R.H. Burdon and V. Gill, Free Rad. Res. Comms. 7, 149-159, (1989).
15. J.R.Hessler, A.L. Robertson Jr., and G.M. Chisolm III, Atherosclerosis. 32, 213-229, (1979).
16. T. Henriksen, S.A. Evensen, and B. Carlander, Scand. J. Clin. Lab. Invest. 39, 361-368, (1979).
17. J.A. Berliner, M.C. Territo, A. Sevanian, S. Ramin, J.A. Kim, B. Bamshad, M. Esterson, and A.M. Fogelman, J. Clin. Invest. in press, (1990).
18. R.G. Gerrity, H.D. Naito, M. Richardson, and C.J. Schwartz, Amer. J. Pathol. 95, 775-785, (1979).
19. A. Faggiotto, R. Ross, and L. Harker, Arteriosclerosis. 4, 323-340, (1984).
20. E.A. Robinson, T. Yoshimura, and E.J. Leonard, S. Tanaka, P.R. Griffin, J. Shabanowitz, D.F. Hunt, and E. Appella Proc. Natl. Acad. Sci. USA. 86, 1850-1854, (1989).
21. A.J. Valente, D.T. Graves, C.E. Vialle-Valentin, R. Delgado, and C.J. Schwartz, Biochemistry. 27, 4162-4168, (1988).
22. D. Metcalf, Nature. 339, 27-30, (1989).
23. T.B. Rajavashisth, A. Andalibi, M.C. Territo, J.A. Berliner, M. Navab, A.M. Fogelman, and A.J. Lusis, Nature. 344, 254-257, (1990).

Role of LDL Oxidation in Foam Cell Formation and Atherogenesis

Urs P. Steinbrecher, Marilee Lougheed, Hanfang Zhang, and Yuzhou Yang

Department of Medicine, University of British Columbia, Vancouver, British Columbia, Canada

SUMMARY

Oxidative modification of LDL has been shown to alter its properties in a way that tends to increase its atherogenicity. The compositional and structural changes that accompany LDL oxidation include increased electrophoretic mobility, increased density, fragmentation of apolipoprotein B, hydrolysis of phosphatidylcholine, derivatization of lysine amino groups, and generation of fluorescent adducts due to covalent binding of lipid oxidation products to apo B. In addition, oxidation of LDL has been shown to result in changes in its biologic properties that could have pathogenetic importance, including accelerated uptake in macrophages, cytotoxicity, and chemotactic activity for monocytes. Cultured artery wall cells can promote LDL oxidation by secreting superoxide or thiols that generate superoxide in the presence of transition metal ions, or by transferring lipoxygenase-derived hydroperoxy fatty acids to LDL. Oxidized LDL can interact with macrophage scavenger receptor(s) and hence is subject to accelerated degradation in these cells. The domain of oxidized LDL that is recognized by scavenger receptors has not been fully characterized, but derivatization of native LDL or unrelated proteins such as bovine albumin with reactive products obtained from autoxidized polyunsaturated fatty acids is sufficient to allow recognition by the scavenger receptor. These reactive products have some features in common with unsaturated carbonyl compounds but derivatization of LDL with simple aldehydes or alkenals does not lead to recognition by the scavenger receptor. In other studies, we showed that the phospholipid hydrolysis that accompanies LDL oxidation is due to platelet activating factor acetylhydrolase, an unusual phospholipase that exists in plasma in association with lipoproteins. This enzyme is specific for glycerophosphocholine with a short-chain acyl group at the *sn*-2 position, and can hydrolyze LDL phosphatidylcholine that has undergone oxidative fragmentation of the *sn*-2 fatty acid. Although oxidized LDL is rapidly degraded in macrophages, it causes less cholesterol ester accumulation than equivalent amounts of acetyl LDL. This can be explained by a much lower cholesterol:protein ratio in oxidized LDL and because the efficiency of degradation of oxidized LDL is less than acetyl LDL. Several recent studies have provided good evidence for the presence of oxidized LDL in atherosclerotic lesions. However, LDL obtained from plaque-free human aortic intima showed variable and usually mild oxidative changes that were insufficient to allow recognition by the scavenger receptor. Nevertheless, these aortic LDL were internalized more rapidly by macrophages than native LDL by a nonsaturable, probably receptor-independent process. The weight of evidence indicates that oxidized LDL occurs in atherosclerotic plaques, and could play a role in lesion progression. Whether LDL oxidation is an essential factor in the pathogenesis of atherosclerosis has not been conclusively answered.

INTRODUCTION

The advances that have been made in the past few decades in defining risk factors that predispose to atherosclerosis have led to improved therapeutic and preventive strategies. Much progress has been made in understanding lipoprotein metabolism, thrombosis, and the biology of arterial wall cells, all of which are involved in the development of the atherosclerotic lesion. One of the important challenges that remains is to go beyond the risk factor concept to a

© 1990 by Elsevier Science Publishing Co., Inc.
Molecular Biology of Atherosclerosis
A.D. Attie, Editor

comprehensive understanding of the biochemical mechanisms responsible for lesion initiation and progression, and in particular to identify factors essential for atheroma development that might be susceptible to therapeutic intervention. One of the pathologic hallmarks of early atherosclerotic lesions is the presence of foam cells, and it seems plausible (although no proof exists) that cholesterol accumulation in foam cells may be a key step in their development. Careful morphologic and immunohistologic chemical studies have shown that fom cells in early lesions are derived predominantly from macrophages, while in more advanced lesions, foam cells derived from smooth muscle cells are also seen [1-7]. The mechanism by which cholesterol accumulates in these macrophages is not readily apparent, because cultured macrophages do not accumulate cholesterol ester even when incubated with very high concentrations of native LDL [8]. One possible explanation was proposed by Goldstein, Brown and colleagues, who demonstrated that acetylation of LDL resulted in rapid uptake in macrophages via a specific receptor termed the scavenger or acetyl-LDL receptor [8-10]. Because this receptor is not regulated by cellular cholesterol content, massive accumulation of cholesterol ester occurs in macrophages exposed to such modified LDL in vitro. These observations gave rise to the concept that an analogous modification of LDL might occur in vivo. Fogelman and colleagues showed that malondialdehyde-modified LDL was a ligand for the scavenger receptor, and as malondialdehyde was known to occur in vivo as a product of enzymatic and nonenzymatic lipid peroxidation reactions, this was proposed as a potential "biologic" LDL ligand for this receptor [11,12]. A further advance was the recognition that certain types of cultured cells, including endothelial cells and smooth muscle cells were capable of modifying LDL in a way that also led to accelerated uptake in macrophages, at least partly by the acetyl LDL receptor [13-15]. The mechanism for the cell-induced modification of LDL was shown to involve free radical peroxidation of LDL [16-19]. Oxidative modification by cultured cells results in a number of compositional and structural changes to LDL, including increased electrophoretic mobility, increased density, fragmentation of apolipoprotein B, decreased content of phosphatidylcholine with increased lysophosphatidylcholine, derivatization of lysine amino groups, and generation of fluorescent adducts due to covalent binding of lipid oxidation products to apo B [14,15,19-21]. Identical changes occur when LDL is oxidized in the absence of cells, by incubation with transition metal ions such as copper [19,20]. Such copper-oxidized LDL is also recognized by the acetyl LDL receptor of phagocytic cells [20].

In the present article, we will review recent developments in the following areas: the mechanism of oxidation of LDL by cells, uptake mechanisms for oxidized LDL in macrophages, the mechanism for the hydrolysis of phosphatidylcholine that occurs during LDL oxidation, biologic actions of oxidized LDL other than interaction with the scavenger receptor, and the evidence that oxidized LDL occurs in vivo.

I: MODIFICATION OF LDL BY CULTURED CELLS

Several different cell types have been shown to be capable of promoting the oxidative modification of LDL in tissue culture, including endothelial cells, smooth muscle cells, monocyte-macrophages, and even fibroblasts [13-15, 22-25]. We compared the ability of 4 different cell types (rabbit endothelial cells, rabbit arterial smooth muscle cells, bovine aortic endothelial cells, and human skin fibroblasts) to modify LDL under identical culture conditions, and found that the rate at which modification of LDL occured was directly correlated with the rate of superoxide secretion by the cells and inversely related to the cellular content of superoxide dismutase and catalase (Figure 1). It was shown by Hiramatsu and coworkers as well as by Cathcart and colleagues that superoxide dismutase can inhibit the initiation of LDL oxidation by cultured monocyte-macrophages [23, 25]. Further studies showed that the inhibition could only be demonstrated if superoxide dismutase was added within four hours of the start of the incubation of LDL with monocytes whereas butylated hydroxytoluene (BHT) inhibited the modification even when added as late as eleven hours after the onset of incubation [26]. This was interpreted as evidence that superoxide was required for the initiation of oxidative modification but that subsequent propagation and amplification of the oxidative modification involved other free radicals, most likely lipid oxy-radicals rather than superoxide. It seems likely that a superoxide-derived intermediate, for example, perferryl or cupryl ion rather than superoxide itself is involved in the reaction with polyunsaturated fatty acids because the reactivity of superoxide itself is low, and superoxide generated by irradiation or by xanthine-xanthine oxidase in metal-free systems was not found to modify LDL [27, 28].

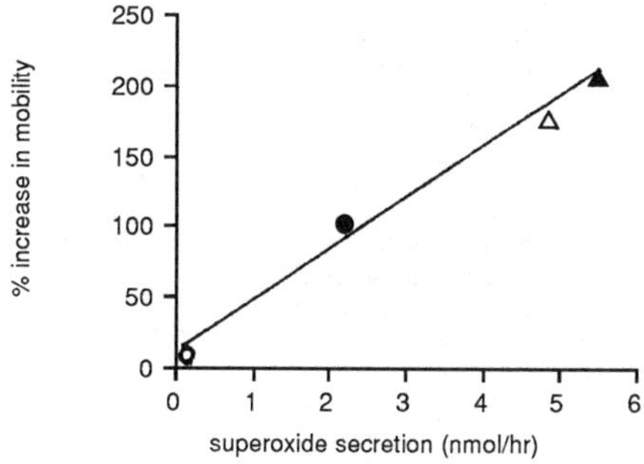

Figure 1. Correlation of the ability of various cultured cell types to modify LDL with their rate of superoxide production. Confluent 60-mm diameter dishes of rabbit aortic smooth muscle cells (▲), rabbit endothelial cells (△), human skin fibroblasts (●), or bovine aortic endothelial cells (○) were incubated in 2 ml serum-free phenol red-free F-10 medium containing 20 uM ferricytochrome c. Superoxide accumulation in the medium was calculated from the superoxide dismutase-inhibitable component of cytochrome c reduction. Parallel dishes from the same plating were incubated for 20 hr in F-10 medium with 200 ug/ml LDL, and the electrophoretic mobility of the LDL was then determined. Values for both parameters represent increase above cell-free control dishes.

There is evidence for more than one process by which different cell types might generate superoxide. The modification of LDL by monocytes only occurs if the cells are treated by an activator to induce the respiratory burst, and therefore it is likely that the NADPH oxidase system is responsible for the production of superoxide that causes LDL modification by these cells. In contrast, smooth muscle cells and endothelial cells produce superoxide continuously albeit at a much lower rate than stimulated monocytes. In these cells, the superoxide production apparently involves the secretion of reduced thiol compounds such as cysteine by the cells, with subsequent formation of a superoxide-like product via interaction with metal ions in the medium [29]. In cultured endothelial cells, superoxide dismutase can only partially inhibit LDL modification, even when present in amounts sufficient to reduce superoxide concentration by over 99% [22]. Parthasarathy and colleagues recently found that endothelial cells can initiate LDL oxidation through a superoxide-independent pathway that involves lipoxygenase [28]. From their work it appears that the lipoxygenase pathway is an important mechanism for the initiation of LDL oxidation in a line of rabbit aortic endothelial cells whereas in arterial smooth muscle cells, the superoxide pathway predominates.

When LDL is exposed to oxidizing conditions, there is typically a lag phase lasting several hours before changes indicating LDL oxidation can be demonstrated [14]. This lag phase appears to be a reflection of the time required to deplete endogenous antioxidants contained within LDL [30]. It is possible that LDL from different individuals may exhibit different susceptibilities to oxidative change depending on the concentration of such endogenous antioxidants within the LDL. Time-course studies suggest that depletion of alpha-tocopherol precedes the depletion of carotene during copper-induced LDL oxidation, suggesting that vitamin E serves as the first line of defense in LDL oxidation (Figure 2).

II: MECHANISMS FOR THE UPTAKE OF OXIDIZED LDL IN MACROPHAGES.

The nature of the interaction of oxidized LDL with cultured cells is greatly influenced by the extent of oxidative modification. LDL that has undergone relatively modest degrees of oxidation (electrophoretic mobility less than 1.5-fold that of native LDL) exhibits a decrease in degradation by the classical LDL receptor evidently because the fragmentation of apolipoprotein B and/or the derivatization of 5-10% of lysine residues is sufficient to abolish interaction with this receptor [20]. However, recognition by the scavenger receptor(s) is typically not seen, and the rate of degradation of such mildly oxidized LDL by cultured macrophages is low. The threshold for recognition by scavenger receptors is reached when oxidation is of sufficient extent to increase the electrophoretic mobility of LDL to about 3-fold that of native LDL. The degradation of such extensively oxidized LDL can be inhibited about 60% by an excess of unlabelled acetyl LDL, and 75 or 80% by scavenger receptor ligands such as polyinosinic acid or fucoidin. This indicates that at least half of the degradation of oxidized LDL can be attributed to a scavenger receptor pathway.

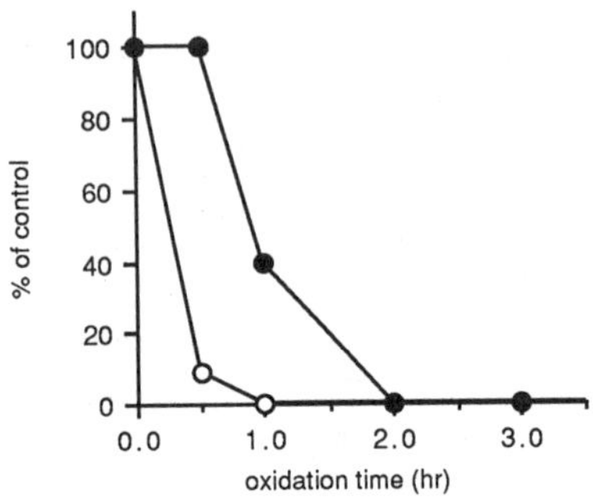

Figure 2. Time course of depletion of intrinsic antioxidants during LDL oxidation. Human LDL (200 ug/ml) was incubated with 5 uM Cu^{++} in Dulbecco's PBS at 37°C for the indicated time periods. Lipids were extracted with hexane following addition of an internal standard of α-tocopherol acetate. The content of α-tocopherol (○) was determined using a Waters 0.4 x 15 cm uBondapak C18 column eluted with methanol:acetonitrile:chloroform (25:60:15) and absorbance detection at 280 nm. β-carotene (●) was measured using the same column eluted with methanol:acetonitrile (25:60) with absorbance detection at 436 nm.

It is well known that chemical modifications of LDL lysine residues that lead to increased net negative charge of LDL allow binding to a scavenger receptor [9,10]. Furthermore, we have shown that oxidation of LDL is accompanied by a decrease in lysine groups, and that binding of lipid peroxidation products to apolipoprotein B occurs during LDL oxidation [21,22]. To determine if the derivatization of apolipoprotein B by lipid peroxidation products is sufficient to allow binding to the scavenger receptor, we performed an experiment in which derivatization of LDL with lipid oxidation products was achieved without other manifestations of oxidative change. This was done by isolating reactive peroxidation products from oxidized fatty acids by reverse-phase HPLC, and then adding these to LDL in the presence of EDTA and BHT such that no oxidation of the LDL itself occurred [31]. It was found that the reactive products were capable of increasing the electrophoretic mobility of the LDL, and also led to recognition by the scavenger receptor (Figure 3).

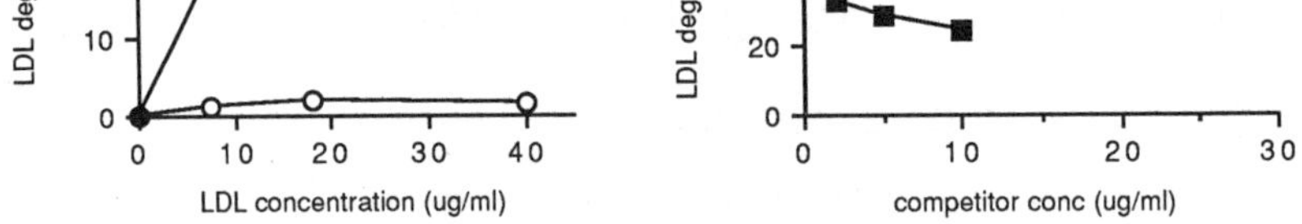

Figure 3. **A.** Degradation by macrophages of LDL modified by fatty acid oxidation products. Reactive products were partially purified from oxidized arachidonic acid by HPLC and mixed with ^{125}I-LDL as described in reference 31. The indicated concentration of native LDL (○) or modified LDL (●) was then incubated with cultured mouse peritoneal macrophages for 5 hr and the amount of LDL degraded was estimated as trichloroacetic acid-soluble noniodide radioactivity. Each point is the mean of triplicate determinations. **B.** Specificity of degradation of LDL modified with arachidonic acid oxidation products. Modified ^{125}I-LDL (10 ug/ml) was incubated with macrophages in the presence of the indicated concentrations of unlabelled native LDL (○), acetyl LDL (●), polyinosinic acid (■), or polycytidylic acid (□), and after 5 hr the medium was assayed for LDL degradation products. Each point is the mean of duplicate dishes.

Of note, the lipid peroxidation products could also modify other proteins (for example, bovine serum albumin) in a way that allowed scavenger receptor uptake. Hence, it appears that suitably derivatized lysine residues on various proteins can bind to this receptor, rather than a specific modified epitope of apolipoprotein B. Preliminary characterization of the reactive products derived from oxidized arachidonic acid revealed evidence for several unsaturated aldehydes, including acrolein, 2-pentenal, and 2-heptenal. However, even though these aldehydes were capable of increasing the electrophoretic mobility of LDL, no recognition of LDL by the scavenger receptor could be demonstrated following modification by these aldehydes [31]. In addition to such short chain aldehydes, the reactive fractions also contained less polar lipids including oxy-derivatives of fatty acids, but full chemical characterization of these substances has not yet been completed.

To ascertain if copper-oxidized LDL exhibited the same epitopes as those on LDL modified with arachidonic acid oxidation products, monoclonal antibodies were generated against LDL modified with arachidonic acid oxidation products. An attempt at immunization with modified mouse LDL failed to generate detectable serum titers against oxidation-product modified LDL. Therefore, mice were immunized with <u>human</u> LDL modified with arachidonic acid oxidation products, and hybridomas were screened against similarly modified bovine albumin to avoid clones directed against apolipoprotein B. Nine hybridoma supernatants were specific for oxidation-product modified proteins and reacted poorly or not at all with oxidized LDL or with LDL modified with various aldehydes. However, 8 hybridoma supernatants reacted strongly with oxidized LDL and most of these also reacted to a variable extent with aldehyde-modified LDLs including acrolein-LDL, crotonaldehyde-LDL, pentenal-LDL, and malondialdehyde-LDL. One of these hybridomas also bound strongly to acetyl LDL but none reacted with methylated LDL or with native LDL.

A candidate scavenger receptor has been purified independently by Via and colleagues and by Kodama and coworkers [32-34]. The purified receptor binds acetyl LDL as well as oxidized LDL and ligands such as polyinosinic acid. This receptor appears to be composed of three identical 77-kD subunits and has an Mr on polyacrylamide gels of about 220,000. The latter group has succeeded in isolating cDNA clones encoding two different forms of the bovine scavenger receptor and have recently reported the nucleotide sequences [35, 36]. One clone encodes a protein of 453 amino acids with a calculated Mr of 49,975; the discrepancy between the calculated Mr and that observed by polyacrylamide electrophoresis was ascribed to glycosylation. Both receptor clones have two extracellular fibrous domains: an α-helical coiled-coil domain and a collagen-like triple helix. The second clone encodes a truncated protein that retains ligand-binding activity despite deletion of a cysteine-rich carboxy-terminal domain. This suggests that one or both of the fibrous domains are responsible for ligand binding.

Other putative receptors with ligand specificity that partly overlaps that of the acetyl LDL receptor have also been reported [37-39]. Sparrow and colleagues recently showed that about 30% of oxidized LDL degradation could not be inhibited by excess unlabelled acetyl-LDL but was fully competed by excess unlabelled oxidized LDL [40]. This was interpreted as evidence for a second receptor with specificity for oxidized LDL but not acetyl LDL. These investigators also showed that a significant portion of the internalized oxidized LDL was not degraded but appeared to accumulate within the cell, in contrast to results with acetyl LDL which was almost completely degraded. Arai and colleagues also found only partial competition between acetyl LDL and oxidized LDL for binding and degradation in cultured macrophages [41]. They concluded that at least three distinct classes of scavenger receptor were involved, one which could interact with both oxidized and acetyl LDL, and additional receptors specific for each modified LDL. We have also found that acetyl LDL does not fully compete for oxidized LDL degradation in macrophages, but the polyanion ligand polyinosinic acid showed essentially complete competition [20]. This could indicate involvement of the receptor for aldehyde-modified proteins described by Horiuchi et al. [38], in that oxidized LDL might be expected to have aldehyde-modified domains and polyinosinic acid interacts with this receptor.

Yokode and colleagues reported that cigarette smoke extract was capable of modifying LDL in a way that led to accelerated uptake in cultured macrophages [42]. The modification was partly inhibited by superoxide dismutase but not by EDTA, and the authors concluded that modification by cigarette smoke extract involved a direct interaction of superoxide with apolipoprotein B. Although some oxidative change was noted after incubation with cigarette smoke extract, this appeared to be insufficient in itself to account for the accelerated uptake. Cigarette smoke is known to contain a number of reactive aldehydes including acrolein, formaldehyde, acetaldehyde, propionaldehyde and butyraldehyde, and it may be that the derivatization of apolipoprotein B by such aldehydes accounts at least in part for the changes induced by cigarette smoke.

III: PHOSPHOLIPID HYDROLYSIS DURING LDL OXIDATION

One of the striking changes that accompanies LDL oxidation is the hydrolysis of phosphatidylcholine; for example, in extensively oxidized LDL up to 50% of phosphatidylcholine is hydrolyzed to lysophosphatidylcholine [19]. This hydrolysis was recently shown to be the result of the action of an unusual phospholipase A_2 called platelet activating factor acetylhydrolase that exists in plasma largely in association with LDL [43]. This phospholipase A_2 is calcium-independent, and shows specificity for short-chain acyl residues at the *sn*-2 position of phosphatidylcholine [44-46]. Although it was previously thought to be specific for platelet activating factor (1-O-alkyl-2-acetyl phosphatidylcholine), recent studies showed it was also capable of acting on other phosphatidylcholine derivatives with short chain, polar substituents at the *sn*-2 position [43,46]. Because the *sn*-2 fatty acid in phosphatidylcholine is usually polyunsaturated, it would be susceptible to oxidative fragmentation. Any fragmentation products that leave a chain length of 6 carbons or less esterified to the glycerophosphocholine backbone could act as substrates for this enzyme. The potential importance of the fatty acid oxidation products liberated in this enzyme reaction has been discussed above, but the lysophosphatidylcholine that is formed probably also has important biological consequences. For example, Quinn and colleagues have recently shown that lysophosphatidylcholine is a potent and specific chemoattractant for human monocytes [47]. Hence, it could play a role in the recruitment of macrophages to sites where LDL oxidation was occuring. Lysophosphatidylcholine as well as oxidized fatty acids have been reported to act as calcium ionophores, and thus could initiate several important calcium-dependent cellular processes including cytotoxicity [48,49]. Furthermore, lysophosphatidylcholine has recently been shown to be the factor that accounts for the impairment of endothelium-dependent vasodilation caused by oxidized LDL. [50].

IV: OTHER ACTIONS OF OXIDIZED LDL

One of the earliest biologic actions of oxidized LDL to be identified was its cytotoxicity to cultured fibroblasts and endothelial cells [16-18, 51,52]. Most of the cytotoxicity is attributable to lipid components of modified LDL. Many of the fatty acid oxidation products that are found in oxidized LDL have potentially cytotoxic effects, including 2-alkenals, 4-hydroxy-2-alkenals, lipid hydroperoxides, and hydroxy fatty acids [53]. These aldehydes can covalently bind to cellular proteins as well as DNA, resulting in toxicity and mutagenic effects. As well, oxidized fatty acids have been shown to be ionophores for divalent cations, and hence could interfere with cellular function by altering calcium permeability.

Although oxidized LDL stimulates cholesterol esterification and cholesterol accumulation in cultured macrophages, it is less potent in this regard than equivalent concentrations of acetyl LDL (Figure 4a). The cholesterol:protein ratio of oxidized LDL is greatly reduced due to the oxidation of cholesterol esters and free cholesterol [21, 54]. We found that the most abundant oxysterol present in extensively oxidized LDL is 7-ketocholesterol but smaller amounts of 7-hydroxycholesterol and 5,6-epoxycholesterol are also present [54]. Although it might have been expected that these oxysterols would tend to stimulate acyl CoA-cholesterol acyltransferase and enhance cholesteol ester formation, this was not the case. In fact, the less effective stimulation of cholesterol esterification by oxidized LDL compared to acetyl LDL could be satisfactorily accounted for by the reduced content of cholesterol per LDL particle and by the fact that more than half of the internalized LDL was not degraded (Figure 4b). The simplest explanation for these findings is that the cholesterol contained within the nondegraded internalized LDL failed to enter the acyl CoA:cholesterol acyltransferase substrate pool, and that the different oxysterols in oxidized LDL had opposing effects on cholesterol esterification [54, 55].

Oxidized LDL can have potentially significant effects on the functions of other cell types involved in the development of atherosclerosis. Incubation of human saphenous vein endothelial cells with oxidized LDL in vitro leads to a concentration-dependent, stimulation of prostacyclin release [56]. In this system, the effects of oxidized LDL were predominantly on prostacyclin production, whereas stimulation of these same cells with ionophore A23187 resulted predominantly in $PGF_{2\alpha}$ production. Yokode et al. found that incubation of oxidized LDL with mouse peritoneal macrophages led to a marked increase in secretion of LTC_4 and PGE_2 [57]. In contrast, LDL containing relatively high levels of lipid peroxide inhibited prostacylin biosynthesis in rat aorta slices and in perfused bovine coronary arteries [58]. It has recently been shown that the effect of oxidized LDL on prostaglandin secretion by cultured smooth muscle cells is determined by the extent of oxidation of LDL [59]. LDL containing relatively low levels of lipid peroxides was found to stimulate prostaglandin synthesis while more extensively oxidized LDL inhibited prostaglandin synthesis. This inhibitory effect of oxidized LDL could not be attributed to a nonspecific toxic effect, but mimicked the inhibition of cyclooxygenase seen with some fatty acid hydroperoxides.

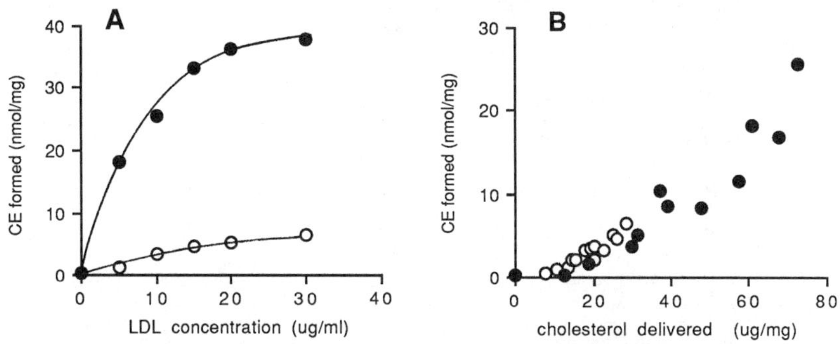

Figure 4. Comparison of the effects of oxidized LDL and acetyl LDL on cholesterol esterification in cultured macrophages. **A.** Varying concentrations of oxidized LDL (○) and acetyl LDL (●) were incubated for 10 hr with macrophages together with 50uM [^{3}H]oleic acid, and then radioactivity in cholesterol ester was determined. **B.** Varying concentrations of ^{125}I-oxidized LDL (○) with cholesterol:protein ratio 0.75±0.11, and ^{125}I-acetyl LDL (●) with cholesterol:protein ratio 1.56± 0.06 were incubated with macrophages for 10 hr together with 50uM [^{3}H]oleic acid. Medium was then assayed for ^{125}I-LDL degradation products and content of radioiodine and cholesteryl [^{3}H]oleate in cells was measured. More than 95% of the cell-associated radioactivity with oxidized LDL was precipitable with 10% trichloroacetic acid. Cholesterol delivery to the cells was calculated as the product of LDL degradation and the cholesterol:protein ratio.

Oxidized LDL can also modulate the production of growth factors and mediators of inflammation by cultured cells. Fox and coworkers found that oxidized LDL or a lipid extract from oxidized LDL inhibited the production of a platelet-derived growth factor-like protein by cultured endothelial cells [60]. As well, Hamilton and colleagues reported that the expression of tumor necrosis factor mRNA was decreased by oxidized LDL [61]. Recent studies by Rajavashisth and coworkers showed that LDL that had been minimally oxidized (to an extent much less than that required to produce altered uptake in macrophages) stimulated the production of several growth factors by cultured endothelial cells, including GM-CSF, M-CSF, and G-CSF [62]. In related studies, these investigators found that minimally modified LDL stimulated production of a specific monocyte chemotactic factor by cultured human endothelial cells and smooth muscle cells, and also caused increased adhesiveness of endothelial cells toward monocytes [63]. Similarly, Frostegard and colleagues found that exposure of human peripheral blood monocytes and U937 cells to extensively oxidized LDL increased their adhesiveness as reflected in self-aggregation or adherence to cultured human umbilical vein endothelial cells [64]. This increased adherence was accompanied by enhanced expression of HLA class II and Leu M3 antigens but decreased expression of CD4 antigen, a pattern suggesting differentiation to a more macrophage-like phenotype.

V: EVIDENCE FOR OXIDIZED LDL IN VIVO

The abundant antioxidant defenses present in blood or whole plasma are generally sufficient to prevent significant oxidation of LDL, and although low levels of thiobarbituric acid-reactive substances have been found in plasma [65], a study using a sensitive chemiluminescence assay found no detectable lipid peroxide in normal human plasma [66]. On the other hand, Morel and coworkers found that VLDL/LDL from streptozotocin-diabetic rats showed evidence of oxidative modification and was cytotoxic to cultured fibroblasts [67]. The cytotoxicity was prevented by treating the animals with vitamin E, probucol, or insulin. Evidence for the presence of oxidatively modified LDL in atherosclerotic lesions has been reported in several studies based on immunologic or immunohistochemical techniques [68-71]. More direct evidence of oxidative modification of LDL in atherosclerotic plaques was obtained by Yla-Herttuala and associates who demonstrated that LDL extracted from aortic lesions of human subjects or Watanabe heritable hyperlipidemic rabbits showed physical and chemical changes indicative of advanced oxidation, and was internalized in macrophages via a scavenger receptor-dependent process [72].

We have performed similar studies on LDL isolated from lesion-free areas of human aortic intima. Our own studies revealed minimal or no evidence of oxidative change in LDL isolated from normal aortic intima obtained at the time of organ harvest from transplantation donors. LDL isolated from plaque-free areas of elderly subjects showed intermediate changes that would be compatible with oxidative change but much less marked than the lesions found by Yla-Herttuala and colleagues. We observed a correlation between the degree of fragmentation of apolipoprotein B and the accumulation of cholesterol esterification when LDL was incubated with cultured macrophages. However, the uptake of aortic LDL in our studies was nonsaturable and was not inhibited by polyinosinic acid, indicating that scavenger receptors were not involved.

Although the weight of the available evidence indicates that LDL oxidation is likely to play a role in atherogenesis, proof of a causal relationship has not yet been obtained. Perhaps the strongest evidence for a causal role is the observation that probucol, a potent antioxidant drug, can retard atheroma progression in Watanabe rabbits [73]. A similar experiment has also been performed in restricted ovulator chickens, which develop marked hyperlipidemia and atherosclerosis on standard poultry feed. Treatment of the mutant chickens with vitamin E had no effect on lipid levels but prevented atherosclerosis in that the aortic intimal thickness of vitamin E supplemented restricted ovulators was the same as that found in normal laying hens [74]. If the protective effect of these agents is confirmed in other animal models and is shown to result specifically from the inhibition of LDL oxidation, then it would be reasonable to consider intervention trials in human subjects.

REFERENCES

1. Fowler, S.; Shio, H.; Haley, W.J. Lab. Invest. 4: 372-378 (1979).
2. Schaffner; T.; Taylor, K.; Bartucci, E.J.; Fischer-Dzoga, K.; Beenson, J.H.; Glagov,S.; Wissler, R. Am. J. Pathol. 100: 57-80 (1980).
3. Gerrity, R.G. Am. J. Pathol. 103: 181-190 (1981).
4. Gerrity, R.G. Am. J. Pathol. 103: 191-200 (1981).
5. Faggiotto, A.; Ross, R.; Harker, L. Arteriosclerosis 4: 323-340 (1984).
6. Aqel, N.M.; Ball, R.Y.; Waldman, H.; Mitchinson, M.J. Atherosclerosis 53:265-271 (1984).
7. Rosenfeld, M.E.; Tsukuda, T.; Gown, A.M.; Ross, R. Arteriosclerosis 7: 9-23 (1987).
8. Goldstein, J.L.; Ho, Y.K.; Basu, S.K.; Brown, M.S. Proc. Natl. Acad. Sci. USA 76: 333-337 (1979).
9. Brown, M.S.; Basu, S.K.; Falck, J.R.; Ho, Y.K.; Goldstein, J.L. J. Supramol. Struct. 13: 67-81 (1980).
10. Brown, M.S.; Goldstein, J.L. Ann. Rev. Biochem. 52: 223-261 (1983).
11. Fogelman, A.M.; Schecter, I.S.; Seager, J.; Hokom, J.M.; Child, S.; Edwards, P.A.. Proc. Natl. Acad. Sci. USA 77: 2214-2218 (1980).
12. Haberland, M.E.; Fogelman, A.M.; Edwards, P.A. Proc. Natl. Acad. Sci. USA 79: 1712-1716 (1982).
13. Henriksen, T.; Mahoney, E.M.; Steinberg, D. Proc. Natl. Acad. Sci. USA 78: 6499-6503 (1981).
14. Henriksen, T.; Mahoney, E.M.; Steinberg, D. Arteriosclerosis 3: 149-159 (1983).
15. Heinecke, J.W.; Baker, L.; Rosen, L.; Chait, A. J. Clin. Invest. 77: 757-761 (1986).

16. Morel, D.W.; Hessler, J.R.; Chisolm, G.M. J. Lipid Res. 24: 1070-1076 (1983).
17. Hessler, J.R.; Morel, D.W.; Lewis, L.J.; Chisolm, G.M. Arteriosclerosis 3: 215-222 (1983).
18. Morel, D.W.; DiCorleto, P.E.; Chisolm, G.M. Arteriosclerosis 4: 357-364 (1984).
19. Steinbrecher, U.P.; Parthasarathy, S.; Leake, D.S.; Witztum, J.L.; Steinberg, D. Proc. Natl. Acad. Sci. USA 81: 3883-3887 (1984).
20. Steinbrecher, U.P.; Witztum, J.L.; Parthasarathy, S.; Steinberg, D. Arteriosclerosis 7: 135-143 (1987).
21. Steinbrecher, U.P. J. Biol. Chem. 262: 3603-3608 (1987).
22. Steinbrecher, U.P. Biochim. Biophys. Acta 959: 20-30 (1988).
23. Hiramatsu, K.; Rosen, H.; Heinecke, J.W.; Wolfbauer, G.; Chait, A. Arteriosclerosis 7: 55-60 (1987).
24. Parthasarathy, S.; Printz D.J.; Boyd, D.; Joy, L.; Steinberg, D. Arteriosclerosis 6: 505-510.
25. Cathcart, M.K.; Chisolm, G.M.; McNally, A.K.; Morel, D.W. In Vitro Cell. Dev. Biol. 24: 1001-1008 (1988).
26. Cathcart, M.K.; McNally, A.K.; Morel, D.W.; Chisolm III, G.M. J. Immunol. 142: 1963-1969 (1989).
27. Bedwell, S.; Dean, R.T.; Jessup,W. Biochem. J. 262: 707-712 (1989).
28. Parthasarathy, S.; Wieland, E.; Steinberg, D. Proc. Natl. Acad. Sci. USA 86: 1046-1050 (1989).
29. Heinecke, J.W.; Rosen, H.; Suzuki, L.; Chait, A. J. Biol. Chem. 262: 10098-10103 (1987).
30. Esterbauer, H.; Jurgens, G.; Quehenberger, O.; Koller, E. J. Lipid Res. 28: 495-509 (1987).
31. Steinbrecher, U.P.; Lougheed, M.; Kwan, W-C.; Dirks, M. J. Biol. Chem. 264: 15216-15223 (1989).
32. Via, D.P.; Dresel, H.A.; Cheng, S-L.; Gotto Jr., A.M. J. Biol. Chem. 260: 7379-7386 (1985).
33. Dresel, H.A.; Friedrich, E.; Via, D.P.; Sinn, H.; Ziegler, R.; Schettler, G. EMBO J. 6: 319-326 (1987).
34. Kodama, T.; Reddy, P.; Kishimoto, C.; Krieger, M. Proc. Natl. Acad. Sci. USA 85: 9238-9242 (1988).
35. Kodama, T.; Freeman, M.; Rohrer, L.; Zabrecky, J.; Matsudaira, P.; Kreiger, M. Nature 343: 532-535 (1990).
36. Rohrer, L.; Freeman, M.; Kodama, T.; Penman, M.; Krieger, M. Nature 343: 570-572 (1990).
37. Haberland, M.E.; Rasmussen, R.R.; Olch, C.L.; Fogelman, A.M. J. Clin. Invest. 77: 681-689 (1986).
38. Horiuchi, S.; Murakami, M.; Takata, K.; Morino, Y. J. Biol. Chem. 261: 4962-4966 (1986).
39. Takata, K.; Horiuchi, S.; Morino, Y. Biochim. Biophys Acta 984: 273-280 (1989).
40. Sparrow, C.P.; Parthasarathy, S.; Steinberg, D. J. Biol. Chem. 264: 2599-2604 (1989).
41. Arai, H.; Kita, T.; Yokode, M.; Narumiya, S.; Kawai, C. Biochem. Biophys. Res. Commun. 159: 1375-1382 (1989).
42. Yokode, M.; Kita, T.; Arai, H.; Kawai, C.; Narumiya, S.; Fujiwara, M. Proc. Natl. Acad. Sci. USA 85: 2344--2348 (1988).
43. Steinbrecher, U.P.; Pritchard, P.H. J. Lipid Res. 30: 305-315 (1989).
44. Wardlow, M.L.; Cox, C P.; Meng, K.E.; Greene, D.E.; Farr, R.S. J. Immunol. 136: 3441-3446 (1986).
45. Stafforini, D.M.; Prescott, S.M.; McIntyre, T.M. J. Biol. Chem. 262: 4223-4230 (1987).
46. Stremler, K.E.; Stafforini, D.M.; Prescott, S.M.; Zimmerman, S.M.; McIntyre, T.M. J. Biol. Chem. 264: 5331-5334 (1989).
47. Quinn, M.T.; Parthasarathy, S.; Steinberg, D. Proc. Natl. Acad. Sci. USA 85: 2805-2809 (1988).
48. Ungemach, F.P. Chem. Phys. Lipids 45: 171-205 (1987).
49. Serhan, C.; Anderson, P.; Goodman, E.; Dumhan, P.; Weissmann, G. J. Biol. Chem. 256: 2736-2741 (1981).
50. Kugiyama, K., Kerns S.A., Morrisett J.D., Roberts R., Henry P.D. Nature 344: 160-162 (1990).

51. Henriksen, T.; Evensen, S.A.; Carlander, B. Scand. J. Clin. Lab. Invest. 39: 361-368 (1979).
52. Hessler, J.R.; Robertson Jr., A.L.; Chisolm, G.M. Atherosclerosis 32: 213-229 (1979).
53. Jurgens, G., H.F. Hoff, G.M. Chisolm, and H. Esterbauer. Chem. Phys. Lipids 45: 315-336 (1987).
54. Zhang, H.; Basra, H.J.K.; Steinbrecher, U.P. J. Lipid Res. in press (1990).
55. Morin, R.J.; Peng, S.K. Ann. Clin. Lab. Sci. 19: 225-237 (1989).
56. Triau, J.E.; Meydani, S.M.; Schaefer, E.J. Arteriosclerosis 8: 810-818 (1988).
57. Yokode, M.; Kita, T.; Kikawa, Y.; Ogorochi, T.; Naruyima, S.; Kawai, C. J. Clin. Invest. 81: 720-729 (1988).
58. Szczeklik, A.; Gryglewski, R.J. Artery 7: 488-495 (1980).
59. Zhang, H.; Davis, W.B; Chen, X.; Jones, K.H.; Whisler, R.L.; Cornwell, D.G. J. Lipid Res. 31: 551-565 (1990).
60. Fox, P.L.; Chisolm, G.M.; DiCorleto, P.E. J. Biol. Chem. 262: 6046-6054 (1987).
61. Hamilton, T.A.; Ma, G.; Chisolm, G.M. J. Immunol. 144: 2343-2350 (1990).
62. Rajavashisth, T.B.; Andalibi, A.; Territo, M.C.; Berliner, J.A.; Navab, M.; Fogelman, A.M.; Lusis, A.J. Nature 344: 254-257 (1990).
63. Berliner, J.A.; Territo, M.C.; Sevanian, A.; Ramin, S.; Kim, J.A.; Bamshad, B.; Esterson, M.; Fogelman, A.M. J. Clin. Invest. 85: 1260-1266 (1990).
64. Frostegard, J.; Nilsson, J.; Hagerstrand, A.; Hamsten, A.; Wigzell, H.; Gidlund, M. Proc. Natl. Acad. Sci. USA 87: 904-908 (1990).
65. Yagi, K. Chem. Phys. Lipids 45: 337-351 (1987).
66. Frei, B.; Yamamoto, Y.; Niclas, D.; Ames, B.N. Anal. Biochem. 175: 120-130 (1988).
67. Morel, D.W.; Chisolm, G.M. J. Lipid Res. 30: 1827-1834 (1989).
68. Haberland, M.; Fong, D.; Cheng, L. Science 241: 215-218 (1988).
69. Palinski, W.; Rosenfeld, M.E.; Yla-Herttuala, S.; Gurtner, G.C.; Socher, S.S.; Butler, S.W.; Parthasarathy, S.; Carew, T.E.; Steinberg, D.; Witztum, J.L. Proc. Natl. Acad. Sci. USA 86: 1372-1376 (1989).
70. Boyd, H.C.; Gown, A.M.; Wolfbauer, G.; Chait, A. Am. J. Pathol. 135: 815-825 (1989).
71. Mowri, H.; Ohkuma, S.; Takano, T. Biophys. Biochim. Acta 963: 208-214 (1988).
72. Yla-Herttuala, S.; Palinski, W.; Rosenfeld, M.E.; Parthasarathy, S.; Carew, T.E.; Butler, S.; Witztum, J.L.; Steinberg, D. J. Clin. Invest. 84: 1086-1095 (1989).
73. Carew, T.E.; Schwenke, D.C.; Steinberg, D. Proc. Natl. Acad. Sci. USA 84:7725-7729 (1987).
74. Smith, T.L., Kummerow, F.A. Atherosclerosis 75: 105-109 (1989).

The Role of Apolipoprotein(a) in Atherosclerosis

Richard M. Lawn

Department of Cardiovascular Research, Genentech, Inc., South San Francisco, California

Abstract. Lp(a) is a lipoprotein particle whose high levels have been determined to be a major inherited risk factor for atherosclerosis. The particle closely resembles low density lipoprotein, with the addition of a single large protein called apo(a). Cloning and sequencing of apo(a) cDNA showed that this protein is closely related to plasminogen, a protein whose functions include the lysis of blood clots. Current research is focusing on the possible functional similarities of apo(a) and plasminogen that could provide a link between the process of thrombosis and atherogenesis.

Atherosclerosis is the leading cause of death in the United States, and the mechanisms of this disease are complex and poorly understood. Since elevated levels of low density lipoprotein (LDL) cholesterol are an established risk factor for this disease, and the proximal event in myocardial infarction is an occlusive blood clot in a coronary artery, mechanistic links between lipoproteins and the blood clotting system have been eagerly sought. It is apparent that cholesterol-laden arterial plaques can become the focus of a thrombotic event, and that the components of LDL particles can be identified in these plaques. However, the details of this process are unclear, and myocardial infarctions can occur in the setting of low plasma cholesterol. In the past few years, details of the structure of another lipoprotein species have focused attention on one possible link between lipoproteins and the clotting cascade.

Lipoprotein(a), or Lp(a), is a lipoprotein first described by K. Berg in 1963 as an antigen detectable in about 30% of a Northern European population (3). Early studies indicated an association between the presence of the particle and increased incidence of heart disease (4-6). With the advent of sensitive quantitative assays of Lp(a), it is now believed that the plasma of virtually all individuals contains this lipoprotein, in concentrations that range from less than 1 to more than 100 mg/dl (1, 12). Numerous studies have confirmed the strong association between high levels of Lp(a) and atherosclerosis (2, 8, 13, 15, 16). People in the top quartile of Lp(a) concentration, 20-30 mg/dl, have a several-fold relative risk of the disease, which is exacerbated by elevated levels of LDL. Although atherogenicity of the particle has yet to be directly demonstrated, and prospective studies have not been completed, the evidence is persuasive that plasma levels of Lp(a) that are less than one-tenth that of LDL represent a risk factor for cardiovascular disease.

The Lp(a) particle closely resembles LDL in lipid composition and in the presence of apolipoprotein B-100 (apoB-100), the ligand by which LDL binds to the LDL receptor (7). The distinguishing feature of Lp(a) is the presence of apolipoprotein(a), (apo(a)), bound to apoB-

© 1990 by Elsevier Science Publishing Co., Inc.
Molecular Biology of Atherosclerosis
A.D. Attie, Editor

100 by disulfide linkage (10, 11, 17). Apo(a) is a highly glycosylated protein whose molecular weight varies from 300,000-800,000 among individuals. As apo(a) is the distinguishing feature of this possibly atherogenic particle, we began a detailed study of its structure, evolution and tissue distribution.

Partial amino acid sequence analysis of apo(a) purified from a single human donor (9) revealed an unexpected homology to the sequence of plasminogen . Plasminogen is a 92,000 Dalton serine protease zymogen of the fibrinolytic system that consists of five homologous and tandemly repeated domains known as kringles, followed by a trypsin-like protease domain. Plasminogen is converted to an active enzyme by cleavage at a specific arginine residue by urokinase and tissue plasminogen activator. Although the partial amino acid sequence obtained for highly purified apo(a) was very similar to plasminogen, the amino terminus of apo(a) did not correspond to the amino terminus of plasminogen, but to the beginning of its fourth kringle domain (9).

We employed synthetic oligonucleotide probes to clone and characterize apo(a) cDNA derived from human liver RNA (14). This procedure revealed the remarkable sequence of apo(a). The 5' untranslated sequence and prepeptide coding region are virtually identical to plasminogen. Following deletion of the amino terminal domains of plasminogen, the apo(a) message contains 37 copies of a 342 base sequence that closely resembles kringle 4 of plasminogen. This is followed by sequences similar to kringle 5, the protease domain, and the 3' untranslated regions of the plasminogen message. The degree of intragenic repetition is striking. Twenty-four of the kringle encoding sequences are identical, and the remaining differ by from 3 to 71 nucleotides (14). This degree of homology is suggestive of recent duplications and deletions caused by out-of-register homologous recombinations. This could lead to a distribution in the population of apo(a) genes containing different numbers of kringle domains, and account for the observed range in size of the protein in individuals. This hypothesis is supported by recent reports of correlation between the size of apo(a) mRNA and protein in individual baboons (18) and humans (19). It is estimated that individual apo(a) genes in the human population contain anywhere from about 15-40 copies of the repeated kringle domain. The effects of individual variants of apo(a) will be the subject of future investigations.

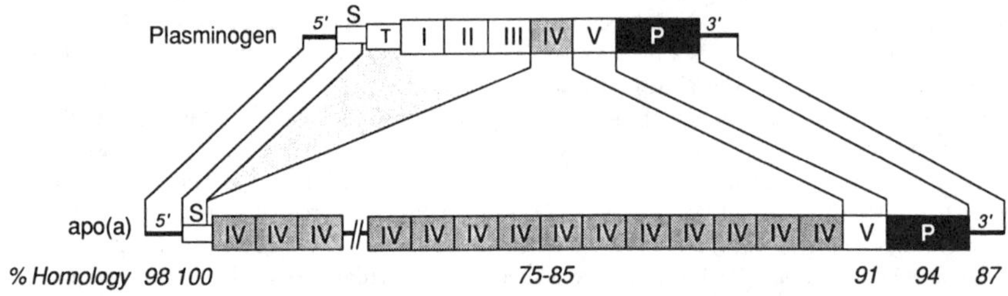

Figure 1. Sequence comparison of plasminogen and apolipoprotein(a). The domains of plasminogen and apo(a) cDNA are compared with S indicating the signal sequence, T the tail or preactivation peptide, I-V the kringles and P the protease domains. Connecting lines indicate regions of homology with shading to represent the domains lacking in apo(a). The percentage of DNA sequence identity for each domain is indicated at the bottom. (Reprinted with permission from Nature, ref. 14.)

It was hoped that the unexpected sequence similarity to plasminogen would yield some clues to the function and possible atherogenicity of apo(a). An obvious candidate is proteolytic activity, since the protease domain of human apo(a) contains 88% amino acid identity to the corresponding domain of plasminogen, and since all three residues of the catalytic triad are present (14). However, the arginine residue of the plasminogen activation site is substituted by serine in apo(a) (9, 14). Neither tissue plasminogen activator, urokinase, or streptokinase were able to promote plasmin-like activity from apo(a), nor did Lp(a) react with diisopropyl fluorophosphate, a compound which covalently binds to the catalytic site of active serine proteases (14). The possibility still exists that Lp(a) has proteolytic activity that does not resemble plasminogen in its substrate specificity (24). The homology of the kringle structures has also promoted the search for binding properties that are similar to plasminogen. Some of the kringles of plasminogen and other kringle-containing proteins bind to macromolecules during the process of clot formation and lysis. If apo(a) shared the fibrin binding capability of plasminogen by virtue of its many kringle domains, the positioning of cholesterol-rich Lp(a) particles at the sites of vessel damage could contribute to the development of atherosclerosis. The ability of Lp(a) to bind to immobilized fibrin has been shown by two groups (20, 25), whereas others have failed to detect fibrin binding utilizing different procedures (23, 26). Harpel et al. reported that partial degradation of the immobilized fibrinogen enhanced the Lp(a) binding (20). In addition, Lp(a) has been shown to bind to fibronectin (24). Since fibronectin can be present in connective tissue and blood clots, this could lead to the deposition of Lp(a) in sites of vessel damage.

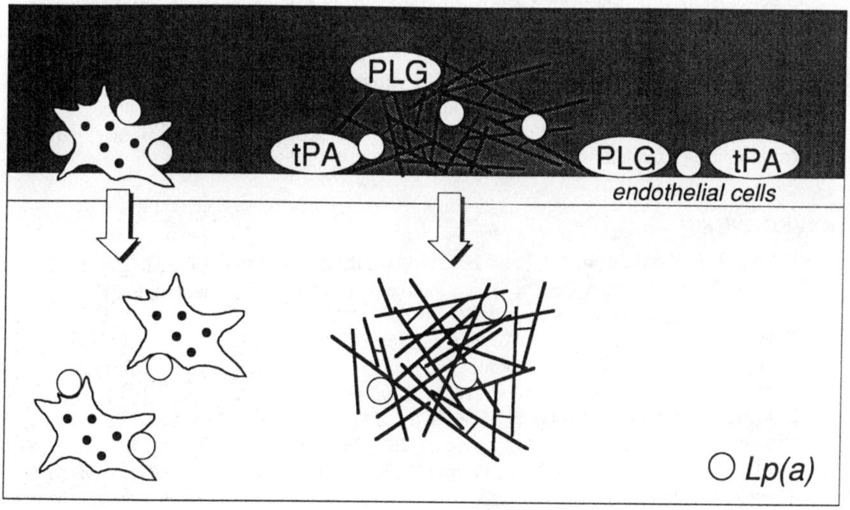

Figure 2. Possible atherogenic properties of Lp(a). Several models are indicated by which Lp(a) could stimulate the growth of an atherosclerotic plaque and become incorporated within the enlarging vessel intima. Binding of Lp(a) to macrophages (left) could lead to the development of lipid-laden foam cells and the stimulation of growth factor activities. Lp(a) can compete with the binding of plasminogen to sites on the endothelial cell surface and impede local plasminogen activation, prolonging the lysis of clots at the cell surface. This might lead to the development of an occlusive thrombis, or the incorporation of the residual thrombis within the growing plaque. Lp(a) may also bind directly to clots via interaction with fibrinectin or partially degraded fibrin.

The homology of apo(a) to plasminogen also suggests that Lp(a) might inhibit the normal process of clot lysis by interfering with plasminogen activators directly or by competing with binding sites on the surface of cells where the components of the fibrinolytic pathway might assemble. Despite the attractive nature of these hypotheses, no consensus has been reached about the function of apo(a) in these settings. Research groups differ in their assessment of the ability of Lp(a) to inhibit the activity of plasminogen activators in solution (21-23, 25). In addition to any effect in solution, the observation that Lp(a) competes with plasminogen for binding to endothelial cells suggests that elevated Lp(a) might interfere with clot lysis at the cellular level. Hence, the nearly 25% of the population with Lp(a) levels in the increased risk range do not appear to have gross clotting abnormalities, but may possess increased residual thrombi at the surface of blood vessels which could lead to the gradual development of atherosclerotic lesions.

Not all of the properties of apo(a) need reflect its sequence similarities with plasminogen. By imunohistochemistry, Lp(a) has been located in atherosclorotic plaques in regions which also contain macrophage derived, lipid laden foam cells (27, 28). We have recently shown that Lp(a) and recombinant apo(a) bind to macrophages via a specific, high affinity receptor (29). This could represent a significant route of entry into the vessel media and contribute to the onset of disease by means that have been proposed for modified LDL (see ref. 30 for review). None of these proposed functions of Lp(a) need be exclusive of others. Perhaps the safest conclusion that can be drawn at this time is that the biochemical properties of Lp(a) may be more subtle and difficult to pinpoint than its ultimate effect of exacerbating the process of atherogenesis.

In conclusion, it is now well established that elevated plasma levels of Lp(a) represent a significant, inherited risk factor for heart disease. Furthermore, these levels are largely determined by inheritance of a single genetic locus, and they are relatively resistant to dietary manipulation or to most cholesterol lowering drugs. We know the composition of this lipoprotein particle, and its site of synthesis in the liver. The current and future challenges are to understand the "normal" function of Lp(a) and its role in precipitating heart disease, with the hope of inhibiting its deleterious effects.

REFERENCES

1. Albers, J. J., Adolphson, J. L., and Hazzard, W. R. *J. Lipid Res.* **18**, 331-338 (1977).
2. Armstrong, V., Cremer, P., Eberle, E., Manke, A., Schulze, F., Wieland, H., Kreuzer, H., and Seidel, D. *Atherosclerosis* **62**, 249-257 (1986).
3. Berg, K. *Acta Path. Microbiol. Scand.* **59**, 369-382 (1963).
4. Berg, K., Borresen, A. L., and Dahlen, G. *Lancet* **i**, 499 (1976).
5. Berg, K., Dahlen, G., and Borresen, A. L. *Clin. Genetics* **16**, 347-352 (1979).
6. Berg, K., Dahlen, G., and Krick, M. H. *Clin. Genetics* **6**, 230-235 (1974).
7. Brown, M. S. and Goldstein, J. L. *Science* **232**, 34-37 (1986).
8. Dahlen, G., Guyton, J., Attar, M., Farmer, J., Kautz, J., and Gotto, A. *Circulation* 74, 758-765 (1986).
9. Eaton, D., Fless, G., Kohr, W., McLean, J., Xu, Q., Miller, C., Lawn, R., and Scanu, A. *Proc. Natl. Acad. Sci. USA* **84**, 3224-3228 (1987).
10. Fless,G. M., Rolih, C. A., and Scanu, A. M. *J. Biol. Chem.* **259**, 11470-11478 (1984).
11. Gaubatz, J. W., Heideman, C., Gotto, A. M., Morrisett, J.D., and Dahlen, G. H. *J. Biol. Chem.* **254**, 4582-4589 (1983).
12. Groener, J. E. M. and Kostner, G. M. *J. Lipid Res.* **28**, 1053-1056 (1987).
13. Költringer, P. and Jürgens, G. *Atherosclerosis* **58**, 187-198 (1985).
14. McLean, J., Tomlinson, J., Kuang, W.-J., Eaton, D., Chen, E., Fless, G., Scanu, A., and Lawn, R. *Nature* **330**, 132-137 (1987).
15. Rhoads, G, Dahlen, G., Berg, K., Morton, N., and Dannenberg, A. *J. Am. Med. Assoc.* **256**, 2540-2544 (1986).
16. Schriewer, H., Assmann, G., and Sandkamp, M. *J. Clin. Chem. Clin. Biochem.* **22**, 591-596 (1984).
17. Utermann, G. and Weber, W. *FEBS Lett.* **154**, 257-261 (1983).

18. Hixson, J. E., Britten, M. L., Manis, G. S. and Rainwater, D. L. *J. Biol. Chem.* **264**, 6013-6016 (1989).
19. Koschinsky, M. L., Beisiegel, U., Henne-Bruns, D., Eaton, D. L., and Lawn, R.M. *Biochemistry* **29**, 640-644 (1990)
20. Harpel, P. C., Gordon, B. R., and Parker, T. S. *Proc. Natl. Acad. Sci. USA* **86**, 3847-3851 (1989).
21. Edelberg, J. J., Gonzalez-Gronow, M., and Pizzo, S. V. *Biochemistry* **28**, 2370-2374 (1989).
22. Hajjar, K. A., Gavish, D., Breslow, J. L., and Nachman, R. L. *Nature* **339**, 303-305 (1989).
23. Lawn, R. M., Tomlinson, J. E., McLean, J. W., and Eaton, D. L. in: Lipoprotein(a), A. Scanu, ed. (Academic Press, San Diego, 1990) In press.
24. Salonen, E. M., Jauhiainen, M., Zardi, L. Vaheri, A., and Enholm, C. *EMBO J.* **8**, 4035-4040 (1989).
25. Loscalzo, J., Weinfeld, M., Fless, G.M. and Scanu, A.M., *Arteriosclerosis* **10**, 240-245 (1990).
26. Kluft, C., Jie, A.F.H., Los, P., de Wit, E., and Havekes, L. *Biochem. Biophys. Res. Comm.* **161**, 427-433 (1989).
27. Rath, M. et al. *Arteriosclerosis* **9**, 579-592 (1989).
28. Cushing, G. L. et al. *Arteriosclerosis* **9**, 593-603 (1989) .
29. Zioncheck, T. F., Lawn, R. M., Rice, G. C., Eaton, D.L., and Powell, L. M. Submitted (1990).
30. Steinberg, D. et al. *New Engl. J. Med.* **320**, 915-924 (1989).

Neutral Lipid Accumulation Accompanies ras-Oncogene Induced Growth Arrest in a Smooth Muscle-Like Cell Line

Scott Lowe,* Tadashi Hirakawa,† Wen Chang,* and H. Earl Ruley*

*Center for Cancer Research and Department of Biology, Massachusetts Institute of Technology, Cambridge, Massachusetts; †Central Research Laboratories, Ajinomoto Co., Inc., Kawasaki, Japan

ABSTRACT

Activated *ras* oncogenes are unable to transform cells of the established REF52 line because expression of the oncogene inhibits cell proliferation. Genes such as adenovirus E1A and SV40 large T antigen enable *ras* to transform REF52 cells by negating cellular controls that cause *ras* to inhibit cell proliferation. Inhibition of cell growth is accompanied by large accumulations of neutral lipids (cholesterol esters, triglycerides, and glycerol ethers). Cholesterol esters were serum-derived, while triglycerides and glycerol ethers appear to be products of cell metabolism. Factors that influence the growth and accumulation of neutral lipids in REF52 cells may contribute to pathological changes observed in vascular smooth muscle cells during the development of atherosclerotic plaque.

INTRODUCTION

Oncogenes are genes implicated in carcinogenesis by virtue of their associations with oncogenic retroviruses, tumor-specific chromosome abnormalities, and DNA sequences that transform cultured cells to a tumorigenic state. Most, if not all, oncogenes encode proteins that participate in signal transduction pathways by which external stimuli regulate cell growth and differentiation [1, 2].

Transformation of cultured cells to a tumorigenic state frequently requires combinations of oncogenes acting in concert [2, 3]. For example, activated *ras* oncogenes transform primary cells (i.e. tissue explants that have not been passaged in culture) poorly, if at all, while genes such as *myc*, adenovirus early region 1A (E1A), and Simian-virus 40 (SV40) large T antigen enable *ras* to transform primary cells to a tumorigenic state. Similarly, *myc* and E1A do not transform but each can promote the establishment of primary cells into lines capable of growing indefinitely in culture. While these results suggest that *in vitro* establishment is a necessary precondition for transformation, E1A and SV40 large T antigen also enable *ras* to transform cells of the established REF52 line [4, 5], demonstrating that *in vitro* establishment alone does not render cells susceptible to transformation by *ras*.

ras genes encode 21 kilodalton proteins (referred to as p21s) thought to propagate or amplify second messenger signals from cell surface growth factor receptors [6]. The oncogenic potential of *ras* is unmasked by point mutations that impair the ability of accessory proteins to stimulate GTP hydrolysis, thus deregulating p21 activities which induce susceptible cells to proliferate [7, 8]. All of the known genes that enable *ras* to transform cultured cells encode nuclear proteins, appear to regulate processes important in transcription and cell cycle control, and by as yet unknown mechanisms, affect controls that regulate transformation by *ras* [3].

Published 1990 by Elsevier Science Publishing Co., Inc.
Molecular Biology of Atherosclerosis
A.D. Attie, Editor

Our laboratory has studied transforming interactions between *ras* and other oncogenes in order to identify relevant biochemical interactions involved in normal growth control and transformation. REF52 cells have proven particularly useful in this regard, since they provide one of the tightest biological systems in which transformation by *ras* strictly requires a second, collaborating oncogene. *ras* fails to transform REF52 cells because expression of even modest levels of oncogenic p21 inhibits cell proliferation. E1A and SV40 large T antigen collaborate with *ras* by inactivating or circumventing cellular controls that cause *ras* to inhibit proliferation [5].

Inhibition of cell growth by *ras* was accompanied by massive accumulations of cholesterol esters and other neutral lipids [9]. The process did not resemble normal adipocyte differentiation, since the cells became arrested in the G2/M phase of the cell cycle, accumulated lipids other than triglycerides, and did not express adipocyte specific genes [5, 9]. However, similarities between REF52 cells and vascular smooth muscle cells raises the possibility that factors which influence the growth and accumulation of neutral lipids in REF52 cells are relevant to pathobiology of atherosclerosis.

RESULTS

Temperature-sensitive mutations in SV40 large T antigen have been isolated and have provided a convenient means to regulate transformation by *ras*. Thus, cells transfected by the T24 Ha-*ras* oncogene, together with plasmids encoding a temperature-sensitive SV40 large T antigen (*tsA58*) produced far more transformed foci at a permissive temperature (33°C) for T antigen expression than at a non-permissive temperature (39°C) [5]. Moreover, as shown in Figure 1, cells transformed at 33°C by *ras* and *tsA58* ceased growing when transferred to 39°C. Growth arrest was seen only when cells transformed with *tsA58* and *ras* were shifted to the non-permissive temperature, and therefore did not result from the sudden temperature shift or toxic breakdown products of T antigen. Cells maintained at 39°C were plated at 33°C to assess whether *ras*-induced growth arrest was reversible. As shown in Figure 1C, growth arrest was reversible for 2 days, but recovery declined thereafter and was largely irreversible after 10 days. Plating efficiencies declined only among Ha-*ras*/*tsA58* co-transformants, but the cells remained metabolically viable for at least 2 weeks at 39°C, as judged by trypan blue dye exclusion (Figure 1B). These results indicate that transformation of REF52 cells by *ras* requires continuous expression of a collaborating oncogene and suggest that the collaborating oncogenes influence cellular responses that cause *ras* to inhibit cell proliferation.

In some experimental systems, expression of the Ha-*ras* oncogene results in cellular differentiation [10, 11]. Thus, phenotypic changes in *tsA*/*ras* transformants were examined to assess whether growth arrest might be accompanied by a program of cellular differentiation. Previous studies have shown that transfer of an activated *ras* oncogene into REF52 cells generates rare clones of transformed cells [4]. However, these clones are only abortively transformed since most fail to survive subsequent sub-culturing. Prior to their eventual loss, abortive transformants became multi-nucleated, accumulated large cytoplasmic vacuoles, and sloughed fragments into the media. The cells also stained prominently with the lipophilic dye, Oil Red O, indicating the cytoplasmic vacuoles were lipid-filled [9]. Similarly, as judged by Oil Red O staining, the majority of clones transformed by *tsA58* and T24 Ha-*ras* accumulated lipid when transferred to 39°C (Table 1). In contrast, the cell lines

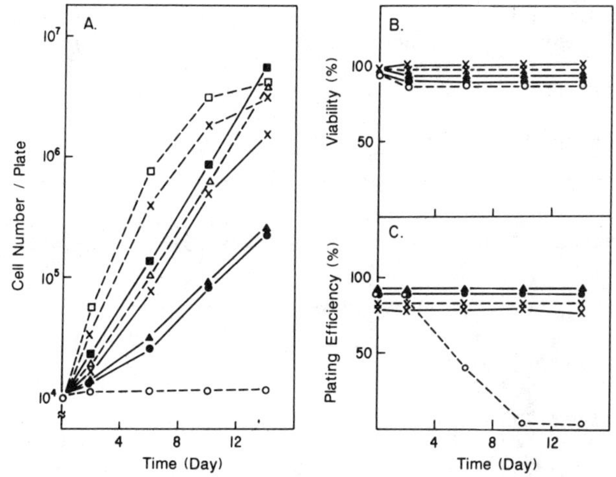

Figure 1. Temperature-dependent growth and survival of transfected REF52 cells. A. Growth potential of transfected clones. Subconfluent cultures maintained at 33°C were trypsinized and 10^4 cells were inoculated into 20 10-cm dishes. Every other day, cells from replica cultures maintained at either 33°C (—) or 39°C (---) were trypsinized and counted. Growth of REF52 cells (x) and derivative lines expressing *tsA58* alone (clone TS-1; ❑,■), *tsA58* and T24 Ha-*ras* (Clone TSR-5; ○,●); and wild-type large T antigen gene and T24 Ha-*ras* (clone WSR-1; Δ,▲) are plotted. B. Viability of transfected clones. Cells harvested for counting in A were stained with 0.2% trypan blue. Cell viability, expressed as the percent of dye-excluding cells, is plotted for each clone as in A. C. Irreversible loss of growth potential of TSR-5 cells maintained at 39°C. Two hundred cells, harvested for counting in A, were seeded into 60 mm dishes and cultured at 33°C. After 7 days, colonies were fixed, stained with crystal violet, and counted. Plating efficiencies, expressed as the percent of cells forming colonies at 33°C, are plotted for each clone as in A. Reprinted from [5].

transfected with T24 Ha-*ras*, wild-type T antigen, *tsA* alone, or transformed by wild-type T antigen and T24 Ha-*ras* did not accumulate lipid at 39°C.

The time-course of lipid accumulation in *tsA*/T24 Ha-*ras*-transformed REF52 cells (clone TSR-5.12) is shown in Figure 2A. Neutral lipids were extracted with methanol-chloroform, fractionated by thin-layer chromatography, and stained with iodine vapor. Aside from free cholesterol, which stains poorly with iodine, TSR-5.12 cells maintained at 33°C contain negligible levels of neutral lipids. However, cells transferred to 39°C accumulated massive levels of several species of non-polar lipids. Several of these lipids were readily identified comparing their mobilities on TLC with known lipid standards. Cholesterol esters accumulated first, and increased by about 1 μg/day (per 75 μg of total cell protein) over a four-day period. Similar levels of triglycerides also accumulated, but with delayed kinetics. In addition,

Table 1. Lipid accumulation in REF52 clones. Cells were co-transfected with the indicated genes and a neomycin resistance gene. After selection for neomycin resistant colonies at the indicated temperatures, stably transfected clones were expanded in mass culture and tested for lipid accumulation upon transfer to 39°C. The number of clones that stained with Oil-Red-O after 4 days at 39°C is indicated. Reprinted from [9] with permission.

Transfected Genes	Temperature Selected (°C)	Number of Clones Tested	Number Stained by Oil Red O
T24 Ha-*ras* + *tsA*	33	9	7
tsA	33	3	0
T24 Ha-*ras*	37	3	0
T24 Ha-*ras* + SVLT	33	3	0
SVLT	33	2	0
neo alone	37	2	0

a relatively non-polar lipid species (with a mobility between that of triglycerides and cholesterol esters) accumulated. Subsequent experiments suggested that these were diacylglycerol ethers (data not shown). Cholesterol esters did not accumulate in cells maintained in human lipoprotein-deficient serum (Figure 2B), but triglyceride accumulation was unaffected, and the accumulation of diacylglycerol ethers was enhanced. These results indicate that cholesterol esters were serum derived, whereas the triglycerides and glycerol ethers were apparent products of cellular metabolism.

Although oncogene-induced lipogenesis appeared to be a highly regulated process, several considerations suggested the phenomenon was not an aberrant form of adipocyte differentiation. First, the combination of neutral lipids was inappropriate, since adipocytes accumulate triglycerides almost exclusively. Second, *tsA/ras* transformants arrested in the G2/M phase of the cell cycle. Finally, the cells did not express any of the four adipocyte-specific markers tested [5, 9].

While *tsA58* provided a convenient means to regulate cellular responses to *ras*, the approach is limited since the cells must initially be transformed. To conclusively demonstrate that growth arrest and lipid accumulation resulted from *ras* expression (rather than the loss of T antigen from transformed cells), it was necessary to develop a direct method to express oncogenic p21 in normal REF52 cells. For this, retrovirus-mediated gene transfer has proven useful for several reasons: (i) genes can be synchronously introduced into a relatively large number of cells, (ii) transduced genes are expressed within hours after infection, and (iii) the retrovirus itself causes minimal cytopathic effects [12].

A retrovirus vector (U3Histkras) expressing the T24 Ha-*ras* oncogene was constructed from a previously described virus (U3Histkneo) by replacing the *neo* gene with a T24 Ha-*ras* cDNA [13]. This vector uses the herpes simplex virus thymidine kinase (tk) promoter to drive constitutive *ras* expression. U3Histkras and U3Histkneo vectors were transfected into NIH 3T3 cells expressing the packaging-defective ψ2 helper virus [14] and cell lines producing high titers of both viruses were isolated. REF52 cells were infected with U3Histkras and U3Histkneo viruses at a high multiplicity of infection and changes in cell density were monitored at various times post-infection. As shown in Figure 3, REF52 cells infected with the U3Histkneo retrovirus

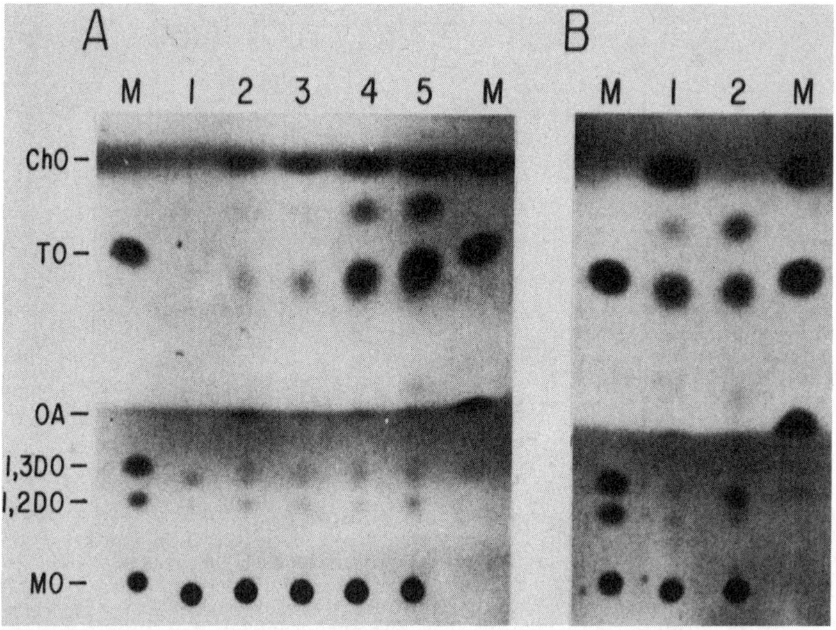

Figure 2. Time course of *ras*-induced lipid accumulation. A. TLC analysis of neutral lipids extracted from 5 x 10^5 TSR5.12 cells maintained at 33°C (lane 1) or transferred to 39°C for 1, 2, 3, and 4 days (lanes 2-5, respectively). Lipid standards (M) on the left contained (5 µg each): TO, triolein; 1,3DO, 1,3, diolein; 1,2DO, 1,2 diolein and MO, monolein. Markers on the right included (5 µg each): ChO, cholesterol oleate; OA, oleic acid and cholesterol (weakly staining and unlabeled). B. Lipid accumulation in lipoprotein-deficient medium. TLC analysis of neutral lipids extracted from 5 x 10^5 TSR5.12 cells maintained at 39°C for three days in medium supplemented with 10% fetal bovine serum (lane 1) or 10% human lipoprotein deficient medium (lane 2). Lipid markers (M) were the same as in A. Reprinted from [9] with permission.

continued to proliferate (with a normal doubling time of approximately24hours) until the cells reached confluence 4 - 5 days post-infection. However, infection with the U3Histkras virus resulted in a rapid inhibition of cell proliferation. While some *ras*-expressing cells became refractile and detached from the plate, the majority of cells acquired a large, flat, morphology. These results provide a further indication that (i) *ras* alone can not transform REF52 cells and (ii), expression of oncogenic p21 *ras* results in a cellular response which inhibits cell proliferation.

To determine if *ras* was sufficient to cause neutral lipid accumulation, uninfected cells and cells infected with U3Histkneo and U3Histkras were fixed and stained with Oil Red O at various times post-infection (Figure 4). In addition, neutral lipids were extracted with methanol-chloroform and analyzed by thin layer chromatography. While normal, proliferating REF52 cells contained prominently staining droplets, the lipid was lost as the cells reached confluence. Levels of neutral lipid were higher in U3Histkras-infected cells two days post-infection than in control cells (Figures 4 and 5), and unlike uninfected and U3Histkneo-infected cells, neutral lipids persisted for at least 14

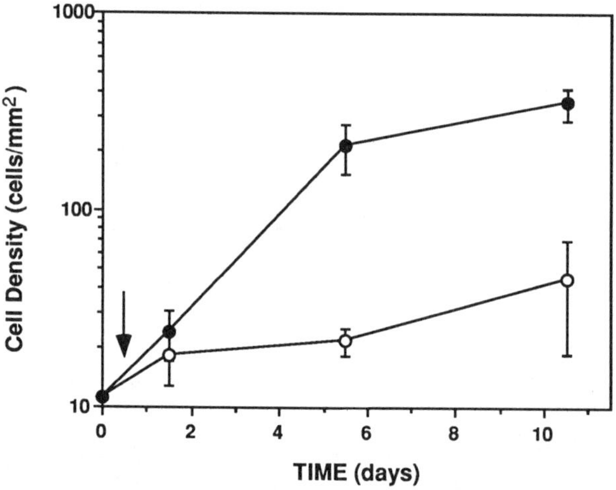

Figure 3. Growth kinetics of REF52 cells expressing T24 Ha-*ras*. REF52 cells were were plated at an initial density of 2 x 10^5/150 mm dish and infected at high multiplicity of infection with the U3Histkneo or U3Histkras retrovirus. Recombinant retroviruses were collected in 5 ml media from approximately 10^8 ψ2-derived virus producers maintained in roller bottles. After 2 hours at 37°C, the virus-containing supernatant was passaged through a 0.2 μm filter to remove cellular debris. Polybrene was added to a final concentration of 8 μg/ml to enhance virus uptake by cells. REF52 cells were infected for 2 hours at 37°C using 5 ml of virus-containing supernatant per dish. At various times post-infection, cell density was estimated by counting cells from a series of photomicrographs taken of random areas of each dish. The mean and standard deviation from 3 separate infections is plotted. (●) REF52 cells expressing the neomycin phosphotransferase gene, and (○) the T24 Ha-*ras* gene at 2 days post-infection. Cells were seeded at the 0 time point, and the vertical arrow indicates the time of infection.

days post-infection (Figure 5 and data not shown). TLC analysis confirmed that the accumulated lipids in normal, proliferating REF52 cells, and U3Histkras-infected cells were similar to those seen in *tsA*/*ras* transformants at 39°C. These results indicate that *ras* alone, in the absence of transformation, is able to cause both growth arrest and lipid accumulation.

DISCUSSION

ras oncogenes fail to transform REF52 cells because expression of the oncogene inhibits cell proliferation. Inhibition of cell growth was accompanied by large accumulations of neutral lipids in cells (i) abortively transformed by *ras*, (ii) conditionally transformed by *ras* and a temperature-sensitive SV40 large T antigen, and (iii) infected by retroviruses that express $p21^{T24Ha\text{-}ras}$. As *ras* is thought to propagate signals that promote cell growth, the effects of *ras* on REF52 cells may seem paradoxical. However, while continuous expression of $p21^{T24Ha\text{-}ras}$ inhibits growth, microinjected $p21^{T24Ha\text{-}ras}$ stimulates quiescent REF52 cells to proliferate [15]. This suggests that controls that

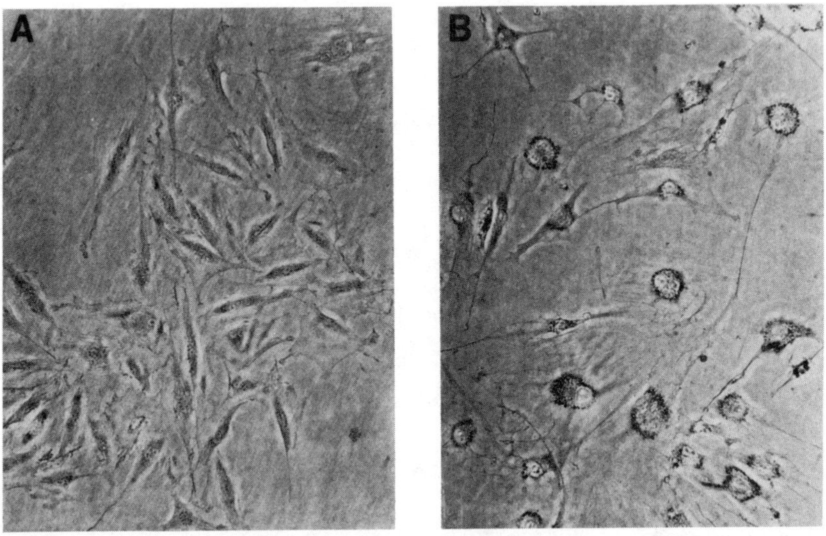

Figure 4. Neutral Lipid Staining of REF52 cells expressing T24 Ha-*ras*. REF52 cells were infected as described in Figure 3. At various times post-infection, cells were fixed in formaldehyde and stained with Oil Red O. REF52 cells expressing (A) the neomycin phosphotransferase gene, and (B) the T24 Ha-*ras* gene at 2 days post-infection.

prevent transformation may be activated by *ras* (and other mitogens) as part of a feedback mechanism that limits the ability of cells to proliferate in response to mitogenic stimuli.

These considerations suggest the following model for *ras*-induced lipid accumulation. Forced expression of the *ras* oncogene stimulates activities at the plasma membrane associated with cell proliferation. These include membrane ruffling, pinocytosis, and increased uptake of LDL. However, with the activation of controls that limit proliferation, neutral lipids accumulate because internalized phospholipids and LDL cholesterol esters are not cycled into newly synthesized membranes as would occur in growing cells. Consistent with this notion, neutral lipids that accumulate in *ras*-expressing cells are similar to those observed in normal proliferating REF52 cells. However, while lipid pools are depleted as normal cells reach confluence and stop proliferating, lipids persist in cells whose growth has been arrested by *ras*. In other words, *ras* appears to affect the normal coupling of neutral lipid pools to the growth state of the cell.

While the tissue of origin is unknown (the line was established from 14 day gestation rat embryos [16]), REF52 cells resemble smooth muscle cells with regard to morphology, growth factor requirements [17] and expression smooth muscle-forms of tropomyosin and α-actin [18]. Moreover, while many established rodent lines are transformed by *ras* alone, two other transformation-resistant lines (A7r5 and A10) that we have identified (A. Lamond, L. Gouw and H.E.R., manuscript in preparation) were derived from rat aortas and resemble vascular smooth muscle cells [19].

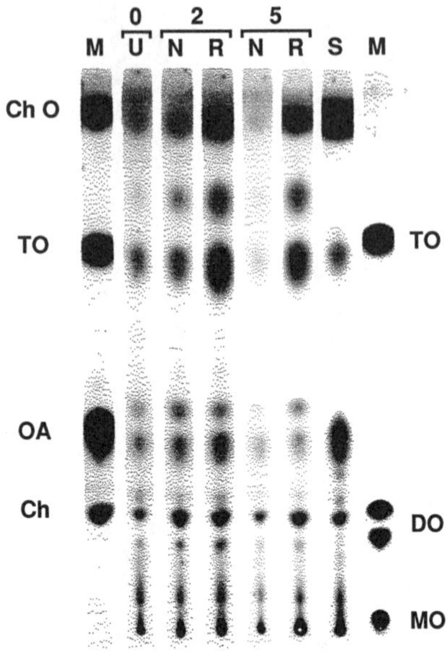

Figure 5. Thin layer chromatography of neutral lipids extracted from REF52 cells. REF52 cells were infected as described in Figure 3. At 2 and 5 days post-infection, neutral lipids were extracted from 3.5 x 10^5 cells using a modification of the Bligh and Dyer method. Samples were spotted on Silica Gel G TLC plates and lipid species were separated in petroleum ether-ethyl ether-glacial acetic acid (80:20:1). Lipid spots were visualized in iodine vapor. M(left), lipid standards: cholesterol oleate (ChO), triolein (TO), oleic acid (OA), and cholesterol (Ch); U, uninfected cells from day 0; N, cells infected with U3Histkneo; R, cells infected with U3Histkras; S, lipids extracted from 0.1 ml fetal bovine serum; M(right), lipid standards: triolein (TO), 1,2- and 1,3-diacyl glycerol (DG), and monolein (MO).

Similarities between REF52 and vascular smooth muscle cells raises the possibility that *ras*-induced lipogenesis is relevant to the pathology of atherosclerosis. While macrophages can accumulate cholesterol esters via receptors that bind and transport altered forms of LDL [20, 21], the present study describes a physiological mechanism whereby mesenchymal cells may be induced to accumulate neutral lipids. Moreover, it is reasonable for smooth muscle cells to possess tight controls which limit their responses to mitogenic stimuli. Renewal of smooth muscle does not involve continuously cycling stem cells; rather, cell divisions are infrequent and dispersed throughout the arterial wall [22, 23], suggesting that mitogenically stimulated cells cycle only once. The fact that some smooth muscle cells *in vivo* become arrested at the G2/M phase of the cell cycle [24, 25, 26] is intriguing, since REF52 cells conditionally transformed by *ras* and *tsA* also arrest at G2/M [5]. Factors such as hypertension, diabetes, and smoking, by increasing the demand for smooth muscle proliferation, may eventually promote neutral lipid accumulation, assuming the lipids persist in cells resistant to further cell divisions. Hypercholesterolemia may promote smooth muscle proliferation [27, 28, 29, 30], or simply enhance the uptake of LDL by growth arrested cells. This model assumes that factors promoting the development of atherosclerosis can stimulate smooth muscle proliferation without specific injury to the vascular wall, but growth promoting factors may be synthesized by the vascular endothelium [31, 32], released by thrombinolysis [33] or synthesized by infiltrating macrophages [34, 35]. Finally, the relevance of this model to all types of atherosclerosis need not be assumed. For example, atherosclerosis in hypertensive smokers with normal serum cholesterol levels is likely to involve different intracellular mechanisms than in the disease resulting from congenital hypercholesterolemia.

In principle, somatic mutations in oncogenes such as *ras* may also constitutively activate growth-promoting stimuli, and could account for the limited clonality of atherosclerotic plaque [36, 37, 38]. Nevertheless, evidence supporting this possibility is limited. While expression of the PDGF B chain is enhanced in plaque, it is not clear whether this is a cause or a consequence of atherosclerotic change [34, 39, 40, 41, 42]. Moreover, an early report suggesting that DNA from athersclerotic plaque was capable of transforming NIH3T3 cells has not be substantiated [43].

ACKNOWLEDGEMENTS

We thank Karen Traite for help preparing this manuscript. This work was supported by Public Health Service grants (CA40602; CA42063) and a Latham Family Career Development Professorship to H.E.R. and partially supported by a Cancer Center "Core" grant (CA14051) to P.A. Sharp.

REFERENCES

1. Bishop, J.M., Science 235, 305-311 (1987).
2. Weinberg, R., Cancer Res. 49, 3713-3721 (1989).
3. Ruley, H.E., Cancer Cells (in press) (1990).
4. Franza, B.R., K. Maruyama, J.I. Garrels and H.E. Ruley, Cell 44, 409-418 (1986).
5. Hirakawa, T. and H.E. Ruley, Proc. Natl. Acad. Sci. (USA) 85, 1519-1523 (1988).
6. Barbacid, M., Ann. Rev. Biochem. 56, 779-827 (1987).
7. Adari, H., D.R. Lowy, B.M. Willumsen, C.J. Der and F. McCormick, Science 240, 518-521 (1988).
8. Cales, C., J.F. Hancock, C.J. Marshall and A. Hall, Nature 332, 548-551 (1988).
9. Hirakawa, T., K. Maruyama, N.E. Kohl, T. Kodama and H.E. Ruley, Oncogene (in press) (1990).
10. Noda, M., *et al.*, Nature 318, 73-75 (1985).
11. Bar-Sagi, D. and R.J. Feramisco, Cell 42, 841-848 (1985).
12. Varmus, H., Science 240, 1427-1435 (1988).
13. von Melchner, H. and H.E. Ruley, J. Virol. 63, 3227-3233 (1989).
14. Mann, R., R.C. Mulligan and D. Baltimore, Cell 33, 153-159 (1983).
15. Feramisco, J.R., M. Gross, T. Kamata, M. Rosenberg and R.W. Sweet, Cell 38, 109-117 (1984).
16. Logan, J., *et al.*, Virology 78, 419-422 (1981).
17. McClure, D.B., M.J. Hightower and W.C. Topp, Cold Spring Harb. Conf. Cell Prolif. 9, 345-364 (1982).
18. Garrels, J.I. and B.R. Franza Jr., J. Biol. Chem. 264, 5283-5289 (1989).
19. Kimes, B.W. and B.L. Brandt, Exp. Cell Res. 98, 349-366 (1976).
20. Goldstein, J.L., Y.K. Ho, S.K. Basu and M.S. Brown, Proc. Natl. Acad. Sci. (USA) 76, 333-337 (1979).
21. Kodama, T., *et al.*, Nature 343, 531-535 (1990).

22. Dilley, R.J., J.K. McGeachie and F.J. Prendergast, Atherosclerosis 63, 99-107 (1987).
23. Schwartz, S.M., G.R. Campbell and J.H. Campbell, Circ. Res. 58, 427-444 (1986).
24. Owens, G.K., P.S. Rabinovitch and S.M. Schwartz, Proc. Natl. Acad. Sci. (USA) 7759, 7763-7767 (1981).
25. Barrett, T.B., P. Sampson, G.K. Owens, S.M. Schwartz and E.P. Benditt, Proc. Natl. Acad. Sci. (USA) 80, 882-885 (1983).
26. Goldberg, I.D., *et al.*, Science 226, 559-561 (1984).
27. Ross, R. and J.A. Glomset, Science 180, 1332-1338 (1973).
28. Libby, P., P. Miao, J.M. Ordovas and E.J. Schaefer, J. Cell Physiol. 124, 1-8 (1985).
29. Fischer-Dzoga, K. and R.W. Wissler, Atherosclerosis 24, 515-525 (1976).
30. Fischer-Dzoga, K., R. Fraser and R.W. Wissler, Exp. Mol. Pathol. 24, 346-359 (1976).
31. Castellot Jr., J.J., L.V. Favreau, M.J. Karnovsky and R.D. Rosenberg, J. Biol. Chem. 257, 11256-11260 (1982).
32. Barrett, T.B., C.M. Gajdusek, S.M. Schwartz, J.K. McDougall and E.P. Benditt, Proc. Natl. Acad. Sci. (USA) 81, 6772-6774 (1984).
33. Friedman, R.J., *et al.*, J. Clin. Invest. 60, 1191-1201 (1977).
34. Ross, R., *et al.*, Science 248, 1009-1012 (1990).
35. Martinet, Y., *et al.*, Nature 319, 158-160 (1986).
36. Benditt, E.P. and J.M. Benditt, Proc. Natl. Acad. Sci. (USA) 70, 1753-1756 (1973).
37. Pearson, T.A., J.M. Dillman, K. Solez and R.H. Heptinstall, Amer. J. Pathol. 93, 93-102 (1978).
38. Pearson, T.A., J.M. Dillman, K. Solez and R.H. Heptinstall, Circ. Res. 43, 10-18 (1978).
39. Fingerle, J., R. Johnson, A.W. Clowes, M.W. Majesky and M.A. Reidy, Proc. Natl. Acad. Sci. (USA) 86, 8412-8416 (1989).
40. Barrett, T.B. and E.P. Benditt, Proc. Natl. Acad. Sci. (USA) 84, 1099-1103 (1987).
41. Barrett, T.B. and E.P. Benditt, Proc. Natl. Acad. Sci. (USA) 85, 2810-2814 (1988).
42. Wang, A.M., M.V. Doyle and D.F. Mark, Proc. Natl. Acad. Sci. (USA) 86, 9717-9721 (1989).
43. Penn, A., S.J. Garte, L. Warren, D. Nesta and B. Mindich, Proc. Natl. Acad. Sci. (USA) 83, 7951-7955 (1986).

PDGF Receptors: What? Where? Why?

Daniel F. Bowen-Pope, Gina Schatteman, and R. A. Seifert

Department of Pathology, University of Washington, Seattle, Washington

During the last two years it has become clear that there is more than one receptor for PDGF (platelet-derived growth factor). In this chapter we will discuss the structure of the PDGF receptors and the ways in which regulation of expression of these receptors may influence or determine normal and pathological processes. Data available to date suggests that regulation of PDGF receptor expression is as important as is regulation of PDGF synthesis in determining the ways in which the PDGF system functions *in vivo*.

THE DISCOVERY OF PDGF AND INITIAL HYPOTHESES ABOUT BIOLOGICAL FUNCTIONS

Platelet-derived growth factor (PDGF) was first recognized as a mitogenic activity released from blood platelets during platelet activation, eg during the clotting of whole blood (Ross et al 1974). Ever since the existence of such a factor in platelets was first suspected, PDGF has been hypothesized to play a role in the regulation of proliferation of smooth muscle cells within the artery wall, and to play a role in the etiology of atherosclerotic lesions (Ross and Glomset, 1976). At first, PDGF was believed to be strictly a platelet product. Development of specific methods for detection of PDGF from other sources led, during the mid 1980's, to the realization that many cultured cells could, under certain circumstances, secrete PDGF into their culture medium. These observations have suggested that PDGF may play a role in regulating growth by many cell types under many different circumstances (reviewed in Ross et al 1986). For example, within a single simple tissue, the large arteries, multiple possible sources of PDGF have been demonstrated, including the endothelial cells which line the vessels, the smooth muscle cells which constitute the vessel wall, the monocyte/macrophages which accumulate in atherosclerotic lesions, and the platelets which adhere and degranulate during acute injury. With the finding that the B-chain of PDGF is homologous to the oncogene of Simian Sarcoma Virus, and many reports that the endogenous PDGF genes are activated during oncogenic transformation by other agents, considerable interest has also been generated in the possible involvement of PDGF in tumorigenesis. Recent findings suggest that roles for PDGF may begin during early embryogenesis.

THE STRUCTURE OF PDGF: MULTIPLE ISOFORMS ARE EXPRESSED IN A TISSUE-SPECIFIC PATTERN

Although little has been proven yet about the actual roles of PDGF, much is now known about PDGF as a molecule (reviewed in Raines et al 1990). Purification and biochemical characterization indicated that PDGF is a disulfide-bonded dimer of two subunit chains, each with a molecular weight of about 15,000. Partial amino acid analysis demonstrated the presence of two different but homologous sequences in preparations of pure PDGF. One sequence is homologous to the oncogene (v-sis) of simian sarcoma virus and is now usually designated the "B-chain" of PDGF. The cloning and sequencing of the human B-chain cDNA and gene was soon followed by the cloning and sequencing of the A-chain cDNA.

© 1990 by Elsevier Science Publishing Co., Inc.
Molecular Biology of Atherosclerosis
A.D. Attie, Editor

This permitted analysis of PDGF gene expression by different cells at the level of mRNA expression. These studies demonstrated that the two PDGF genes are independently regulated. Situations have been reported in which A-chain or B-chain or both are expressed, and levels can change independently in response to certain stimuli.

CHANGING CONCEPTS OF THE STRUCTURE OF THE PDGF RECEPTOR

Up until this point, studies of PDGF binding had yielded results which were interpreted in terms of a single monomeric PDGF receptor. This receptor was described as a single 170-180 kDa membrane glycoprotein which has an extracellular ligand-binding domain and an intracellular tyrosine kinase domain (eg Glenn et al 1982; Heldin et al 1983; Pike et al 1983; Williams et al 1984; Daniel et al 1987). The publication (Yarden et al 1986) of the cDNA sequence of a mouse PDGF receptor and of the homologous human PDGF receptors (Gronwald et al 1988; Claesson-Welsh et al 1988) confirmed the biochemical results and showed that the PDGF receptor has a "split" tyrosine kinase domain comparable to that of the CSF-1 receptor and the c-kit proto-oncogene.

The cloning of the two PDGF genes allowed the two homodimeric isoforms of PDGF (PDGF-AA and PDGF-BB) to be expressed by recombinant technology. Chain-specific antisera allowed the PDGF-AB heterodimer to be purified from human platelets (Hart et al 1990). The availability of these pure isoforms of PDGF yielded binding data which necessitated a reevaluation of our concepts of PDGF receptor structure and properties. Binding studies performed using these isoforms and a monoclonal anti-receptor antibody indicated that they were not all binding to a single PDGF receptor molecule. To explain the observed pattern of binding competition, we initially proposed that there were two forms of PDGF receptor on human fibroblasts, an abundant form (designated the "B-receptor) which binds only PDGF-BB and is recognized by PRa7212, and a much less abundant form which binds PDGF-AA, PDGF-AB, and PDGF-BB (designated the A/B receptor Hart et al 1988 and the A receptor by Heldin et al 1988). The estimate of the differential abundance of the two classes of receptor was supported by direct measurements of saturable ligand binding which indicated that the number of ^{125}I-PDGF-BB binding sites was about 7 fold greater than the number of ^{125}I-PDGF-AB binding sites, and by the observation that PDGF-BB stimulated much higher levels of tyrosine phosphorylation than did PDGF-AA or PDGF-AB.

THE RECEPTOR SUBUNIT HYPOTHESIS

When we began to extend our studies to additional cell types, we found cell types, eg MG-63 human osteosarcoma cells and mouse 3T3 cells, which bind much more ^{125}I-PDGF-AA than do fibroblasts. This allowed better evaluation of the hypothesized A/B receptor. We obtained patterns of cross-competition, saturation binding, etc which were not explicable by the original two-receptor model. According to the two receptor model PDGF-AA and PDGF-AB should behave identically since they both bind only to the "A-receptor". This was not always the case. To explain the more complete data set we proposed that each PDGF receptor consists of a dimer of two possible subunits: a beta-subunit which binds only a B-chain and is recognized by monoclonal PR7212, and an alpha-subunit which can bind either an A- or a B-chain but which is not recognized by monoclonal PR7212. In the absence of ligand the subunits exist as monomers. In the presence of ligand, two receptor subunits associate to form a high-affinity PDGF binding site, with each subunit binding one of two chains of the disulfide bonded dimeric PDGF molecule (Seifert et al 1989). This model is diagrammed below.

This model of PDGF receptor structure and function made two major testable predictions: that a second PDGF receptor protein ("subunit") should exist, and that receptor subunits dimerize while binding PDGF. These two predictions have been verified. It is now clear that the initially cloned and identified receptor protein has the properties of the putative beta subunit of the receptor. We have obtained an additional monoclonal antibody (PR292) which specifically recognizes a cell surface protein with the properties of the putative alpha subunit. It is somewhat smaller (170,000 vs 180,000 daltons) than the beta subunit and binds ^{125}I-PDGF-AA. Claesson-Welsh et al (1988a) found a human clonal glioma line which expressed no beta-subunit transcripts and which had the binding properties of an alpha-subunit-only cell line and identified a 170,000 dalton component as the putative alpha subunit. The cDNA encoding the PDGF receptor alpha subunit has now been cloned from human (Matsui et al 1989; Kelly et al unpublished; Claesson-Welsh et al 1989) rat (Lee et al 1990) and mouse (Mercola et al 1990). The cDNA encodes a protein similar in structure to the beta subunit, with a highly conserved intracellular split tyrosine kinase domain and an extracellular putative ligand binding domain in which the spacing of the 10 cysteines is exactly conserved but which shows surprisingly low sequence similarity (about 30%) to the extracellular domain of the beta subunit.

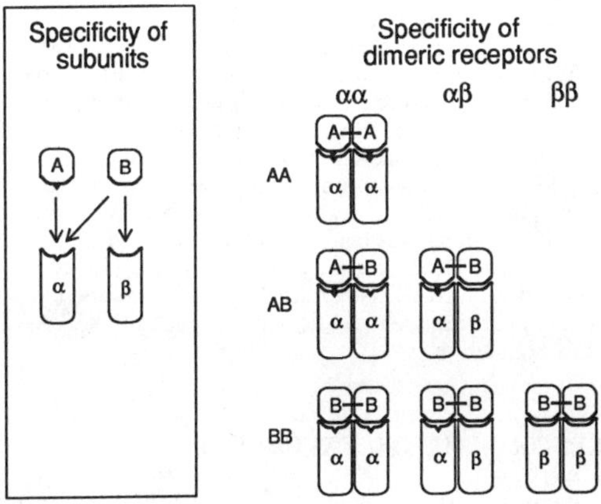

FIGURE 1: The subunit model of PDGF receptor structure and specificity.

The second prediction of the receptor subunit model, that high-affinity PDGF binding involves dimerization of subunits, has also been confirmed in several labs. Seifert et al (1989) showed that detergent solubilized receptor subunits from mouse and human could be coimmunopricipitated by a monoclonal antibody against human receptors, but only after the addition of an isoform of PDGF predicted to be able to form interspecific dimers. Bishayee et al (1989) and Heldin et al (1989) used crosslinking agents, density gradient centrifugation, and gel filtration to demonstrate the the presence of PDGF could cause a doubling of the apparent molecular weight of the receptor.

DO THE DIFFERENT PDGF RECEPTOR SUBUNITS MEDIATE DIFFERENT BIOLOGICAL RESPONSES?

The alpha and beta subunits distinguish between the different chains of PDGF and differ significantly in their intracellular domains, especially the interkinase domain which has been implicated in interacting with second messenger systems (Reviewed in Williams, 1989). Have they evolved to generate different intracellular signals? Several studies have demonstrated differences in the responses of specific cell types to different isoforms of

PDGF and these differences seem to reflect the ability of the different isoforms to bind to different forms of PDGF receptor. For example, Nister et al (1988) and Hammacher et al (1989) reported that forms of PDGF-AA were much less mitogenic than PDGF-AB on AG1523 and did not cause circular ruffel formation or cause actin reorganization or induce chemotaxis. This suggested that the PDGF receptor alpha subunit (which is the only receptor subunit to which PDGF-AA can bind) is not competent (or not as competent) to stimulate these processes. This was interpreted to indicate that the alpha and beta subunits are qualitatively different in their signal transduction pathways. Although this is possible, there is a simpler explanation for the data. The lower potency of PDGF-AA may reflect quantitative differences in levels of expression of the two receptor subunits. This is supported by the observations that although PDGF-AA is indeed less mitogenic than PDGF-BB for human fibroblasts, these cells express many more beta- than alpha-subunits and thus bind much more PDGF-BB than PDGF-AA. Cell types which express equal numbers of the two subunits and bind comparable amounts of the two PDGF isoforms are equally mitogenically responsive to the two isoforms (Seifert et al 1989). When the two subunits are expressed by transfection into receptor-negative host cells they both confer mitogenic and chemotactic responsiveness (Matsui et al 1990; Ferns et al in press). At present, therefore, we feel that although it is possible (and possibly even probable) that the two receptor subunits differ qualitatively in some aspects of intracellular signalling, a specific example of this has not been demonstrated. Why then are there more than one form of PDGF receptor? Possibly they serve to permit a more finely tuned regulation over the functioning of PDGF *in vivo*. At the level of the whole organism or tissue, the combination of the differing specificities of the two receptor subunits and the secretion of different isoforms of PDGF by different cells at different times, allows the PDGF system to function as though it consisted of a set of partially overlapping and partially distinct regulatory networks. For example, expression of receptor alpha subunits (or alpha plus beta) would permit a cell to respond to any isoform of PDGF. A second cell type expressing only beta subunits could respond to PDGF-BB but not to PDGF-AA or PDGF-AB. This permits PDGF-BB to function as a "universal ligand" and stimulate all PDGF-responsive cells while allowing PDGF-AA and PDGF-AB to target subsets of this population.

REGULATION OF RECEPTOR SUBUNIT EXPRESSION

We will briefly describe four systems or situations in which differences in PDGF receptor expression are found. We will speculate on the potential biological significance of these differences.

Only certain cell types express PDGF receptors. The general pattern of receptor expression was established by studies with cultured cells. Cultured connective tissue cell types are usually receptor positive. These include fibroblasts and fibroblastoid cell lines (eg 3T3), vascular smooth muscle cells, glial cells, chondrocytes. Other cell types that are receptor negative include epithelial, endothelial, hematopoietic, and neuronal cells. This suggests that the activities of PDGF in adult animals may be largely restricted to connective tissue maintenance and repair. In general (although much less information is available) the same general cell type distribution of receptor expression is found *in vivo* when tissues are examined for receptor expression by immunocytochemistry or by *in situ* hybridization techniques. However, one particularly interesting difference between *in vivo* and *in vitro* receptor expression has already been found. Cultured vascular smooth muscle cells and dermal fibroblasts were two of the first cell types found to express receptors. Immunocytochemical studies, however, demonstrate only very low levels of receptors *in vivo*. Terracio et al (1988) demonstrated that the level of receptor expression by freshly isolated dermal fibroblasts increases from low to high levels with time in culture. This suggests that receptor expression *in vivo* in some normal tissues may be relatively low but that it can be increased in response to external variables.

Changes in receptor expression in vivo in response to injury. One well characterized experimental model of response of arteries to injury uses an inflated balloon catheter to damage the wall of the rat carotid artery. Within the two weeks following this injury the smooth muscle cells in the artery wall more than double in number (Clowes et al 1983). Even after two weeks, replication remains high in the most luminal layer of smooth muscle cells. It has been widely speculated that PDGF (eg released from platelets or synthesized by activated smooth muscle or other cells) may play a role in stimulating these processes (reviewed in Ross et al 1986). Determination of PDGF receptor expression by Northern blot and *in situ* hybridization shows that levels of beta subunit are transiently decreased following the injury and then increase dramatically in the most luminal (ie most proliferatively active) layer (Majesky et al Submitted). Other examples of increased expression of PDGF receptors by cells proliferating in response to a pathological stimulus have also been found, including vascular smooth muscle cells and kidney mesangial cells during inflamation (Rubin et al 1988; Fellstrom et al 1989). It is possible, but not proven, that this increased expression of PDGF receptors contributes to the proliferation by increasing the responsiveness of the cells to PDGF.

PDGF receptor expression during embryogenesis. mRNA for the A-chain of PDGF has been detected in preimplantation mouse blastocysts (Rappolee et al 1988) and as a maternally encoded transcript in Xenopus oocytes (Mercola et al 1988). This expression of the ligand gene suggests that the PDGF system may be functioning early in development. Since expression of the PDGF receptor alpha subunit protein is necessary for a cell to be able to respond to isoforms of PDGF containing an A-chain, we have begun to evaluate the pattern of PDGF receptor subunit expression during embryogenesis. We have found that the relative abundance of the two PDGF receptor subunits changes during development (Mercola et al 1990). In early embryos, mRNA for the alpha subunit is abundant in 6.5-8.5 day mouse embryos. mRNA for the beta subunit could be detected only by the end of this period. When receptor expression by cultured cells is examined, mouse 3T3 cell lines prepared from late gestation mouse embryos express the two subunits at more or less equal levels (Seifert et al 1989). In cultured adult cells the beta subunit is 5-20 fold more abundant than the alpha subunit (eg see Seifert et al 1989). Although the phenomenon has not yet been systematically investigated, the data noted above suggests that the PDGF receptor alpha subunit is the predominant form expressed during embryogenesis whereas the beta subunit is the predominant form expressed by adult cells.

The reversal in the relative abundances of the two receptor subunits presumably reflects some change in the relative roles or targets of PDGF-AA. The nature of these roles is unclear, but two approaches may provide some insight: evaluating the cell-type specificity of receptor expression during development, and determining the effects of loss of receptor expression on the processes of development. 1) To determine which type of cells express PDGF receptors at different stages of development, we have begun to use *in situ* hybridization to follow a-subunit mRNA expression. In mid-gestation mouse embryos an alpha subunit riboprobe detects high levels of alpha-subunit transcripts in many mesenchymal areas but not in the developing brain and liver (Schatteman et al unpublished observations). This suggests that during that period PDGF receptor alpha subunit function may be involved in mesenchyme development and differentiation but probably not in brain or liver development. 2) To determine whether alpha subunit expression is necessary for early development, or is only correlated with it, we are using a genetically defined mouse mutatant called "Patch" (Ph). We have recently found that the Ph allele includes a deletion of the PDGF receptor alpha subunit gene (Stephenson et al submitted) and speculate that the phenotypic defects in Ph reflect the loss of PDGF receptor alpha subunit expression. Mice that are heterozygous for Ph have characteristic patch of white hair on their stomach and sides, but have no other discernable defects (Gruneberg and Truslove, 1960). Mice that are homozygous for Ph die before birth with a variety of developmental abnormalities which all seem to be related to a defect in tissue fluid regulation. Exactly how this phenotype would result from deficient PDGF receptor espression is not yet clear, but "experiments of nature" of this sort have often proven in the past to be very useful in elucidating or testing causal relationships *in vivo.*

Changes in PDGF and PDGF receptor expression also occur during the post-embryonic period of development. We will mention two systems which have been studied in culture. In the first system, smooth muscle cells cultured from the aorta of newborn rats, but not from 2 month old rats, were shown to express high levels of PDGF B-chain mRNA and secrete PDGF. This suggested that the proliferation of smooth muscle cells in the aorta during this period might be driven, in part, by autocrine stimulation by PDGF, and that growth stopped when PDGF production was shut off (Seifert et al 1984). However, it is not clear that these changes occur *in vivo* (Majesky et al 1988). In the second system, the rat optic nerve around the time of birth, it apears that secretion of PDGF-AA by type-1 astrocytes drives the proliferation, and inhibits premature differentiation of O-2A precursors into oligodendrocytes and type-2 astrocytes (reviewed in Raff 1989).

Regulation of PDGF receptor expression by defined factors. It will be important to determine the factors that regulate expression of the two PDGF receptor subunits. Since receptor expression is cell-type specific it is clear that factors that cause cells to differentiate from receptor positive to receptor negative cell types (or vice versa) will be *de facto* regulators of receptor expression. For example, mouse skeletal satellite cells lose PDGF receptors when they participate in myotube formation (Yablonka-Reuveni et al In Press and unpublished). Embryo stem cell lines begin to express PDGF receptor alpha subunits if differentiation is induced by retinoic acid (Rizzino and Bowen-Pope, 1985; Mercola et al 1990). In addition to changes in expression concommitant with differentiation, regulation of receptor expression can also occur as part of more subtle and reversible cell responses to environmental signals. Exposure to transforming growth factor beta (TGF-beta) causes mouse 3T3 cells to loose virtually all of their receptor alpha subunits within 12 hrs while slightly increasing the level of beta subunit expression (Gronwald et al 1989). This causes a decrease in their responsiveness to PDGF-AA without loss of response to PDGF-BB. This type of regulation in a culture model system may be an example of the type of regulation that occurs *in vivo* to allow levels of receptor expression to be rapidly adjusted to suit the changing needs of the body.

CONCLUSIONS

Previous research into the biochemistry and physiology of PDGF has largely focused on three areas: the structure of PDGF itself, the structure of the PDGF receptor, and the regulation of PDGF synthesis in model systems. The latter area has turned out to be unexpectedly rich and is still developing rapidly. We believe that it is now critical to obtain comparable information about regulation of <u>receptor</u> expression. It is becoming clear that different cell types express different proportions; and absolute amounts of the two PDGF receptor subunits and that these differences seem to be correlated with differences in mitogenic and chemotactic responses to the different isoforms of PDGF. These initial findings suggest that regulation of the level and type of PDGF receptor expressed may be as important as regulation of PDGF synthesis in determining the role of PDGF in culture and *in vivo*. We propose that the role(s) of PDGF during development and in pathological changes are regulated to a significant extent by changes in the cell type distribution of receptor expression and that the magnitude of the responses are determined by changes in levels of receptor expression.

LITERATURE CITED

Bishayee, S., Majumdar, S., Khire, J., and Das, M. (1989) Ligand-induced dimerization of the platelet-derived growth factor receptor J. Biol. Chem. 264:11699-11705.

Bowen-Pope, D. F., Vogel, A., and Ross, R. (1984) Production of Platelet-derived Growth Factor-like molecules and reduced expression of Platelet-derived Growth Factor receptors accompany transformation by a wide spectrum of agents. Proc. Natl. Acad. Sci. USA 81:2396-2400

Bowen-Pope, D.F., Hart, C.E., and Seifert, R.A. (1989) Sera and conditioned media contain different isoforms of PDGF which bind to different classes of PDGF receptor. <u>J. Biol. Chem.</u> 264:2502-2508.

Briggs, M.R., Kadonaga, J.T., Bell, S.P., and Tjian, R. (1986) Purification and biochemical characterization of the promoter-specific transcription factor, Sp1. Science 234:47-52

Claesson-Welsh, L., Hammacher, A., Westermark, B., Heldin, C.H., and Nister, M. (1988a) Identification and structural analysis of the A type receptor for platelet-derived growth factor J. Biol. Chem. 1742-1747.
Claesson-Welsh, L., Ericksson, A., Severinsson, A., Ek, B., Ostman, A., Betsholtz, C., and Heldin, C.H.(1988b) cDNA cloning and expression of a human platelet-derived growth factor receptor specific for a B-chain-containing PDGF molecule. Molec. Cell. Biol. 8:3476-3486.
Claesson-Welsh, L., Ericksson, A., Westermark, B., and Heldin, C.H. (1989) cDNA cloning and expression of the human A-type platelet-derived growth factor (PDGF) receptor establishes structural similarity to the B-type PDGF receptor. PNAS 86:4917-4922.
Clowes, A.W., Reidy, M.A., and Clowes, M.M. (1983) Kinetics of cellular proliferation after arterial injury. Lab. Invest. 49:327-333.
Daniel, T.O., Milfay, D.F., Escobedo, J., and Williams L.T. (1987) Biosynthetic and glycosylation studies of cell surface Platelet-Derived Growth Factor receptors. Journal of Biological Chemistry 262:9778-9784
Fellstrom, B., Klaereskog, L., Heldin, C-H., Larsson, E., Ronnstrand, L., Terracio, L., Tufveson, G., Wahlberg, J., and Rubin, K. (1989) PDGF receptors in the kidney--upregulated expression in inflamation. Kidney international 36:1099-1102.
Ferns, G.A.A., Sprugel, K.H., Seifert, R.A., Bowen-Pope, D.F., Kelly, J.D., Murray, M., Raines, E.W., and Ross, R. Relative platelet-derived growth factor receptor expression determines cell migration to different dimeric forms of PDGF. Growth Factors In Press 4/1990
Glenn, K., Bowen-Pope, D. F., and Ross, R. (1982) Platelet-derived Growth Factor III. Identification of a Platelet-derived Growth Factor receptor by affinity labeling. The Journal of Biological Chemistry 257:5172-5176
Gronwald, R.G.K., Grant, F.J., Haldeman, B., Hart, C.E. O'Hara, P., Hagen, F.S., Ross, R., Bowen-Pope, D.F. and Murray, M. (1988) Cloning and expression of the human PDGF receptor. Proc. Natl. Acad. Sci. 85:3435-3439.
Gronwald, R,K.G., Seifert, R.S., and Bowen-Pope, D.F. (1989) Differential regulation of two PDGF receptor subunits by TGF-beta. (1989) J. Biol. Chem. 264:8120-8125.
Gruneberg, H. and Truslove, G.M. (1960) Two closely linked genes in the mouse Genet. Res. Camb. 1:69-90
Hammacher, A., Mellstrom, K., Heldin, C.-H., and Westermark, B. (1989) Isoform-specific induction of actin reorganization by platelet-derived growth factor suggests that the functionally active receptor is a dimer EMBO J. 8:2489-2495
Hart, C. E.., Seifert, R. A., Ross, R. R., and Bowen-Pope, D. F. (1987) Synthesis, phosphorylation, and degradation of multiple forms of the Platelet-derived Growth Factor receptor studied using a monoclonal antibody. The Journal of Biological Chemistry 262:10780-10785
Hart, C.H., Forstrom, J.W., Kelley, J.D., Seifert, R.A., Smith, R.A., Ross, R., Murray, M.J., and Bowen-Pope, D.F. (1988) Two classes of PDGF receptor recognize different isoforms of PDGF. Science 240:1529-1531.
Hart, C.E., Bailey, D.A., Curtis, D.A., Osborn, S., Raines, E.W., Ross, R., and Forstrom, J.W. (1990) Purification of PDGF-AB and PDGF-BB from platelet extracts and the identification of all three PDGF dimers in human plarelets. Biochemistry 29:166-172.
Heldin, C-H., Ek, B., and Ronnstrand, L. (1983) Characterization of the receptor for platelet-derived growth factor on human fibroblasts: demonstration of an intimate relationship with a 185,000-Dalton substrate for the platelet-derived growth factor-stimulated kinase. The Journal of Biological Chemistry 258:10054-10061
Heldin, C.H., Backstrom, G., Ostman, A., Hammacher, A., Ronstrand, L., Rubin, K., Nister, M., and Westermark, B. (1988) Binding of different dimeric forms of PDGF to human fibroblasts: evidence for two separate receptor types. EMBO Journal 7:1387-1393.
Heldin, C.-H., Ernlund, A., Rorsman, C. and Ronstrand, L. (1989) Dimerization of B-type platelet-derived growth factor receptors occurs after ligand binding and is closely associated with receptor kinase activation. J. Biol. Chem. 264:8905-8912

Hermansson, M., Nister, M., Betsholtz, C., Heldin, C.-H., Westermark, B. and Funa, K. (1988) Endothelial cell hyperplasia in human glioblastoma: Coexpression of mRNA for platelet-derived growth factor (PDGF) B chain and PDGF receptor suggests autocrine growth stimulation. Proc. Nat. Acad. Sci. U.S.A. 85:7748-7752

Kelly, J., Haldeman, B., Grant, F., Seifert, R., Murray, M., and Bowen-Pope, D. Cloning and properties of the human PDGF receptor a-subunit. Ms. (In preparation)

Lee, K.-H., Bowen-Pope, D.F., and Reed, R. R. (1990) Isolation and characterization of the alpha-PDGF receptor from rat olfactory epithelium Molec. Cell Biol. 10:2237-2249.

Majesky, M.W., Reidy, M.A. Bowen-Pope, D.F., Hart, C.E., Wilcox, J.N., Schwartz, S.M., (Submitted) PDGF ligand and PDGF receptor gene expression during repair of arterial injury.

Majesky, M.W., Benditt, E.P., and Schwartz, S.M. (1988) Wxpression and developmental control of PDGF A-chain and B-chain/sis genes in rat aortic smooth muscle cells PNAS 85:1524-1528.

Matsui, T. Heidaran, M., Miki, T., Popescu, N., La Rochelle, W., Kraus, M., Pierce, J. and Aaronson, S. (1989) Isolation of a novel receptor cDNA establishes the existence of two PDGF receptor genes. Science 243:800-804

Matsui, T., Pierce, J.H., Flemming, T.P., Greenberger, J.S., LaRochelle, W.J., Ruggiero, M., and Aaronson, S.A. (1990) Independent espression of human alpha or beta platelet-derived growth factor cDNAs in a native hematopoietic cell leads to functional coupling with mitogenic and chemotactic signalling pathways PNAS 86:8314-8318.

Mercola, M., Melton, D.A., and Stiles, C.D. (1988) platelet-derived growth factor A-chain is maternally encoded in Xenopus embryos Science 241:1223-1225.

Mercola, M., Wang, C., Kelly, J., Brownlee, C., Jackson-Grusby, L., Stiles, C., and Bowen-Pope, D. Selective Expression of PDGF A and its receptor during early mouse embryogenesis. (1990) Developmental Biology 138:114-122.

Nister, M., Hammacher, A., Mellstrom, K., Siegbhan, A Ronnstrand, L., Westermark, B., and Heldin, C.-H. (1988) A glioma-derived PDGF A chain homodimer has different functional properties from a PDGF AB heterodimer purified from human platelets. Cell 52:791-799.

Pike, L.J., Bowen-Pope, D.F., Ross, R., and Krebs. E.G. (1983) Characterizarion of platelet-derived growth factor-stimulated phosphorylation in cell membranes J. Biol. Chem. 258:9383-9390.

Raff, M.C. (1989) Glial cell diversification in the rat optic nerve Science 243:1450-1455.

Rappolee, D.A., Brenner, C.A., Schultz, R., Mark, D. and Werb, Z. (1988a) Developmental expression of PDGF, TGF-alpha, and TGF-beta genes in preimplantation mouse embryos. Science 241:1823-1825

Raines, E.W. Bowen-Pope, D.F., and Ross, R. (1990) "Platelet-derived growth factor" In: Handbook of Experimental Pharmacology, Volume 95/1 (M.B. Sporn and A.B. Roberts, ed.s) Heidelberg: Springer Verlag.

Rizzino, A. and Bowen-Pope, D.F. (1985) Production of PDGF-like growth factors by embryonal carcinoma cells and binding of PDGF to their endoderm-like differentiated cells. Developmental Biology 110:15-22

Ross, R., Glomset, J., kariya, B., and Harker, L. (1974) A platelet-dependent serum factor that stimulates the proliferation of arterial smooth muscle cells *in vitro*. Proc. Natl. Acad. Sci. USA 71:1207-1210

Ross, R., and Glomset, J.A. (1976) The pathogenesis of atherosclerosis NEJM 295:369-377, 420-425.

Ross, R., Raines, E. W., and Bowen-Pope, D. F. (1986) The Biology of Platelet-derived Growth Factor. Cell 46:155-169

Rubin, K., Hansson, G.K., Ronnstrand, L., Claesson-Welsh, L., Fellstrom, B., Tinstrom, A., Larsson, E., Klareskog, L., Heldin, C-H., and Terracio, L. (1988) Induction of B-type receptors for platelet-derived growth factor in vascular inflammation: possible implications for development of vascular proliferation lesions. Lancet June 18:1353-1356

Seifert, R.A., Schwartz, S.M., and Bowen-Pope, D.F. (1984) Developmentally regulated production of platelet-derived growth factor-like molecules. Nature 311:669-671

Seifert, R.A., Hart, C.A., Phillips, P.E., Ross, R., Forstrom, J., Murray, M.J., and Bowen-Pope, D.F. (1989) Two different subunits associate to create isoform-specific PDGF receptors. J. Biol. Chem. 264:8771-8778.

Terracio, L., Ronnstrand, L., Tinstrom, A., Rubin, K., Claesson-Welsh, L., Funa, K., and Heldin, C-H. (1988) Induction of platelet-derived growth factor receptor expression in smooth muscle cells and fibroblasts upon tissue culturing. J. Cell Biology 107:1947-1957

Williams, L.T. (1989) Signal transduction by the PDGF receptor. Science 243:1565-1570.

Williams, L. T., Tremble, P. M., Lavin, M. F., and Sunday, M. E. (1984) Platelet-derived growth factor receptors form a high affinity state in membrane preparations. The Journal Of Biological Chemistry 259:5287-5294

Yarden, Y., Escobedo, J.A., Kuang, W.-J., Yang-Feng, T.L., Daniel, T.O., Tremble, P.M., Chen, E.Y., Ando, M.E., Harkins, R.N., Francke, U., Fried, V.A., Ullrich, A., and Williams, L.T. (1986) Structure of the receptor for platelet-derived growth factor helps define a family of closely related growth factor receptors. Nature 323:226-232

Characterization of a Non-Tyrosine Kinase FGF-Binding Protein

Laura Burrus, Mike Zuber, Bruce Lueddecke, and Brad Olwin

Department of Biochemistry, University of Wisconsin-Madison, Madison, Wisconsin

Abstract

Fibroblast growth factors function as cell type dependent repressors or promoters of cellular differentiation. To understand the molecular mechanisms involved in transducing biologically diverse signals mediated by FGF, we have identified a putative FGF receptor from embryonic chick. FGF receptor purified from day 7 chick embryo membranes by either FGF-affinity or immunoaffinity chromatography yields three polypeptides that migrate at 150, 70, and 45 kDa when resolved by SDS-PAGE. To identify the FGF-binding protein, the 150, 70, and 45 kDa proteins were separated by SDS-PAGE, transferred to Immobilon (Millipore) membranes, and probed with ^{125}I-FGF. Only the 150 kDa polypeptide bound ^{125}I-FGF demonstrating the 70 and 45 kDa polypeptides are not necessary for FGF binding. Screening of a chick embryonic brain cDNA expression library with monoclonal antibodies that recognize the 150 kDa protein yielded several cDNAs. One 3.5 kb cDNA clone encodes an open reading frame of 1142 amino acids. The predicted amino acid sequence exhibits characteristics expected of a receptor. These include a signal peptide, a cysteine-rich extracellular domain, and a membrane-spanning sequence. Unlike other recently identified members of the FGF receptor family (cek, *bek*, and *flg*), this clone does not contain tyrosine kinase domains. Further studies including expression of the cDNA and immunolocalization of the putative FGF receptor are in progress.

Introduction

Polypeptide growth factors are implicated in both the regulation of vascular development and in the maintenance of the vascular system. Basic fibroblast growth factor (bFGF), a member of the FGF family, which is comprised to date of 7 related polypeptides stimulates angiogenesis and healing of wounds in healing-compromised animals[4,11,40]. *In vitro*, bFGF and acidic FGF (aFGF) are potent mitogens for cell types from all three germ layers including ectoderm, mesoderm and endoderm[4, 23]. These growth factors are also implicated in the regulation of several developmental processes that include repression of skeletal muscle[6, 16], cardiac muscle[14], adipocyte[22], and chondrocyte differentiation[12]. aFGF and bFGF promote neuronal outgrowth and enhance neuronal survival[10, 20, 34, 39, 41, 42]. Furthermore, aFGF, bFGF, and k-FGF stimulate mesoderm induction in the amphibian embryo[13, 27, 37] and mitogenesis in Swiss 3T3 cells at similar relative

Published 1990 by Elsevier Science Publishing Co., Inc.
Molecular Biology of Atherosclerosis
A.D. Attie, Editor

concentrations, suggesting the use of common receptors[27]. These data argue that FGFs are crucial mediators of embryonic development. Although seven distinct polypeptides comprise the FGF family (Table 1), differences in the biological activities, sites of action, and metabolism of these related factors has not been established.

Several aspects of FGF biology are unique to this family of growth factors. aFGF and bFGF, the best characterized FGFs, possess no signal peptide sequence yet are widely distributed and are often localized in the extracellular matrix[4]. Several different forms of bFGF have been identified that arise from alternative translational initiation at CUG codons upstream of the Kozak consensus site for AUG translational initiation[9, 28]. These forms appear to be differentially distributed within the cell; AUG-initiated translational products are found in the cytoplasm, while some CUG-initiated bFGF forms appear to be localized to the nucleus[1, 9, 28]. The relationship of cellular localization to the biological activities of FGF has not been established. Int-2, an FGF family member, is similar to aFGF and bFGF as it has a weak signal peptide sequence that is inefficiently cleaved and is found in both the cytoplasm and nucleus of cells, again as a result of alternative translational initiation at upstream CUG codons[1]. Of the remaining 4 FGF family members, 3 have "traditional" signal peptide sequences and appear to be secreted via described mechanisms involving recognition and cleavage of signal peptide sequences[4].

Table 1
Structural Characteristics of the FGF Family

Growth Factor	M_r (kDa)	Sequence Identity to bFGF
acidic FGF (HBGF-1)[17, 38]	16-19	53%
basic FGF (HBGF-2)[3, 17]	18-24	100%
Int-2 (HBGF-3)[8]	(231 aa)	42%
k-FGF/HST (HBGF-4)[7]	21	42%
FGF-5 (HBGF-5)[43]	(267 aa)	43%
FGF-6 (HBGF-6)[19]	?	?
KGF (HBGF-7)[32]	28	39%

FGF-binding proteins can be grouped into three distinct classes (Table 2) including three membrane-associated tyrosine kinases (cek 1 or flg, cek 2, and cek 3 or bek)[15, 18, 26, 30, 33], heparan sulfate proteoglycans [29,35], and a membrane-associated protein that retains high affinity for aFGF and bFGF[5]. The tyrosine kinase containing FGF receptors are most similar to ret tyrosine kinase, the platelet-derived growth factor receptors, and the CSF-1 receptor [15, 18, 25, 26, 30]. This group of FGF-binding proteins is likely to represent "classical" growth factor receptors for several FGFs. The second distinct class of FGF-binding proteins are the heparan-sulfate proteoglycans[21, 31, 35, 36]. Although it is likely that several types of HSPG interact with FGF, to date one membrane-bound HSPG[29] (syndecan), and an extracellular matrix HSPG have[35] been shown to bind bFGF. HSPGs are proposed to function as storage depots for FGF[4, 23, 31], since the affinity of these proteins for FGF is several orders of magnitude less than that of the tyrosine kinases (Table 2). The participation of the HSPGs in FGF signal transduction is unclear as is the relationship between FGF binding HSPGs in the extracellular matrix vs. those in the plasma membrane. An example of the third class of FGF-binding proteins was identified and first characterized by our group[5]. This membrane-associated protein exhibits high affinity binding of aFGF and bFGF yet, contains no homology to other proteins including tyrosine or serine/threonine kinases. Data from sequencing cDNA clones that encode p150 has revealed a signal peptide, and a membrane-spanning region within the open reading frame, suggesting the protein is oriented within the plasma membrane and may function as a FGF receptor. Further details including the complete primary amino acid sequence and structural analysis will be described elsewhere. The significance of all three classes of FGF-binding proteins as well as their respective contributions to transducing FGF-mediated biological processes is not known. The recent identification of these molecules should serve to greatly increase our understanding of their roles in FGF biology.

Table 2
FGF-Binding Proteins

Binding Protein	Protein Structure	FGFs Bound	Affinity for FGF
cek 1 (*flg*) [15, 25]	tyrosine kinase	bFGF, aFGF	100 pM
cek 2 [26]	tyrosine kinase	?	?
cek 3 (*bek*) [18, 26]	tyrosine kinase	bFGF, k-FGF	100 pM
p150 [5]	unknown membrane	bFGF, aFGF	?
syndecan [29]	heparan/chondroitin-sulfate proteoglycan	bFGF	≥ 300 nM

Results

The presence of high levels of FGF and FGF-binding proteins in embryonic tissues strongly suggests that these factors play crucial roles in the developing organism. During chick embryogenesis, FGF-binding can be detected as early as 2 days following fertilization (day 2) and remains relatively constant until organogenesis is completed by day 7 (Figure 1)[24]. From day 7 to day day 13 the FGF-binding drops precipitously, and has disappeared from both heart and skeletal muscle by day 19, but is retained in brain, eye, and liver, although at lower levels than in early development[24]. Crosslinking of FGF to chick embryonic membranes reveals at least two proteins that appear to decline in parallel with the loss of FGF-binding[5, 24].

Because of the relatively high levels of FGF-binding proteins present during chick embryogenesis, we chose to use embryonic chick for the isolation of these proteins. Two FGF-binding proteins have been purified from embryonic chick, a 120 kDa membrane-bound tyrosine kinase (flg or cek 1)[15] and a 150 kDa membrane-bound non-tyrosine kinase[5]. Crosslinking of ^{125}I-aFGF or ^{125}I-bFGF to crude preparations of day 7 chick embryo membranes reveals a major product that migrates at 165 kDa and appears to bind both aFGF and bFGF (Figure 2)

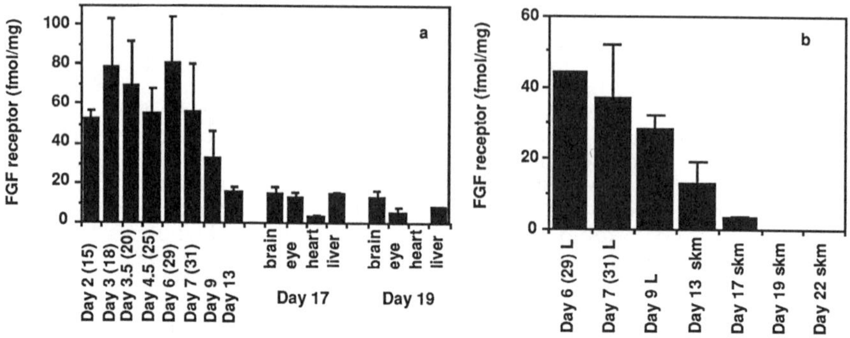

Figure 1: FGF receptor levels in embryonic chick. **(a).**FGF receptor levels in whole chick embryo from day 2 through day 13 and in brain, eye, heart, and liver from day 17 and 19 embryonic membranes. **(b)** FGF receptor levels in limbs [L] from day 6 to day 9 and in skeletal muscle (skm) from day 13 to day 22 (one day post-hatching). Reprinted with permission from[24]

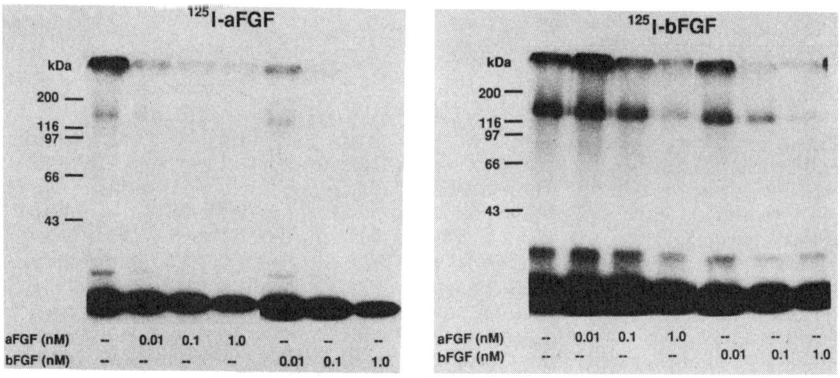

Fig. 2. **Crosslinking of ^{125}I-aFGF and ^{125}I-bFGF to chick membranes.** Chick membranes (200 µg) were incubated with 100 pM ^{125}I-aFGF *[top)]* or ^{125}I-bFGF (*bottom*) for 1 hr at 22°C and then covalently crosslinked with disuccinimidyl suberate as described in [5]. Increasing concentrations of unlabeled aFGF or bFGF were used to specifically compete for binding of ^{125}I-FGF to FGF receptor. Molecular weight standards are indicated at the left. Reprinted with permission from [5]

To purify the 165 kDa product (150 kDa after subtraction of 15 kDa for FGF) membranes were solubilized with 1% Triton X-100, applied to a wheat germ lectin affinity column, and glycoproteins eluted with N-acetylglucosamine. FGF-binding proteins were further purified over aFGF or bFGF affinity columns. Crosslinking of either ^{125}I-aFGF or ^{125}I-bFGF to the eluted fractions demonstrated purification of a major FGF-binding complex migrating at 165 kDa, as well as minor complexes migrating at 120 kDa and at the top of the separating gel[5]. Analysis of the protein content of FGF-affinity purified fractions by coomassie/silver staining of SDS-polyacrylamide gels revealed three major polypeptides migrating at 150, 70 and 45 kDa (p150, p70, and p45)[5]. The 150 kDa protein contains N-linked carbohydrate, but does not contain detectable covalently linked heparan sulfate[5]. Neither p70 nor p45 contain detectable N-linked carbohydrate or heparan sulfate, suggesting they may be intracellular proteins that co-purify with p150[5]. Since the FGF-binding protein is a component of a 165 kDa complex and is a membrane glycoprotein, the logical candidate for binding FGF is p150.

To identify the FGF-binding proteins present in the purified pool, a ligand blotting technique was performed. Fractions purified by aFGF-Sepharose affinity chromatography were subjected to SDS-PAGE at 4°C in the absence of a reducing agent. Fractions were then transferred to Immobilon (Millipore, Inc.) membranes, and incubated with ^{125}I-aFGF or ^{125}I-bFGF in the presence or absence of excess unlabeled aFGF, bFGF, or epidermal growth factor[5]. Two additional Immobilon strips were incubated with or without a monoclonal antibody to p150 and visualized using alkaline phosphatase(Lueddecke & Olwin, unpublished data). These results (Figure 3) unequivocally identify p150 as the FGF-binding protein present in the purified fractions. Additional experiments utilizing the monoclonal antibody to remove p150 from wheat germ lectin fractions suggests that p150 is the major FGF-binding protein present(Burrus and Olwin, unpublished data).

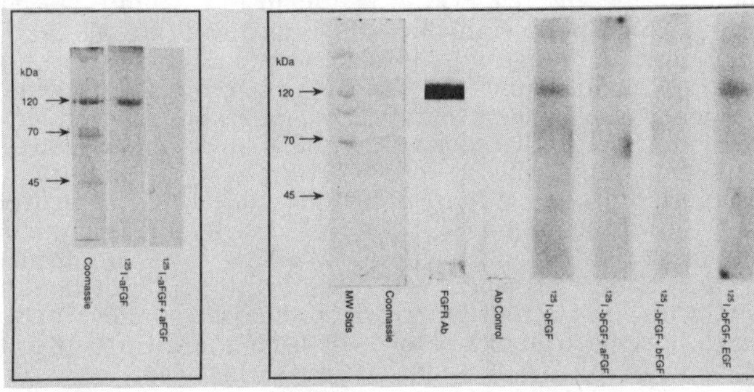

Fig. 3. **Ligand blotting of FGF receptor with ^{125}I-aFGF and ^{125}I-bFGF.** Highly purified FGF receptor fractions were separated by SDS-PAGE under nonreducing conditions and electroblotted onto Immobilon membranes at 4°C. Strips of Immobilon containing MW standards and FGF receptor fractions were stained with Coomassie. Immobilon strips were developed as described previously [5]. The 150 kDa polypeptide shown in Figure 2 migrates at 120 kDa when electrophoresed under nonreducing conditions. This polypeptide binds ^{125}I-aFGF and ^{125}I-bFGF with high affinity. Unlabeled aFGF and bFGF, but not EGF, compete for binding of ^{125}I-FGF to the polypeptide, demonstrating appropriate specificity for a FGF receptor. Two strips of Immobilon used for the ligand blot were also incubated with a monoclonal antibody that immunoprecipitates ^{125}I-FGF/FGF receptor complex.

Discussion

We have isolated and characterized a 150 kDa polypeptide present in chick embryos that specifically binds aFGF and bFGF with high affinity. Starting with 40 dozen chick embryos, approximately 15 μg of purified p150 is recovered with an overall fold purification of 28,000 (Table 4)[5].

Table 4.
FGF Receptor Purification

Fraction	FGF receptor (μg)	FGFR (μg/mg protein)	Purification-fold	Yield (%)
Membranes	38	0.015	1	100
Wheat Germ Lectin Pool	42	5.6	470	110
aFGF-Sepharose Pool	15	330	28,000	39

Sequencing of p150 cDNAs has identified a signal peptide, N-linked carbohydrate attachment consensus sites, and a membrane spanning domain, but no tyrosine or serine/threonine conserved protein kinase catalytic domains. Thus, these data support our hypothesis that p150 is a FGF receptor, however, the mode of signal transduction from the extracellular to the intracellular milieu is unclear. The co-purification of p70 and p45, which are most likely intracellular proteins, with p150 suggests these proteins form a complex that may be involved in FGF-mediated signal transduction. Purification of p70 and p45 and sequencing of their respective cDNAs may help to elucidate the possible mechanism by which p150 transduces FGF-mediated signals across the plasma membrane. Although we speculate that p150 functions as a FGF receptor, other plausible functions can be proposed. The protein could function as a "scavenger" or clearance receptor for extracellular FGF. Several groups have recently reported that bFGF and int-2 are targeted to the nucleus depending on the site of translational initiation. An additional report provides evidence that internalized FGF is delivered to the nucleus during the G_1-phase of the cell cycle[2]. It is possible that p150 functions to internalize FGF for mediation of unknown FGF-dependent intracellular biological processes, with p150 functioning in a manner analogous to steroid transport proteins. Finally, p150 may function as a specific transporter of FGF from the intracellular to the extracellular environment. This possibility seems least likely as p150 appears to undergo standard routing through the Golgi apparatus, revealed by the presence of a defined signal peptide sequence and mature N-linked carbohydrate. It thus remains unclear how FGF, without a signal peptide, gains access to the Golgi cisternea for binding and transport by p150.

The relationship of p150 to other FGF-binding proteins is unknown. Two additional distinct classes of FGF-binding proteins include the transmembrane tyrosine kinases (3 known members) and the heparan sulfate proteoglycans that reside both in the plasma membrane (syndecan) and in the extracellular matrix. Experiments are in progress to determine whether p150 associates with the tyrosine kinases or heparan sulfate proteoglycans. Obviously, the number of FGFs and FGF-binding proteins argues for a large number of complex interactions to generate the diversity of biological activities ascribed to the FGFs.

References

1. Acland, P., M. Dixon, G. Peters and C. Dickson. Subcellular fate of the Int-2 oncoprotein is determined by choice of initiation codon. Nature. **343**(6259): 662-665 (1990).

2. Baldin, V., A. M. Roman, B. I. Bosc, F. Amalric and G. Bouche. Translocation of bFGF to the nucleus is G1 phase cell cycle specific in bovine aortic endothelial cells. Embo J. **9**(5): 1511-1517 (1990).

3. Bohlen, P., A. Baird, F. Esch, N. Ling and D. Gospodarowicz. Isolation and partial molecular characterization of pituitary fibroblast growth factor. . Proc Natl Acad Sci U S A. **81**(17): 5364-8 (1984).

4. Burgess, W. H. and T. Maciag. The heparin-binding (fibroblast) growth factor family of proteins. . Annu Rev Biochem. **58**: 575-606 (1989).

5. Burrus, L. W. and B. B. Olwin. Isolation of a receptor for acidic and basic fibroblast growth factor from embryonic chick . J Biol Chem. **264**(31): 18647-18653 (1989).

6. Clegg, C. H., T. A. Linkhart, B. B. Olwin and S. D. Hauschka. Growth factor control of skeletal muscle differentiation: commitment to terminal differentiation occurs in G1 phase and is repressed by fibroblast growth factor. . J Cell Biol. **105**(2): 949-56 (1987).

7. Delli-Bovi, P., A. M. Curatola, K. M. Newman, Y. Sato, D. Moscatelli, R. M. Hewick, D. B. Rifkin and C. Basilico. Processing, secretion, and biological properties of a novel growth factor of the fibroblast growth factor family with oncogenic potential. . Mol Cell Biol. **8**(7): 2933-41 (1988).

8. Dickson, C. and G. Peters. Potential oncogene product related to growth factors [letter]. . Nature. **326**(6116): (1987).

9. Florkiewicz, R. Z. and A. Sommer. Human basic fibroblast growth factor gene encodes four polypeptides: three initiate translation from non-AUG codons. . Proc Natl Acad Sci U S A. **86**(11): 3978-81 (1989).

10. Gensburger, C., G. Labourdette and M. Sensenbrenner. Brain basic fibroblast growth factor stimulates the proliferation of rat neuronal precursor cells in vitro. . Febs Lett. **217**(1): 1-5 (1987).

11. Greenhalgh, D. G., K. H. Sprugel, M. J. Murray and R. Ross. PDGF and FGF stimulate wound healing in the genetically diabetic mouse. Am J Pathol. **136**(6): 1235-1246 (1990).

12. Kato, Y. and M. Iwamoto. Fibroblast growth factor is an inhibitor of chondrocyte terminal differentiation. J Biol Chem. **265**(10): 5903-5909 (1990).

13. Kimelman, D. and M. Kirschner. Synergistic induction of mesoderm by FGF and TGF-beta and the identification of an mRNA coding for FGF in the early Xenopus embryo. . Cell. **51**(5): 869-77 (1987).

27. Paterno, G. D., L. L. Gillespie, M. S. Dixon, J. Slack and J. K. Heath. Mesoderm-inducing properties of INT-2 and kFGF: Two oncogene-encoded growth factors related to FGF . Development. **106**(1): 79-83 (1989).

28. Prats, H., M. Kaghad, A. C. Prats, M. Klagsbrun, J. M. Lelias, P. Liauzun, P. Chalon, J. P. Tauber, F. Amalric, J. A. Smith and a. l. et. High molecular mass forms of basic fibroblast growth factor are initiated by alternative CUG codons. . Proc Natl Acad Sci U S A. **86**(6): 1836-40 (1989).

29. Krufka, A., Olwin, B.B & Rapreager, A., (unpublished data).

30. Reid, H. H., A. F. Wilks and O. Bernard. Two forms of the basic fibroblast growth factor receptor-like mRNA are expressed in the developing mouse brain. Proc Natl Acad Sci Usa. **87**(4): 1596-1600 (1990).

31. Rifkin, D. B. and D. Moscatelli. Recent developments in the cell biology of basic fibroblast growth factor. . J Cell Biol. **109**(1): 1-6 (1989).

32. Rubin, J. S., H. Osada, P. W. Finch, W. G. Taylor, S. Rudikoff and S. A. Aaronson. Purification and characterization of a newly identified growth factor specific for epithelial cells. . Proc Natl Acad Sci U S A. **86**(3): 802-6 (1989).

33. Ruta, M., W. Burgess, D. Givol, J. Epstein, N. Neiger, J. Kaplow, G. Crumley, C. Dionne, M. Jaye and J. Schlessinger. Receptor for acidic fibroblast growth factor is related to the tyrosine kinase encoded by the fms-like gene (FLG) . Proc Natl Acad Sci Usa. **86**(22): 8722-8726 (1989).

34. Rydel, R. E. and L. A. Greene. Acidic and basic fibroblast growth factors promote stable neurite outgrowth and neuronal differentiation in cultures of PC12 cells. . J Neurosci. **7**(11): 3639-53 (1987).

35. Saksela, O., D. Moscatelli, A. Sommer and D. B. Rifkin. Endothelial cell-derived heparan sulfate binds basic fibroblast growth factor and protects it from proteolytic degradation. . J Cell Biol. **107**(2): 743-51 (1988).

36. Saksela, O. and D. B. Rifkin. Release of basic fibroblast growth factor-heparan sulfate complexes from endothelial cells by plasminogen activator-mediated proteolytic activity. J Cell Biol. **110**(3): 767-775 (1990).

37. Slack, J. M., B. G. Darlington, J. K. Heath and S. F. Godsave. Mesoderm induction in early Xenopus embryos by heparin-binding growth factors. . Nature. **326**(6109): 197-200 (1987).

38. Thomas, K. A., C. M. Rios and S. Fitzpatrick. Purification and characterization of acidic fibroblast growth factor from bovine brain. . Proc Natl Acad Sci U S A. **81**(2): 357-61 (1984).

14. Kohtz, D. S., N. R. Dische, T. Inagami and B. Goldman. Growth and partial differentiation of presumptive human cardiac myoblasts in culture. . J Cell Biol. **108**(3): 1067-78 (1989).

15. Lee, P. L., D. E. Johnson, L. S. Cousens, V. A. Fried and L. T. Williams. Purification and complementary DNA cloning of a receptor for basic fibroblast growth factor. . Science. **245**(4913): 57-60 (1989).

16. Linkhart, T., C. Clegg and S. Hauschka. Myogenic differentiation in permanent clonal myoblast cell lines: regulation by macromolecular growth factors in the culture medium. Dev. Biol. **86**: 19-30 (1981).

17. Lobb, R. R. and J. W. Fett. Purification of two distinct growth factors from bovine neural tissue by heparin affinity chromatography. . Biochemistry. **23**(26): 6295-9 (1984).

18. Mansukhani, A., D. Moscatelli, D. Talarico, V. Levytska and C. Basilico. A murine fibroblast growth factor (FGF) receptor expressed in CHO cells is activated by basic FGF and Kaposi FGF. Proc Natl Acad Sci Usa. **87**(11): 4378-4382 (1990).

19. Marics, I., J. Adelaide, F. Raybaud, M. G. Mattei, F. Coulier, J. Planche, L. O. de and D. Birnbaum. Characterization of the HST-related FGF.6 gene, a new member of the fibroblast growth factor gene family. . Oncogene. **4**(3): 335-40 (1989).

20. Morrison, R. S., A. Sharma, V. J. de and R. A. Bradshaw. Basic fibroblast growth factor supports the survival of cerebral cortical neurons in primary culture. . Proc Natl Acad Sci U S A. **83**(19): 7537-41 (1986).

21. Moscatelli, D. Metabolism of receptor-bound and matrix-bound basic fibroblast growth factor by bovine capillary endothelial cells. . J Cell Biol. **107**(2): 753-9 (1988).

22. Navre, M. and G. M. Ringold. Differential effects of fibroblast growth factor and tumor promoters on the initiation and maintenance of adipocyte differentiation . J Cell Biol. **1**(1857): 1857-1863 (1989).

23. Olwin, B. Heparin-Binding Growth Factors and Their Receptors. Cytotechnology. **2**: 351-365 (1989).

24. Olwin, B. B. and S. D. Hauschka. Fibroblast growth factor receptor levels decrease during chick embryogenesis. J Cell Biol. **110**(2): 503-509 (1990).

25. Pasquale, E. B. A Distinctive Family of Embryonic Protein-Tyrosine Kinase Receptors. Proc. Natl. Acad. Sci. USA. **87**: 5812-5816 (1990).

26. Pasquale, E. and S. Singer. Identification of a developmentally regulated protein-tyrosine kinase by using anti-phosphotyrosine antibodies to screen a cDNA expression library. Proc. Natl. Acad. Sci. USA. **86**: 5449-5453 (1989).

39. Togari, A., G. Dickens, H. Kuzuya and G. Guroff. The effect of fibroblast growth factor on PC12 cells. . J Neurosci. **5**(2): 307-16 (1985).

40. Tsuboi, R. and D. B. Rifkin. Recombinant basic fibroblast growth factor stimulates wound healing in healing-impaired db/db mice. J Exp Med. **172**(1): 245-251 (1990).

41. Unsicker, K., P. H. Reichert, R. Schmidt, B. Pettmann, G. Labourdette and M. Sensenbrenner. Astroglial and fibroblast growth factors have neurotrophic functions for cultured peripheral and central nervous system neurons. . Proc Natl Acad Sci U S A. **84**(15): 5459-63 (1987).

42. Walicke, P., W. M. Cowan, N. Ueno, A. Baird and R. Guillemin. Fibroblast growth factor promotes survival of dissociated hippocampal neurons and enhances neurite extension. . Proc Natl Acad Sci U S A. **83**(9): 3012-6 (1986).

43. Zhan, X., B. Bates, X. G. Hu and M. Goldfarb. The human FGF-5 oncogene encodes a novel protein related to fibroblast growth factors. . Mol Cell Biol. **8**(8): 3487-95 (1988).

Subject Index